Delmar's
CLINICAL
HANDBOOK
for the
MEDICAL OFFICE

Third Edition

Michelle Heller, CMA (AAMA), RMA
Medical Assisting Faculty for Columbus State
Community College, Columbus, Ohio

Connie Krebs, CMA-C, BGS

DELMAR
CENGAGE Learning

Australia • Brazil • Canada • Mexico • Singapore • United Kingdom • United States

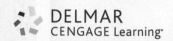
DELMAR
CENGAGE Learning·

**Delmar's Clinical Handbook
for the Medical Office, Third
Edition**
Michelle E. Heller

Vice President, Careers &
Computing: Dave Garza

Director of Learning Solutions:
Matthew Kane

Executive Editor: Rhonda
Dearborn

Managing Editor: Marah
Bellegarde

Product Manager: Lauren
Whalen

Vice President, Marketing:
Jennifer Baker

Marketing Director: Wendy E.
Mapstone

Senior Marketing Manager:
Nancy Bradshaw

Marketing Coordinator:
Piper Huntington

Production Manager: Andrew
Crouth

Content Project Manager:
Allyson Bozeth

Art Director: Jack Pendleton

For product information and technology assistance, contact us at
Cengage Learning Customer & Sales Support, 1-800-354-9706

For permission to use material from this text or product,
submit all requests online at **www.cengage.com/permissions.**
Further permissions questions can be e-mailed to
permissionrequest@cengage.com

Library of Congress Control Number: 2012934354

ISBN-13: 978-1-133-69156-3

ISBN-10: 1-133-69156-0

Delmar
5 Maxwell Drive
Clifton Park, NY 12065-2919
USA

Cengage Learning is a leading provider of customized learning
solutions with office locations around the globe, including
Singapore, the United Kingdom, Australia, Mexico, Brazil, and Japan.
Locate your local office at: **www.cengage.com/global**

To learn more about Delmar, visit **www.cengage.com/delmar**

Purchase any of our products at your local college store or at our
preferred online store **www.cengagebrain.com**

Printed in Mexico
Print Number: 04   Print Year: 2021

CONTENTS

Section One

ABBREVIATIONS, SYMBOLS, AND COMMON MISSPELLED TERMS

Section Two

DOCUMENTATION AND IN-OFFICE SCREENINGS

Section Three

TELEPHONE SCREENINGS

Section Four

ROUTINE CLINICAL PROCEDURES PERFORMED IN THE MEDICAL OFFICE

Section Five
PEDIATRIC SCREENINGS AND PROCEDURES

Section Six
ASSISTING IN AN OB-GYN PRACTICE

Section Seven
PHARMACOLOGY PROCEDURES

Section Eight

LABORATORY NORMAL VALUES AND PROCEDURES

Section Nine

X-RAY AND DIAGNOSTIC EXAMINATIONS (PREPARATION)

Section Ten

EMERGENCY PROCEDURES

Section Eleven

HUGS IN THE HALLWAY

DEDICATION

This book is dedicated to my former co-author Connie Krebs. Connie passed away between the second and third editions of this book. She was a wonderful mentor, professional, and friend. Connie shared her love with many and cared deeply about those less fortunate. She loved helping students reach their potential, and her students loved and admired her. She is deeply missed!

—Michelle E. Heller

PREFACE

Delmar Learning's Clinical Handbook for the Medical Office, Third Edition, provides a quick and easy reference for individuals considering employment in the health field and those already employed in a medical office. The handbook can serve as a reference tool for medical assisting learners, individuals beginning an externship or internship, recent medical assisting graduates, nurses, physician assistants, and medical office personnel. Office managers can use the handbook as a tool to promote continuity among staff members. The information in this handbook is geared toward family practice, internal medicine, pediatrics, and obstetrics-gynecology (OB-GYN) offices.

Organization of the Clinical Handbook

The handbook is organized in an easy-to-read table format for quick retrieval of pertinent medical information and includes 11 sections. New to this edition are color tabs for quick referencing, the addition of several more procedures, and the inclusion of many illustrations. Sections now include electronic medical record (EMR) applications and great field tips to help users work in an efficient manner. The Hugs in the Hallway section has been expanded to include more feel-good stories straight from the classroom and industry.

Section 1 presents common medical abbreviations for diseases and conditions, charting and diagnostic areas, and the laboratory, as well as common medication abbreviations and symbols. Abbreviations appearing on the Joint Commission's "Do Not Use" list or "Not Recommended" list are color-coded in each chart to alert users that these abbreviations should not be used in any type of orders. This section also includes a list of commonly misspelled everyday terms and commonly misspelled medical terms.

Section 2, Documentation and In-Office Screenings, provides users with elemental steps to assist in documenting accurately and efficiently in patient charts. Fundamental documentation of medications and prescriptions, patient screenings, referrals, pre-certifications, procedures, telephone screenings, and patient education are a few of the types of documentation addressed. Several charting examples appear in the documentation section and throughout the handbook. This section includes the most abundant use of EMR applications to help users transcend to the electronic world of medical records.

In Section 3, Telephone Screenings, each table begins with quick facts about a condition that the screener should know before proceeding with questioning. This is especially useful for screeners who are not familiar with specific conditions. The screening portion of each table is presented in a simplified three-column format. The first column lists common questions that should be asked about a specific complaint. The patient's response is noted in the second column. The third column directs the screener to advise the patient on the action to take based on the patient's response. Each screening table should be reviewed and approved by the provider before implementation.

Section 4, Routine Clinical Procedures Performed in the Medical Office, is one of the largest sections in the book. Vital sign measurement, instrument identification, and assisting with surgical procedures are just a few of the procedures covered in this section. This part of the book also includes normal value charts and field tips that will help simplify procedures and save time. Specialty procedures such as medication administration, laboratory procedures, and pediatric and OB-GYN procedures are covered in other specialty sections of the book.

Section 5, Pediatric Screenings and Procedures, includes routine procedures performed at different ages for well-baby and child examinations, recommended childhood and adolescent immunizations, and common pediatric diseases and disorders. A quick-glance screening table that can be used in telephone screenings for pediatric patients is also included.

Section 6, Assisting in an OB-Gyn Practice, addresses procedures routinely performed in the OB-GYN practice. Common tray setups, assessment information, common diseases, common laboratory testing, and charting examples are included.

Section 7, Pharmacology Procedures, presents drug classifications, information regarding the 200 most commonly prescribed drugs, information on over-the-counter medications, and a list of the most common injectable medications. Medication procedures and a complete explanation of the information required when writing prescriptions are also covered in this section.

Section 8, Laboratory Normal Values and Procedures, includes normal chemistry and hematology test values with related abbreviations, reference ranges and their clinical significance, and laboratory procedures and the significance of specific critical laboratory values.

Section 9, X-Rays/Diagnostic Examinations (Preparation) presents descriptions of common radiographic and outside diagnostic procedures, related abbreviations, and tips on information to provide to patients before the procedure.

Section 10, Emergency Procedures, instructs users on what to do when an emergency occurs in the medical office.

Section 11, Hugs in the Hallway, features heart-warming stories from health educators in the classroom and practitioners in the field. The authors wish to convey to all readers that the practice of medicine is more than performing technical tasks. These stories convey the importance of caring and demonstrating compassion toward patients.

New to the Third Edition

We listened! The changes and additions made in the third edition are a direct result of suggestions from consultants, reviewers, graduates of medical assisting programs, and individuals employed in medical offices across the country. Major changes include:

- Section 1: This section now includes abbreviations that are listed as "Do Not Use" or "Not Recommended" by the Joint Commission.

- Section 2: This section now includes Field Tips and EMR Applications and updated documentation samples.

- Section 3: This section now includes Field Tips and EMR Applications.

- Section 4: This section now covers routine clinical procedures as well as instrument identification. Several procedures have been added to this section.

- Section 5: This section now includes pediatric injections as well as a procedure for obtaining length, weight, and height on an infant. Charting examples and EMR Applications were added to this section as well as new information on immunization schedules and obtaining vital signs.

- Section 6: This section now includes expanded step-by-step procedures for assisting with examinations. Patient education for a breast self-examination was also added to the section.

- Section 7: This section now includes updated lists of the top 200 drugs, top over-the-counter medications, and top injectable medications. New information on common measurements and dosage calculations were added as well as procedures for preparing and administrating medications.

- Section 8: 24 step-by-step laboratory procedures have been added to this section.

- Section 9: New information on several radiologic procedures, including positron emission tomography (PET) scans, barium series, cardiac catheterizations, and bone density testing have been added to this section.

- Section 10: This is a completely new section and contains detailed, step-by-step procedures on how to deal with emergency situations as they arise.

- The sections have been reorganized for easier comprehension. Routine clinical procedures have been moved to the front of the handbook, and specialty procedures such as medication administration, laboratory procedures, pediatric, and OB-GYN procedures are grouped together in the second half of the handbook.

- More Field Tips and Charting Examples have been added to the book.

- The inclusion of EMR Applications is a new feature that will assist health care workers transition from paper charts to electronic health records.

- The book now includes color tabs for easier referencing and is full-color with the addition of many new photos and illustrations.

- The book includes many new stories for the Hugs in the Hallway section.

ACKNOWLEDGMENTS

I would like to thank everyone at Delmar, Cengage Learning for their hard work on this exciting project. I would particularly like to thank Lauren Whalen and Rhonda Dearborn for their encouragement and support throughout the project. Lauren—you did a stupendous job in your role as a product manager. Your attention to detail and creativity added significantly to the finished product. Two new major contributors to this edition are Cheryl Baxter, NP, and Ann Zeller, AAS, CMA (AAMA). Without the both of you, this project would have been much more difficult.

I also want to thank my Columbus State family for the opportunity to teach and expand my knowledge and my great students, who teach me so much. And of course, family members of authors sacrifice a great deal during the research and writing phase of a book—a big thank you to all of my family members for their love and support throughout this process!

—Michelle E. Heller

Major contributors include:

Cheryl Baxter, RN, MS, Certified Nurse Practitioner—Nationwide Children's Hospital

Nancy Ford, RN, MS, CPNP—Nationwide Children's Hospital

Ann Zeller, AAS, CMA (AAMA), GxMO—Columbus State Community College

Reviewers

Vicki L. Crabtree, MEd
Chair, School of Technology
Rio Grande Community College
Rio Grande, Ohio

Laurie Dennis, CBCS
HIBC Instructor
Florida Career College
Clearwater, Florida

Vonda R. Godette, RN, MSN, CMA (AAMA)
Program Director
Carteret Community College
Morehead City, North Carolina

Marta Lopez
Program and Clinical Coordinator and Professor
Miami Dade College–Medical Center Campus
Miami, Florida

Judy D. Mackey, CMA, AAS
Director, Medical Assistant Program
International Business College
Indianapolis, Indiana

Tamara E. Mottler, BA, CMA (AAMA)
Program Manager and Assistant Chair
Daytona State College
Daytona Beach, Florida

June M. Petillo, MBA, RMC, NCP
Adjunct Instructor
Capitol Community College
Hartford, Connecticut

Wanda D. Strayhan, MS, CCMA, CBCS
Program Chair Allied Health Science
Florida Career College
Clearwater, Florida

Christina Thomas, CPC, CMA-A, CCMA, CBCS
Lead Instructor
Florida Career College
Clearwater, Florida

Caryn Ziegler, CMA (AAMA), MT (AMT)
Director, Medical Assisting Program
Minneapolis Business College
Roseville, Minnesota

Standard Precaution Icons

Each procedure in this handbook begins with icons that represent standard precautions. The following key presents each icon included in the procedures.

Icons	Description
	GLOVES
	HAND WASH
	BIOHAZARD
	GOWN
	NO NEEDLE RECAPPING
	UTILTITY GLOVES
	SHARPS CONTAINER
	MASK / GOGGLES ICON / FACE SHIELD

Section One
ABBREVIATIONS, SYMBOLS, AND COMMON MISSPELLED TERMS

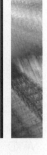

Section 1-1
COMMON MEDICAL ACRONYMS AND ABBREVIATIONS

Abbreviations have been used extensively in the medical field—that is, until the last few years. The use of some medical abbreviations has been banned as a result of the rise in medical errors associated with their use. Some accrediting agencies such as the Joint Commission now have a "Do Not Use" list for abbreviations that carry the largest risk for error. The "Do Not Use" list applies to abbreviations used in orders, such as medication and laboratory orders. Some analysts predict that abbreviations will be dropped entirely in the next few years, especially with the influx of electronic medical records, but until then you should be familiar with their use.

Table 1-1
COMMON DISEASES AND CONDITIONS

AAA	Abdominal aortic aneurysm; acute anxiety attack
ABE	Acute bacterial endocarditis
ACVD	Acute cardiovascular disease
ADD	Attention deficit disorder
ADHD	Attention deficit/hyperactivity disorder
AHD	Atherosclerotic heart disease
AIDS	Acquired immune deficiency syndrome

(continues)

(continued)

ALL	Acute lymphocytic leukemia; acute lymphoblastic leukemia
ALS	Amyotrophic lateral sclerosis
AML	Acute myeloblastic leukemia; acute myelocytic leukemia
AOD	Arterial occlusive disease
APKD	Adult polycystic kidney disease
ARC	AIDS-related complex
ARD	Acute respiratory disease
ARDS	Acute respiratory distress syndrome
ARF	Acute respiratory failure; acute renal failure; acute rheumatic fever
ARI	Acute respiratory infection
AS	Aortic stenosis
ASCVD	Arteriosclerotic cardiovascular disease
ASD	Atrial septal defect
ASHD	Arteriosclerotic heart disease
BBB	Bundle branch block
BCC	Basal cell carcinoma
BD	Bipolar disease
BPH	Benign prostatic hypertrophy
CA	Cancer, carcinoma
CAD	Coronary artery disease
CAG	Closed-angle glaucoma
CBS	Chronic brain syndrome
CE	Cardiac enlargement
CF	Cystic fibrosis
CHD	Coronary heart disease; congenital hip dislocation; congenital heart disease
CHF	Congestive heart failure
CIN	Cervical intraepithelial neoplasia

CIS	Carcinoma in situ
CKD	Chronic kidney disease
CLD	Chronic liver disease; chronic lung disease
COPD	Chronic obstructive pulmonary disease
CP	Cerebral palsy; chest pain
CPD	Cephalopelvic disproportion
CRF	Chronic renal failure
CT	Coronary thrombosis
CT; CTS	Carpal tunnel syndrome
CVA	Cardiovascular or cerebrovascular accident
CVD	Cardiovascular disease
Decub	Decubitus ulcer
DJD	Degenerative joint disease
DKA	Diabetic acidosis
DM	Diabetes mellitus
DOE	Dyspnea on exertion
DTs	Delirium tremens
Dub	Dysfunctional uterine bleeding
DVT	Deep vein thrombosis
EBV	Epstein-Barr virus
ED	Erectile dysfunction
EHT	Essential hypertension
EOM	Extraocular movement
EPS	Extrapyramidal symptoms
ESLD	End-stage liver disease
ESRD	End-stage renal disease
Exp	Expired
FAS	Fetal alcohol syndrome
FB	Foreign body
FTP	Failure to progress

(continues)

(continued)

FTT	Failure to thrive
FUO	Fever of undetermined origin
Fx, fx	Fracture
GAD	Generalized anxiety disorder
GBD	Gallbladder disease
GERD	Gastroesophageal reflux disease
GGE	Generalized glandular enlargement
GU	Gastric ulcer
HA	Headache; hemolytic anemia
HAV	Hepatitis A virus
HBV	Hepatitis B virus
HBC	Hepatitis C virus
HBP	High blood pressure
HC	Huntington's chorea
HCVD	Hypertensive cardiovascular disease
HD	Hodgkin's disease
HDN	Hemolytic disease of the newborn
Hemi	Hemiplegia, hemiplegic
HF	Heart failure
HH	Hiatal hernia
HI	Head injury
HIV	Human immunodeficiency virus
HL	Hearing loss
HLHS	Hypoplastic left heart syndrome
HOH or HoH	Hard of hearing
HPV	Human papillomavirus
HSV-1	Herpes simplex virus type 1
HSV-2	Herpes simplex virus type 2
HTN	Hypertension
IBD	Inflammatory bowel disease

IBS	Irritable bowel syndrome
IDDM	Insulin-dependent diabetes mellitus
IHD	Ischemic heart disease
IM	Infectious mononucleosis
ISVD	Intraventricular septal defect
LAV	Lymphadenopathy-associated virus
LTB	Laryngotracheobronchitis
LVH	Left ventricular hypertrophy
MBD	Minimal brain dysfunction
MD	Muscular dystrophy, manic depression, myocardial disease
MDD	Major depressive disorder
MI	Myocardial infarction
Mono	Mononucleosis
MS	Mitral stenosis; multiple sclerosis
MVP	Mitral valve prolapse
NAD	No acute distress
NIDDM	Non–insulin-dependent diabetes mellitus
OA	Osteoarthritis
OAG	Open-angle glaucoma
OBS	Organic brain syndrome
OCD	Obsessive-compulsive disorder
PA	Pernicious anemia
PAV	Premature atrial contraction
PAT	Paroxysmal atrial tachycardia
PCD	Polycystic disease
PDA	Patent ductus arteriosus
PE	Pulmonary edema, pulmonary embolism
PID	Pelvic inflammatory disease
PIH	Pulmonary induced hypertension

(continues)

(continued)

PKU	Phenylketonuria
PMS	Premenstrual syndrome
PTSD	Posttraumatic stress disorder
PUD	Peptic ulcer disease
PVC	Premature ventricular contraction
RA	Rheumatoid arthritis
RDS	Respiratory distress syndrome
REM	Rapid eye movement
RHD	Rheumatic heart disease
SAB	Spontaneous abortion
SAD	Seasonal affective disorder
SAH	Subarachnoid hemorrhage
SBE	Shortness of breath on exertion; subacute bacterial endocarditis
SBO	Small bowel obstruction
SC	Sickle cell
SCC	Squamous cell carcinoma
SI	Sinus infection
SIDS	Sudden infant death syndrome
SLE	Systemic lupus erythematosus
STD	Sexually transmitted disease
STI	Sexually transmitted infection
SUI	Stress urinary incontinence
TSD	Tay-Sachs disease
UAO	Upper airway obstruction
URI	Upper respiratory infection
UTI	Urinary tract infection
V/D	Vomiting and diarrhea
VSD	Ventricular septal defect

Table 1-2

COMMON CHARTING AND DIAGNOSTIC ABBREVIATIONS (Anything marked in red comes from the ISMP's List of Error Prone Abbreviations, Symbols, and Dose Designations and thus should not be used in any type of order.)

ABO	Abortion
Abd	Abdomen
a.c.	Before meals
AD	Right ear
ADL	Activities of daily living
ADM	Admit, admission, admitted
AI	Allergy index
AF	Atrial fibrillation
AK	Above the knee
AKA	Above the knee amputation
AM, a.m., AM	Before noon
AMA	Against medical advice
Amt	Amount
Ant	Anterior
AP	Anterior/posterior; apical pulse
AS	Left ear
ASAP	As soon as possible
AU	Both ears
AV	Atriovenous, atrioventricular
A&W	Alive and well
Ax	Axillary
Ba, BaE, BE	Barium, barium enema
BAEP	Brainstem auditory evoked potential
BAER	Brainstem auditory evoked response
BBT	Basal body temperature
BC	Birth control

(continues)

(continued)

Bi	Biopsy
BK	Below the knee
BKA	Below the knee amputation
BLA	Both lower extremities
BM	Bowel movement
BMI	Body mass index
BO	Body odor
bol	Bolus
BP	Blood pressure
BPD	Biparietal diameter
BSA	Body surface area
BSE	Breast self-examination
Bx	Biopsy
c̄,/c, w/	With
C, kcal	Calorie
CA, Ca	Cancer
CABG	Coronary artery bypass graft
CAPD	Continuous ambulatory peritoneal dialysis
CAT	Computerized axial tomography
CBI	Continuous bladder irrigation
CC	Chief complaint
CCU	Coronary care unit
CICU	Cardiac (coronary) intensive care unit
CHO	Carbohydrate
c/o	Complains of
CP	Chest pain
CPAP	Continuous positive airway pressure
CPE, CPX	Complete physical examination
CPR	Cardiopulmonary resuscitation
CT	Computerized tomography

Cx	Canceled
CXR	Chest x-ray
D&C	Dilation and curettage
D/C	Discharge
D&E	Dilation and evacuation
def	Deficiency
disch	Discharged
DNS	Did not show
DNR	Do not resuscitate
DOA	Date of admission; dead on arrival
DOB	Date of birth
DOI	Date of injury
DRE	Digital rectal examination
Drg or Drsg	Dressing
DVA	Distance visual acuity
Dx	Diagnosis
EBL	Estimated blood loss
ECG, EKG	Electrocardiogram
ECHO	Echocardiogram
ED	Emergency department
EDC	Expected date of confinement
EDD	Expected date of delivery
EEG	Electroencephalogram
EENT	Eye, ear, nose, and throat
EEP	End expiratory pressure
EF	Ejection fraction
EGD	Esophagogastroduodenoscopy
EMG	Electromyography
EMS	Emergency medical services
ENT	Ear, nose, and throat

(continues)

(continued)

EPAP	Expiratory positive airway pressure
ER	Emergency room
ERCP	Endoscopic retrograde cholangiopancreatography
ESWL	Extracorporeal shockwave lithotripsy
ETD	Estimated time of death
EUS	Endoscopic ultrasonography
Ex	Examination
ex, exam	Examination
expl lap	Exploratory laparoscopy
FB	Foreign body
FDLMP	First day of last menstrual period
FEV	Forced expiratory volume
FF	Force fluids
FH	Family history
FHS	Fetal heart sounds
Flu	Fluoroscopy
FTND	Full-term normal delivery
FTT	Failure to thrive
F/U	Follow-up
FUO	Fever of undetermined origin
Fx, fx	Fracture
Ga	Gastric analysis
GB, gb	Gallbladder
GI	Gastrointestinal
Grav	Gravida (number of pregnancies)
GSW	Gunshot wound
GTT	Glucose tolerance test
GU	Genitourinary
GYN	Gynecology

HA	Headache; hearing aid
HBP	High blood pressure
HC	Head circumference
HEENT	Head, eyes, ears, nose, throat
HI	Head injury
H/O	History of
HOH	Hard of hearing
hosp	Hospital
H&P	History and physical
HPI	History of present illness
HR	Heart rate
HSG	Hysterosalpingogram
Ht	Height
HTN, htn	Hypertension
Hx, hx	History
IABP	Intra-aortic balloon pump
ICD	Implantable cardioverter defibrillator
ICP	Intracranial pressure
ICU	Intensive care unit
I&D	Incision and drainage
imp	Impression
I&O	Intake and output
IQ	Intelligence quotient
IVC	Intravenous catheter; intravenous cholangiogram
IVP	Intravenous pyelogram
KOH	Potassium hydroxide
KUB	Kidneys, ureters, and bladder
$L_1, L_2, \ldots$	Lumbar first, second, etc.
L&A	Light and accommodation

(continues)

(continued)

Lab	Laboratory
Lac	Laceration
LASIK	Laser-assisted in situ keratomileusis
Lat	Lateral
LAVH	Laparoscopic-assisted vaginal hysterectomy
lb	Pound
LBW	Low birth weight
LEEP	Loop electrosurgical excision procedure
LLETZ	Large-loop excision of transformation zone
LLQ	Left lower quadrant
LMP	Last menstrual period
LRQ	Lower right quadrant
LS	Lumbar spine
LSS	Lumbar sacral spine
Lt or Ⓛ	Left
LUQ	Left upper quadrant
L&W	Living and well
mA	Milliampere
met	Metastasis
mm Hg	Millimeters of mercury
MP	Metacarpophalangeal joint
MPI	Myocardial perfusion scan
MRA	Magnetic resonance angiography
MRI	Magnetic resonance imaging
MUGA	Multiple-gated acquisition (scan)
MVA	Motor vehicle accident
NAD	No acute distress
NB	Newborn
N/C	No complaints

neg	Negative
NG (T)	Nasogastric tube
NH (P)	Nursing home placement
NKA	No known allergies
NKDA	No known drug allergies
NL	Normal limits
NMT	Nebulizing mist treatment
N/O	No complaints
Noc	Night
NPO	Nothing by mouth
NSR	Normal sinus rhythm
N/V, N&V	Nausea and vomiting
NVA	Near visual acuity
O_2, O_2 sat	Oxygen, oxygen saturation
OB	Obstetrics
OCP	Oral contraceptive pill
OD	Right eye
OH	Occupational history
OP	Operation, operative; outpatient
OR	Operating room
Ortho	Orthopedics
OS	Left eye
OT	Occupational therapy
OTC	Over-the-counter
OU	Both eyes
OV	Office visit
P	Pulse; plan; posterior
PA	Posterior/anterior
P&A	Percussion and auscultation

(continues)

(continued)

$PaCO_2$	Partial pressure of carbon dioxide
PaO_2	Partial pressure of oxygen
Pap	Papanicolaou (smear)
PARA, para	Number of births (nullipara, primipara, Para I, Para II, etc.)
PAT	Preadmission testing
Path	Pathology
p.c.	After meals
PCI	Percutaneous coronary intervention
PE	Physical examination; pelvic examination
PED	Pediatric
PEFR	Peak expiratory flow rate
Per	By or through
PERRLA	Pupils equal, round, react to light and accommodation
PET	Positron emission tomography
PFT	Pulmonary function test
pH	Potential of hydrogen
PH	Past history
PI	Present illness
PICC	Peripherally inserted central catheter
PM, p.m., PM	Afternoon
PMH	Past medical history
POL	Physician's office laboratory
POMR	Problem-oriented medical record
post-op	Postoperative
PN	Parenteral nutrition
PP	Postpartum; postprandial
Preg	Pregnant
Pre-op	Preoperative

Prep	Prepare
PRN, p.r.n, prn	As needed
Prog	Prognosis
Psych	Psychiatry
Pt, pt	Patient
PT	Physical therapy
PTA	Prior to admission
PTCA	Percutaneous transluminal coronary angioplasty
Pulm	Pulmonary
Px	Prognosis
PX or PE	Physical examination
P/Y; PY	Pack-years
R	Respiration
® or RT	Right
Reg	Regular
RGP	Retrograde pyelogram
RLQ	Right lower quadrant
R/O	Rule out
ROM	Range of motion
ROS	Review of systems
RR	Respiratory rate; recovery room
Rt or ®	Right
RT	Respiratory therapist; radiation therapy
RUQ	Right upper quadrant
℞	Prescription
S	Subjective
$\bar{s}$	Without
SaO_2	Oxygen saturation level
SH	Social history

(continues)

(continued)

Sig:	Instructions to patient
SMWD	Single, married, widowed, divorced
SNF	Skilled nursing facility
SOAP	Subjective, objective, assessment, plans
SOB	Shortness of breath
spec	Specimen
SR	Systems review
$\bar{s}$	Without
$\bar{ss}$	Half
S&S	Signs and symptoms
ST	Speech therapist
STAT	Immediately
surg	Surgical, surgery
Sx or sx	Symptom
Sz	Seizure
T, temp	Temperature
T&A	Tonsillectomy and adenoidectomy
TAB	Therapeutic abortion
TAH	Total abdominal hysterectomy
TEDS	Thromboembolic disease stockings
TEE	Transesophageal echocardiogram
TENS	Transcutaneous electrical nerve stimulation
TM	Tympanic membrane
TO	Telephone order
TPN	Total parenteral nutrition
TPR	Temperature, pulse, respiration
tr, trt, tx	Treatment
TSE	Testicular self-examination
TURB	Transurethral resection of the bladder
TURP	Transurethral resection of the prostate

TV	Tidal volume
TVS	Transvaginal sonography
TWE	Tap water enema
Tx	Treatment
UAO	Upper airway obstruction
UCHD	Usual childhood diseases
UGI	Upper gastrointestinal (series)
ULQ	Upper left quadrant
UNK	Unknown
UOP	Urinary output
URQ	Upper right quadrant
US, U/S	Ultrasound
UV	Ultraviolet
VA	Visual acuity
VC	Vital capacity
VCU, VCGU	Voiding cystourethrogram
V/D	Vomiting and diarrhea
VF	Ventricular fibrillation
V/O	Ventilation/perfusion
VO	Verbal order
VS	Vital signs
$\bar{w}$	With
WB	Weight bearing
WDWN	Well-developed, well-nourished
wk	Work
wk(s)	Weeks
WNL	Within normal limits
w/o	Without
Wt, wt	Weight
W/U, w/u	Workup
yr	Year

Table 1-3

COMMON LABORATORY ABBREVIATIONS

A1c or A1C	Hemoglobin A_{1c}
ABG	Arterial blood gases
ACTH	Adrenocorticotropic hormone
ADH	Antidiuretic hormone
ALB	Albumin
ALP	Alkaline phosphatase
ALT	Alanine aminotransferase
ANA	Antinuclear antibodies
Bi or bx	Biopsy
BG	Blood glucose
BMP	Basal metabolic panel
BS	Blood sugar
BT	Bleeding time
BUN	Blood, urea, nitrogen
Ca	Calcium
CBC	Complete blood count
CEA	Carcinoembryonic antigen
Chem	Chemistry
Chol	Cholesterol
CL⁻	Chloride
CO	Carbon monoxide
CO_2	Carbon dioxide
CMH	Comprehensive metabolic panel
CPK	Creatine phosphokinase
CrCl	Creatinine clearance
Creat	Creatinine
C&S	Culture and sensitivity
CSF	Cerebrospinal fluid

Diff	Differential
EBV	Epstein-Barr virus
ELISA	Enzyme-linked immunosorbent assay
EPO	Erythropoietin
ESR	Erythrocyte sedimentation rate
ETOH	Ethyl alcohol
FBS	Fasting blood sugar
Fe	Iron
FS	Frozen section
FSH	Follicle-stimulating hormone
GC	Gonorrhea culture
GFR	Glomerular filtration rate
GH	Growth hormone
Glob	Globulin
GTH	Gonadotropic hormone
GTT	Glucose tolerance test
hb, hgb	Hemoglobin
HbA1c, HgA1c, A1c	Hemoglobin A_{1c}
hCG	Human chorionic gonadotropin hormone
HCl	Hydrochloric acid
Hct, hct	Hematocrit
HDL	High-density lipoprotein
hGH	Human growth hormone
HIV	Human immunodeficiency virus
H&H	Hematocrit and hemoglobin
HLA	Human leukocyte antigen
hpf	High-power field
H. pylori	*Helicobacter pylori* bacterium
Ig	Immunoglobulin

(continues)

(continued)

INR	International normalized ratio
ISG	Immune serum globulin
K	Potassium
KCl	Potassium chloride
Lab	Laboratory
LDH, LD	Lactic dehydrogenase
LDLs	Low density lipoproteins
LFT	Liver function test
LH	Luteinizing hormone
Lpf	Low-power field
Lytes	Electrolytes
Mag	Magnesium
MCH	Mean corpuscular hemoglobin
MCHC	Mean corpuscular hemoglobin concentration
MCV	Mean corpuscular volume, mean cell volume
mEq/L	Milliequivalent per liter
Mg	Magnesium
Mm^3	Cubic millimeters, millimeters cubed
Mono, mono	Mononucleosis
MSH	Melanocyte-stimulating hormone
Na	Sodium
O_2	Oxygen
P	Phosphorus
$PaCO_2$, PaO_2	Partial pressure of carbon dioxide
Pap	Papanicolaou test
PAT	Preadmission testing
Path	Pathology
PBI	Protein-bound iodine
PCV	Packed cell volume
PKU	Phenylketonuria

PLT	Platelet
POL	Physician's office laboratory
PPE	Personal protective equipment
PSA	Protein specific antigen
PT	Pro-time
PTH	Parathyroid hormone
PTT	Partial thromboplastin time
QA	Quality assurance
QC	Quality control
Qns	Quantity nonsufficient
Qs	Quantity sufficient
RBC, rbc	Red blood cell
RBS	Random blood sugar
SG, Sp gr	Specific gravity
Staph	Staphylococcus
Strep	Streptococcus
STS	Serological test for syphilis
T_3	Triiodothyronine
T_4	Thyroxine
Tb	Tubercle bacillus
TC	Throat culture
T&C	Type and cross match
TG	Triglyceride
TIBC	Total iron-binding capacity
TP	Total protein
TPA	Tissue plasminogen activator
TSA	Tumor specific antigen
TSH	Thyroid-stimulating hormone
UA	Urinalysis; uric acid
UC	Urine culture

(continues)

(continued)

VDRL	Venereal Disease Reference Laboratory
VRSA	Vancomycin-resistant *Staphylococcus aureus*
WBC, wbc	White blood cell
WNL	Within normal limits
X-match	Cross match

Table 1-4

COMMON MEDICATION ABBREVIATIONS

Any abbreviation that appears on the ISMP's List of Error-Prone Abbreviations, Symbols, and Dose Designations does not appear in Tables 1-4 through 1-6.

$\bar{a}$	Before
a.c.	Before meals
ad lib	As desired
AM, a.m., AM	Before noon or morning
Amp	Ampule
Aq	Water
BC	Birth control
BID, b.i.d, bid	Twice per day
$\bar{c}$	With
Cap	Capsule
DAW	Dispense as written
Dil	Dilute
DS	Double strength
D/W	Distilled water
Fl	Fluid
h, hr	Hour
Hypo	Hypodermic

ID	Intradermal
IM	Intramuscular
Inj	Injection
IT	Inhalation therapy
IV	Intravenous
IVP	Intravenous push
IVPB	Intravenous piggyback
Meds	Medication
NKDA	No known drug allergies
Noc	Night
NPO	Nothing by mouth
p̄	After
p.c.	After meals
PDR	*Physicians' Desk Reference*
PO, po	By mouth
PR	Per rectum
PRN, p.r.n., prn	As needed
q	Every
q.i.d, qid	Four times a day
℞	Prescription
s̄	Without
Sig	Let it be labeled
Sol	Solution
STAT	Immediately
Subcut	Subcutaneous
Supp	Suppository
Syr	Syrup
tab(s)	Tablet(s)
t.i.d, tid	Three times daily

(continues)

(continued)

Tinc	Tincture
Ung	Ointment
W/O	Without

Table 1-5
COMMON MEASUREMENT ABBREVIATIONS

g, gm	Gram
gt	Drop
gtt	Drops
Kg	Kilogram
lb	Pounds
L	Liter
Mcg	Microgram
mEq	Milliequivalent
Mg	Milligram
ml, mL	Milliliter
Ng	Nanogram

Table 1-6
COMMON SYMBOLS

Δ,^{d}	Change
✓	Check
↓	Decrease
O or ♂	Female
′	Foot

"	Inch
↑	Increase
Ⓛ	Left
⊙–	Lying
☐ or ♂	Male
⊖	Negative
∅	None or negative
#	Number
⊕	Positive
®	Right
⊙=	Sitting
♀	Standing

Section 1-2

COMMONLY MISSPELLED EVERYDAY TERMS

The following is a list of everyday terms that are commonly misspelled! Always double-check your documentation to ascertain you have the correct spelling.

absence	analysis	benefited
accidentally	analyze	business
accommodate	annual	calendar
accumulate	appearance	candidate
achievement	ascend	capital
acquaintance	assure	capitol
acquire	balance	category
advice	belief	changeable
advise	believe	choose
affect	beneficial	chose

coarse	February	personal
conscience	foreign	personnel
conscious	formerly	perspiration
coming	forty	physical
commission	fourth	possibility
complement	generally	possible
compliment	grammar	practically
course	grievous	precede
definition	height	precedence
describe	humorous	preference
description	immediately	preferred
desperate	incidentally	prejudice
device	independence	preparation
devise	inevitable	prevalent
disappearance	insure	principal
disappoint	intelligence	principle
disastrous	knowledge	privilege
discipline	laboratory	probably
dissatisfied	laid	procedure
effect	led	proceed
eighth	maintenance	profession
eligible	maybe	professor
eliminate	necessary	prominent
embarrass	ninety	pronunciation
ensure	noticeable	pursue
environment	occasionally	quantity
equipped	occurred	quizzes
especially	occurrence	recede
exaggerate	omitted	receive
excellence	opinion	receiving
existence	opportunity	recommend
existent	optimistic	reference
experience	paid	referring
explanation	particular	repetition
familiar	performance	rhyme
fascinate	permissible	rhythm

salary	stationary	transferring
schedule	stationery	tries
seize	statue	truly
sense	studying	unnecessary
separate	succeed	until
separation	succession	usually
severely	technique	weird
similar	temperamental	whether
sincerely	tendency	
specifically	tragedy	

Section 1-3

COMMONLY MISSPELLED MEDICAL TERMS

The following is a list of medical terms that are commonly misspelled! Always double-check your documentation to ascertain you have the correct spelling.

abscess	humerus	phlegm
aneurysm	ischium	pneumonia
anemia	ilium	pruritus
arrhythmia	ileum	psychiatrist
brachial	illicit	pyrexia
calcaneus	inflammation	rheumatic
catheterization	ischemia	roentgenology
cirrhosis	larynx	sagittal
clavicle	malaise	specimen
conscious	melanoma	sphygmomanometer
curettage	mucous	staphylococcus
diaphragm	mucus	tetanus
elicit	ophthalmology	tonsil
endometriosis	palliative	trachea
epididymis	paralysis	unconscious
hemorrhage	paralyze	vein
hemorrhoids	parenteral	vesicle
homeostasis	pharynx	

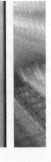

Section Two
DOCUMENTATION AND IN-OFFICE SCREENINGS

INTRODUCTION

Throughout this handbook, the term *provider* may refer to a physician, nurse practitioner, or physician assistant.

Documentation is one of the most important tasks that you will perform in the medical office. It is also one of the most controversial because of its subjectivity. Most health care professionals document the way that they were taught during their training programs.

It is not our intention to determine who is right in their documentation practices and who is wrong. We want to give our readers the fundamentals that are necessary to avoid legal ramifications and to document to the degree of thoroughness set forth by the insurance industry.

After all, those who benefit the most from complete and accurate documentation are the patients!

WHO IS REVIEWING YOUR DOCUMENTATION?

Only in the last several years, with the implementation of managed care, and now with health care reform, have charts been open to the scrutiny of a wide range of health care professionals. Before managed care, the only people viewing charts were those directly affiliated with the practice. On some occasions, a chart was reviewed by an insurance company or in a court of law, but that usually involved alleged wrongdoing.

Today, many outsiders are reviewing charts—especially with the implementation of electronic medical records (EMRs). With the click of a button, parts of patients' EMRs are now shared with a multitude of sources, including insurance companies, providers to whom patients are being referred, emergency departments, and the patients themselves.

This section includes information regarding the types of medical documentation that are performed in ambulatory care. It also includes many documentation samples.

Another feature of this section is the in-office screening charts, which provide readers with a list of questions that should be asked when the patient presents with specific symptoms.

DOCUMENTATION BASICS

The following principles will help with good documentation:

- **Right Chart:** Many patients have the same name, which can lead to incorrect documentation in a chart that does not belong to the patient. Be certain that you have the right chart when documenting information into a patient's chart. Double-check by asking patients their birth date or last four digits of their Social Security number, as well as their name.

- **Document All Patient Encounters:** Document each office visit, all procedures, each telephone call, and all appointment-related changes, such as broken appointments, canceled appointments, and rescheduled appointments. This can help to show noncompliance on the part of the patient should a lawsuit arise.

EMR Application

Many EMR programs are linked to the appointment application, so if a patient calls to cancel an appointment, the cancellation and reason for cancellation is saved at the time the appointment is canceled, thus there is no need to document the cancellation in the patient's progress note. The information is permanently stored in a designated area of the chart. An audit of these cancellations or no-shows can be printed and sent to the patient to verify the dates and reasons for the cancellations, in the event the patient is terminated due to excessive missed appointments.

- **Document Accurately and Objectively:** Document only factual information. Avoid assumptions and opinions.

- **Document Completely:** Don't leave out pertinent facts such as location and when symptoms started. Some patients will admit to negligence in passing conversation, for example, "Since I had the foot surgery, I run my foot into everything." This type of statement might sound humorous, but if infection sets in, and complications arise it can demonstrate negligence on the part of the patient.

- **Document the Date and Time at the Beginning of Each Entry:** This could be very important in legal matters.

- **Write in Black Ink When Recording in Paper Charts:** Because the chart is a legal document, black ink is preferred.

- **Correct Spelling:** Use correct spelling. If you don't know the spelling, use a synonym that you do know how to spell or leave space and look it up in a pocket dictionary when you leave the patient's room. Even in the EMR, not all spell-check programs catch every spelling error. Always double-check your spelling.

- **Use Standard Abbreviations:** The Joint Commission and other federal agencies are steering health care professionals away from the use of abbreviations, particularly when documenting medication procedures and orders. This is due to the number of errors that occur with their use. If you work in a facility that still uses medical abbreviations, avoid using the abbreviations that appear on the Joint Commission's "Do Not Use" list or the Institute for Safe Medication Practices (ISMP) "Error-Prone" Abbreviation list, or abbreviations that are not universal.

EMR Application

The following is a statement from the Joint Commission:
Currently, the requirement not to use abbreviations that appear on the "Do Not Use" list does not apply to preprogrammed health information technology systems (for example, electronic medical records or computerized physician order entry [CPOE] systems), but this application remains under consideration for the future. Organizations contemplating introduction or upgrade of such systems should strive to eliminate the use of dangerous abbreviations, acronyms, symbols, and dose designations from the software.

- **Positive and Negative Symbols:** Circle all positive ⊕ and negative ⊖ symbols when working in paper charts. Circling helps the symbols stand out so that they are not mistaken for something else.

- **Document Specifics:** Don't forget to include the *date or time of onset* or *duration; specific locations* (e.g., R. ear, L. calf); *colors* when applicable (e.g., yellow purulent discharge, black stool); *odors* (e.g., strong ammonia odor; *size* (e.g., the knot is the size of a dime); *temperature* when there is a chance for infection. List *related symptoms* when they apply. *Rate all pain* on a scale from 1 to 10 when responsible for developing the history of the present illness.

- **Document on Every Line:** There shouldn't be any blank lines be-tween entries. This prohibits someone from changing the entry. In cases in which the entry stops before the right margin, make certain that the last line of your entry extends all the way to the end of the right margin by inserting a line following your name and credential.
- **Signature:** Be sure to sign all entries with an approved closing sig-nature (i.e., first initial, last name, and credential).

Documentation Don'ts

- **Don't Procrastinate:** Document while the information is fresh. Accuracy is essential! Details are much clearer right after working with the patient.
- **Don't Diagnose:** List symptoms only. If patients state they think they have a urinary tract infection (UTI) or migraine, place what the patient said in quotations to show that it was the patient's own words.
- **Don't Document for Someone Else and Don't Allow Others to Document for You:** This could cause serious legal problems.
- **Don't Scribble Over or Use Correction Fluid in Paper Charts:** It may look like you are hiding something. Draw a single line through the error, initial it, date it, and write in the new entry.

EMR Application

Once an entry is officially entered in the patient's electronic medical record (EMR), it is there for the life of the record. In most EMRs, you will need to make an addendum to the original entry if an error is spotted following submission. Both the original entry and addendum will be available for future viewing.

Section 2-1
PATIENT SCREENINGS

Each time a patient comes into the office, a screening will be performed. The depth of screening will be determined by the reason for the visit and the role of the individual performing the screening. The provider will usually develop the history of the present illness, but other ancillary team members such as the medical assistant will start the screening. Each screening should start with a review and update of the patient's medications and a review and update of the patient's allergies, particularly drug and latex allergies.

Brief Patient Screenings

A brief patient screening usually begins with an update of the patient's medications and allergies and a recording of the patient's chief complaint. The chief complaint is a description of what is wrong with the patient, usually in the patient's own words. A brief screening may also include the duration of the problem.

Table 2-1

COMPONENTS OF A BRIEF PATIENT SCREENING AND CHIEF COMPLAINT

Parts of the Complaint	Description or Tips
1. Today's date and time	Many facilities use military time. Always check with a supervisor when starting a new position.
2. Review and update the patient's medication list.	Patients often see multiple providers. Check to see if any medications were added or deleted from the list, including regular over-the-counter (OTC) medications. This may be recorded in the progress note or in a table somewhere else in the chart.
3. Review and update the patient's drug allergies.	The patient may have developed a drug allergy or some other type of drug sensitivity since the last visit. Drug allergies should be written in red.
4. Patient's chief complaint	This is a brief description of what is wrong with the patient. Use the patient's own words in this part of the screening. Avoid using medical terms. You may use standard abbreviations to shorten the complaint.
5. Date of onset or duration of the problem	When did the incident occur or when did the patient first notice the symptoms?
6. Closing signature	First initial, last name, followed by credential

CHARTING EXAMPLE 1

04/05/XXXX	Medications and Allergies: No changes since last visit.
9:45 a.m.	CC: "My head has been killing me for the past 6 hours."
	T. Smith, CMA (AAMA) ————————————————

CHARTING EXAMPLE 2

10/23/XXXX	Medications and Allergies: Levoxyl, 125 mg per day
12:15 p.m.	and one multivitamin each day. Drug allergy to
	codeine. CC: Pt. c/o a "sore throat" × 3 days. J. Davis,
	LPN ————————————————————————

CHARTING EXAMPLE 3

08/19/XXXX	Medications and Allergies: Sildenafil, 25 mg as
10:10 a.m.	needed. NKDA. CC: Pt cut the bottom of his left foot
	on a broken bottle 2 hours ago. "Wound will not stop
	bleeding." Last tetanus, 3 years ago. M. Brown, RMA

EMR Application

Most EMR software programs have a medication section where you can add and delete medications. If you accidentally delete a medication that should not have been deleted, you can usually get it back by clicking on a "reactivation" tab beside the name of the medication that you accidentally deleted.

Field Tip

When patients have puncture injuries or other injuries that break the skin, always inquire about the patient's last tetanus vaccine. If it has been longer than 10 years, the patient will probably need a new tetanus vaccine. Always get an order before administering any medication.

Comprehensive Patient Screenings

A comprehensive patient screening is an in-depth look at the patient's presenting symptoms. Performing a comprehensive screening will cut down on the amount of writing that the provider has to do, although providers may need to review the information with the patient and ask their own questions to obtain full reimbursement from the insurance company. Performing a comprehensive screening also provides the medical assistant or nurse with anticipation skills necessary for properly preparing the patient and setting up the room before the provider's entrance.

Table 2-2 provides the necessary information for documenting findings from a comprehensive screening.

Table 2-2
COMPONENTS OF A COMPREHENSIVE PATIENT SCREENING

Parts of the Complaint	Description
1. Today's date and time	Many facilities use military time. Always check with a supervisor when starting a new position.
2. Review and update the patient's medication list.	Patients often see multiple providers. Check to see if any medications (prescribed and regular over-the-counter (OTC) medications were added or deleted from the list. This may be recorded in the progress note or in a table somewhere else in the chart. OTCs that are just being taken for current symptoms should be recorded beside "Therapeutic Measures" or "Home Treatment" within the complaint itself.
3. Review and update the patient's drug allergy status.	The patient may have developed a drug allergy or some other type of drug sensitivity since the last visit. Drug allergies should be written in red.
4. Chief complaint	This is a brief description of what is wrong with the patient. Use the patient's own words in this part of the complaint and enclose them in quotation marks. Avoid using medical terms. You may use standard abbreviations to shorten the complaint.
5. Date of onset or duration	How long have the symptoms been present or when did the incident occur?
6. Severity or character	How bothersome is the problem? Does it keep the patient from sleeping? Does it wake the patient up? Does it interfere with physical activity? When pain is involved, rate the pain on a scale from 1–10. The number "1" would indicate mild pain and the number "10" intense pain.

(continues)

(continued)

Parts of the Complaint	Description
7. Location or radiation of pain	Where is the pain located? Does it radiate to any other structures?
8. Any related symptoms?	Symptoms that may be related to the general complaint (Refer to Table 2-3 for a list of related symptoms for various types of complaints.)
9. Any home treatment or therapeutic measures taken?	What makes symptoms better? A different position, OTC medications, etc.
10. Closing signature	First initial, last name, and credential

Field Tip

Some providers will want you to list the last monthly period (LMP) for all female patients of child-bearing age, even in cases in which the patient has no urogenital symptoms. Some offices complete a social history each time the patient comes in as well. Social history questions may include items such as tobacco use, alcohol or drug use, caffeine consumption and seatbelt information. Other providers may request you to list all patient allergies, not just drug allergies. It is important to document and highlight any latex allergies because some offices still use latex products.

CHARTING EXAMPLE 1

| 02/25/XXXX 1:15 p.m. | Current ℞: None, Regular OTC: One-a-Day Vitamin Women's/Daily; ⊖ Drug or Latex Allergies. CC: "It hurts when I go to the bathroom × 4 days." Pain level "9" (1 to 10 scale) ⊕ frequency (especially at night), ⊕ burning, ⊖ fever, ⊖ N/V, ⊖ back pain, ⊖ Abd pressure/pain, ⊖ vaginal symptoms, LMP 01/19/XXXX, Therapeutic Measures: Urostat, 3 doses (little relief.). J. Crawford, CMA (AAMA) —————— |

CHARTING EXAMPLE 2

04/15/XXXX 11:25 a.m.	Current ℞: Imitrex Inj (6 mg as needed for pain), Paxil (20 mg/day), Regular OTC: None, Drug Allergy: Codeine, No Latex Allergy. CC: "I have a migraine headache." Pain level "10" (1–10 scale). Duration (6 hours) ⊕ N/V (3 episodes), ⊕ light sensitivity, ⊕ aura before HA, ⊕ Hx of migraines, No other symptoms. Therapeutic Measures: Imitrex injection 3 hours ago (No relief). T. Brown, RMA ————————

CHARTING EXAMPLE 3

06/16/XXXX 4:10 p.m.	Current ℞: None, Regular OTC: None, Drug Allergies: Sulfa Products. CC: "I have a cold" × 5 days, ⊕ sore throat "10" (1–10 scale), ⊕ L. ear pain "4" (1–10 scale) ⊕ head pressure (right side of forehead), ⊕ productive cough (yellow-green phlegm), ⊕ fever. ("100–101 degrees F") Home Treatment: 2 Regular Strength Tylenol Cold Tabs every 6 hours × 3 days (little to no relief). C. Riffle, CMA (AAMA) ————————

Gathering Questions for the History of the Present Illness

This handbook features two types of screenings: in-office and telephone screenings. In this section we discuss in-office screenings. To learn more about telephone screenings, refer to Section 3.

The purpose of the Quick Glance History of the Present Illness (HPI) and Anticipation Table is to train medical personnel to develop their screening skills by learning what symptoms routinely correspond to particular conditions.

Developing the chief complaint will aid health care workers in knowing how to properly set up the patient's room and how to have the patient disrobe. It also alerts the medical assistant or nurse to the possibility for diagnostic testing when the patient displays specific symptoms.

How to Use the Chart

The reader will start the in-office screening by asking the questions found in Table 2-2. When the reader gets to question 8 in the table, he or she will turn to the History of the Present Illness (HPI) table (Table 2-3) and find the condition that best matches the patient's presenting symptoms. The reader will then proceed by asking the questions found underneath the related symptoms. Medical assisting students or new medical assistants may want to use the anticipation column to see how to set up the room and patient before the examination. (The anticipation column is a list of suggestions reflecting what the provider may want when the patient presents with certain symptoms.) The reader will then return to Table 2-2 and start with question 9 and proceed until all questions in the table have been asked.

In cases in which pretesting can save time, the medical assistant can alert the provider of the patient's symptoms to see if the provider wants any preliminary testing performed before the actual examination (e.g., urinalysis for urinary symptoms or rapid strep test for a sore throat). These test and procedure alerts can be found in the anticipatory guidance column of Table 2-3 under "Provider's Call." Medicare and other insurance companies may not allow testing until a full examination has been performed. *Never perform any diagnostic test without a specific order from the provider. Even if you cannot perform the test before examination, you can set everything up in the event that the testing or procedure is ordered.*

Table 2-3
RELATED SYMPTOMS AND ANTICIPATORY GUIDANCE

Related Symptoms or Questions	Anticipatory Guidance
Complaint: Abdominal or Stomach Pain	
1. Rate pain on a scale of 1 to 10 and give exact location of pain.	• *Disrobing Instructions:* If symptoms appear to be above the waist, disrobe from waist up. If symptoms appear to be below the waist, disrobe from waist down. Give patient a gown.
2. Does patient have any nausea or vomiting?	
3. Have there been any changes in bowel habits? (List last bowel movement and texture.)	• *Vital Signs:* TPR and BP
4. Are there any signs of dehydration? (e.g., dry mouth, last urination greater than 8–10 hours ago, etc.)	• *Comfort Instructions:* If patient has nausea and vomiting, offer an emesis basin. Do not allow patient to eat or drink anything.
5. Does patient have a fever? (List the last reading and route.)	***Provider's Call:*** *(Possible Diagnostic Testing and Tray Setups)*
6. Are there any penile or vaginal symptoms? (List LMP for females.)	• *Urinary Symptoms:* Collect a clean-catch urine sample for a possible urinalysis and culture.
7. Does patient have any urinary symptoms?	• *Vaginal Symptoms:* Pelvic tray and cultures
8. Does patient have lower back pain?	• *Penile Symptoms:* Appropriate cultures

Complaint: Allergic Reactions

1. Any shortness of breath or swelling of the tongue, throat, or bronchial tubes?
2. Does patient have hives? (Give location.)
3. Rash? (Give location and appearance.)
4. Any changes in detergents, soaps, or medications?
5. Any nausea or vomiting or diarrhea?
6. Any headache or dizziness?
7. Any history of prior reactions?

- *Disrobing Instructions:* Expose affected areas.
- *Vital Signs:* TPR and BP (Avoid applying BP cuff over rash.)

Provider's Call: *Possible Meds*
In the event of anaphylaxis the following should be ready: Epinephrine, crash tray, and oxygen. Always have patients wait a minimum of 20–30 minutes following all injections.

Complaint: Anxiety or Stress

1. Any history of prior attacks?
2. Any shortness of breath?
3. Any heart irregularities?
4. Any psychotic or delusional behavior?
5. Any visual or auditory hallucinations?
6. Any trembling, shaking, or crying?
7. Is there a decrease in ability to concentrate?
8. Any decrease in appetite or weight loss?

- *Disrobing Instructions:* None
- *Vital Signs:* TPR and BP
- *Comfort Instructions:* Talk calmly and softly to patient. Offer tissue if patient starts to cry. Avoid facial expressions or gestures that may appear to be judgmental. If patient hyperventilates, have patient take slow deep breaths into a paper bag. Alert provider of any breathing or cardiac irregularities.

Complaint: Back Pain

1. Rate pain on a scale of 1 to 10 and give exact location.
2. Is pain related to an injury?
3. Does pain radiate to any other parts of the body?
4. Any numbness or tingling in association with pain?

- *Disrobing Instructions:* Have patient disrobe from waist up for symptoms above the waist and waist down for symptoms below the waist. Give patient a gown.
- *Vital Signs:* TPR and BP

(continues)

(continued)

Related Symptoms or Questions	Anticipatory Guidance
Complaint: Back Pain	
5. Any urinary symptoms? 6. Any loss of bowel or bladder control? 7. Any abdominal pain? 8. Any fever?	• *Comfort Instructions:* Place patient in position that provides comfort. **Provider's Call:** *(Possible Diagnostic Testing)* If patient has lower back pain or urinary symptoms, collect a clean catch urine sample for a possible urinalysis (UA) and culture. If pain is related to an injury, anticipate an x-ray of the affected area.
Complaint: Burns	
1. List type of burn and give approx. diameter. (May refer to coin sizes.) 2. What color is the skin where the burn occurred? 3. Any blistering? 4. Any drainage? (List color and odor.) 5. Any edema? 6. Any heart palpitations or respiratory distress?	• *Disrobing Instructions:* Expose affected area. • *Vital Signs:* TPR and BP (Do not apply cuff over burned area.) • *Comfort Instructions:* **Provider's Call:** Apply sterile 4 × 4s saturated with cool sterile saline or sterile water over burned area to provide temporary relief. • *Possible Tray Setup* *Debridement Supplies:* Sterile 4 × 4s, sterile saline, and forceps. Burn ointment such as Silvadene and sterile bandaging supplies.
Complaint: Chest Pain	
1. Rate pain on a scale of 1 to 10. 2. Does pain radiate to any other parts of the body? 3. Any shortness of breath? 4. Any nausea or vomiting? 5. Any changes in skin color? 6. Any hiccoughs?	• *Disrobing Instructions:* Disrobe from waist up. • *Vital Signs:* TPR and BP • *Important Note:* All patients with chest pain should be taken to an examination room immediately by wheelchair. Patient should be placed in a room with a crash tray,

7. Any gastrointestinal (GI) distress?

8. Any history of heart problems?

electrocardiogram (ECG) unit, and oxygen unit. Notify provider right away. Check patient's vital signs and make sure all equipment is ready. Cardiopulmonary resuscitation (CPR) may need to be administered.

Complaint: Colds and Flu

1. Any nasal stuffiness or drainage? (List color of drainage.)

2. Any head or facial pain? (Rate pain and give location.)

3. Any light sensitivity?

4. Does patient have a sore throat?

5. Does patient have a cough? Is the cough productive? (List color of drainage.)

6. Any ear pain? (List which ear and rate on a scale from 1 to 10.)

7. Does patient have a fever? (List exact temp. and route.)

• *Disrobing Instructions:* From waist up

• *Vital Signs:* TPR and BP

Provider's Call: *(Possible diagnostic testing)*

Sore Throat: Rapid strep test/throat culture

Productive Cough: Possible chest x-ray or sputum culture

Complaint: Constipation

1. Record last bowel movement (LBM) and texture.

2. Does patient have a history of constipation or other bowel problems?

3. Is patient able to pass gas?

4. Any nausea or vomiting?

5. Any abdominal or back pain? (Rate pain on a scale from 1 to 10.)

6. Any fever?

7. List any dietary changes.

• *Disrobing Instructions:* Provider may want patient to disrobe from waist down.

• *Vital Signs:* TPR and BP

Provider's Call: *Possible Tray Setups or Procedures*

Laxative or Suppository/Enema

Tray Setup: Rectal examination tray (anoscope or proctoscope with lubricant and occult blood tests)

(continues)

(continued)

Related Symptoms or Questions	Anticipatory Guidance
Complaint: Depression	
1. Any prior history of depression? 2. Is patient on antidepressant therapy? 3. Any auditory or visual hallucinations? 4. Any concentration problems? 5. Any history of substance or alcohol abuse? 6. Any change in sleep pattern? 7. Has or is patient currently in counseling? 8. Has patient ever considered or attempted suicide?	• *Disrobing Instructions:* None • *Vital Signs:* TPR and BP • *Comfort Instructions:* Be a good listener. Have tissue available in case patient starts to cry. A simple pat on the shoulder or in some cases even a hug may be indicated.
Complaint: Diarrhea	
1. List approximate number of episodes since onset. 2. Any blood in stool? 3. Any dizziness or fainting? 4. Any abdominal pain, tenderness, or swelling? (Rate the pain on a scale from 1 to 10). 5. Any nausea or vomiting? (List number of episodes.) 6. Any signs of dehydration? (Dry mouth, last urination greater than 8 hours, sunken eyeballs, etc.) 7. Any fever? 8. Any new medications in the last 3 months? 9. Any recent travel outside the United States?	• *Disrobing Instructions:* Up to provider. May want to have patient disrobe from waist down • *Vitals:* TPR and BP ***Provider's Call:*** *Possible Tray Setup and Diagnostic Testing* Stool culture and ova and parasite (O&P) studies. Tray Setup: Rectal examination tray (anoscope or proctoscope with lubricant and occult blood test)
Complaint: Ear Pain	
1. List which ear and rate pain on a scale from 1 to 10. 2. Any trauma to ear?	• *Disrobing Instructions:* None • *Vital Signs:* TPR and BP

3. Is there a possible foreign body in the ear?

4. Any drainage coming from ear? (List color of drainage.)

5. Any swelling in or around the ear?

6. Does patient have any dizziness?

7. Any nasal stuffiness or drainage? (List color of drainage.)

8. Does patient have a sore throat?

9. Any fever?

10. Any nausea or vomiting? (List how many episodes.)

Provider's Call: Possible Tray Setups and Procedures

• *Tray Setup:* Ear tray (otoscope, ear curette, ear drops/oil, 4 × 4s)

• *Possible Procedures:* If a foreign body is in the ear or patient has a buildup of wax, provider may want an ear irrigation performed. If patient is experiencing hearing loss, doctor may order audiometry testing.

Complaint: Eye Disorder

1. Which eye is affected?

2. Was the disorder the result of an injury or chemical? (List what happened.)

3. Any drainage? (List color and consistency.)

4. Any visual changes?

5. Any redness or swelling?

6. Any light sensitivity?

7. Any other eye disorders?

8. Date of last professional eye examination.

• *Disrobing Instructions:* None

• *Vital Signs:* T and BP

• *Possible Tray Setup and Diagnostic Testing*

• *Tray Setup:* Eye tray (ophthalmo-scope, numbing drops, medications ordered by provider, and slit or ultraviolet lamp.)

Provider's Call: Visual acuity test. Possible irrigation when debris is embedded in the eye.

• *Comfort Instructions:* Cover affected eye with 4 × 4 and turn down lights until provider examines patient.

Complaint: Fainting

1. Any history of fainting episodes in the past?

2. List events before episode.

3. Did patient actually lose con-sciousness and, if so, for how long?

4. Any heart irregularities? How long?

• *Vital Signs:* TPR and BP

• Place patient in Trendelenburg posi-tion if he or she feels faint or does faint.

Provider's Call: May need to call emergency medical services (EMS) if patient does not regain consciousness.

(continues)

(continued)

Related Symptoms or Questions	Anticipatory Guidance
Complaint: Fainting	
5. Any shortness of breath or heart palpitations before or after the episode?	
6. Did patient sustain any other injuries as a result of the fainting episode?	
7. How does patient feel now?	
Complaint: Fever	
1. List exact temperature and route.	• *Disrobing Instructions:* Disrobe according to related symptoms.
2. Has patient had any seizures in conjunction with fever?	• *Vital Signs:* TPR and BP
3. Does patient have any pain in conjunction with fever? (i.e., head, abdominal, back, etc.) Remember to rate the pain on a scale from 1 to 10.	**Provider's Call:** *Possible diagnostic testing* According to patient's related symptoms, e.g., urinary symptoms: Urinalysis (UA) and culture and sensitivity (C&S) sore throat (rapid strep), etc.
4. Any cold or flu symptoms?	
5. Does patient have a stiff neck?	
6. Any nausea or vomiting? (List how many episodes)	
7. Any diarrhea?	
8. Any urinary, vaginal, or penile symptoms?	
Complaint: Headache	
1. Give exact location.	• *Disrobing Instructions:* None
2. Does patient have a history of migraines or cluster headaches?	• *Vital Signs:* TPR and BP
3. Any neck pain?	• *Comfort Instructions:* Turn down lights and provide emesis basin if nausea is present.
4. Any visual disturbances or light sensitivity?	**Provider's Call:** Provider may order analgesic for pain.
5. Any nausea or vomiting? (List how many episodes.)	
6. Any fever?	
7. Any history of hypertension?	

Complaint: Head Trauma

1. Give a brief description of what happened.
2. Did patient lose consciousness? How long?)
3. Any drainage from wound, ears, nose, or mouth? (Describe drainage.)
4. Any neck pain, tingling, or paralysis?
5. Any change in mental status?
6. Any facial swelling?

- *Disrobing Instructions:* Remove any hats, scarfs, or bandage material.
- *Vital Signs:* TPR and BP

Provider's Call: Tray Setups or Diagnostic Procedures

If wound is gaping, set up a suture tray. If wound is bleeding, apply direct pressure with sterile gauze. Check patient's status on last tetanus shot. If patient starts to feel faint, place in Trendelenburg position.

Complaint: Insect Bites or Stings

1. Describe what bite or stung patient.
2. Did patient see or remove stinger?
3. Any history of local or systemic reactions in the past?
4. Any shortness of breath, swelling of the tongue, throat, or bronchial tubes?
5. Is area red or swollen or is any drainage coming from the area? (Describe drainage.)
6. Any itching?
7. Does patient have a rash?
8. Is area painful? Rate on a scale from 1 to 10.
9. Any nausea or vomiting?

- *Disrobing Instructions:* Expose affected area.
- *Vital Signs:* TPR and BP

Provider's Call: Possible Tray Setups or Procedures

Have epinephrine and crash tray ready in case patient goes into anaphylaxis. Hypersensitivity reactions usually (but not always) occur within the first hour of the sting or bite. *Always have a direct order from the physician before administering any medications.*

Complaint: Nosebleeds

1. Give a brief estimate of the amount of blood loss. (May describe in relationship to the amount of teaspoons.)
2. Any dizziness or confusion?
3. Any visual problems?

- *Disrobing Instructions:* May want to have patient remove outer clothing and put on a gown to protect clothing.
- *Vital Signs:* TPR and BP

(continues)

(continued)

Related Symptoms or Questions	Anticipatory Guidance
Complaint: Nosebleeds	
4. Any history of nosebleeds? 5. Any history of hypertension? 6. Is patient on any type of anti-coagulation therapy or does patient have any blood clotting disorders? 7. Describe other possible causes of nosebleed, such as trauma, allergies, etc.	***Provider's Call:*** • *Tray Setup or Possible Diagnostic Testing:* Plenty of gauze and a cautery unit. Some providers may use silver nitrate sticks to stop the bleeding. • *First Aid: Have* patient sit straight up and pinch nostrils with several 4 × 4s. *(Do not allow patient to lean head back or lie down; this will cause blood to run down the back of the throat.)* Placing a cold pack at the bridge of the nose may help to constrict blood vessels.
Complaint: Rash, Skin Tags, Moles, or Warts	
Describe skin condition and give exact location. *If mole:* Any change in size, color, or shape? *If rash:* Any swelling, itching, erythema, or exudate coming from the area? Any change in laundry detergents or lotions? Any new medications? Any fever, headache, sore throat, or stiff neck? Does anyone else in the family have a similar rash?	• *Disrobing Instructions:* Expose affected area. • *Vital Signs:* T and BP (Do not place BP cuff over rash.) ***Provider's Call:*** Tray Setups and Possible Procedures • Some skin disorders such as ringworm of the scalp will require the use of an ultraviolet light. • In cases of a suspicious mole, have excision tray or electric cautery unit ready with anesthetic and biopsy containers. • Warts can be removed with instruments found on an excision tray, or frozen with a cryotherapy unit, such as the Histofreeze.
Complaint: Sprains, Strains, Fractures	
1. Give exact location and explain how injury occurred. 2. Any pain? (Rate on a scale from 1 to 10.) 3. Any loss of feeling or tingling? 4. Any swelling?	• *Disrobing Instructions:* Expose affected area. • *Vital Signs:* TPR and BP • *Wheelchair:* If patient injured lower extremity, transport to room in wheelchair.

5. Is patient able to bear weight on extremity?
6. Any discoloration to area?

Provider's Call:

* *Possible Tray Setup and Diagnostic Testing:* Have patient immobilize, elevate, and apply ice to the site until provider is available.

X-rays: Many providers will want an x-ray of an injured extremity. Be prepared! Never perform an x-ray without a direct order from the provider.

Complaint: Urinary Tract Infections

1. Any history of UTIs?
2. Any pain on urination? (Rate on a scale from 1 to 10.)
3. Any frequency?
4. Any blood or pus in the urine?
5. Any abdominal or back pain?
6. Any vaginal or penile symptoms? (List LMP for females.)
7. Any fever?
8. Any nausea or vomiting?

* *Disrobing Instructions:* If vaginal or penile symptoms are present, disrobe from waist down; otherwise patient does not have to disrobe.
* *Vital Signs:* T and BP

Provider's Call: *Tray Setups and Possible Diagnostic Testing*

Collect a clean-catch urine sample for a complete UA and C&S

* Pelvic tray with sexually transmitted infection (STI) cultures in conjunction with vaginal symptoms. STI cultures in conjunction with penile symptoms. (When an STI is suspected in the male patient, the health care worker should not obtain a urine sample until the cultures have been collected.)

Complaint: Vaginal or Penile Discharge

1. Any discharge? (List color, texture, and odor.)
2. Any vaginal redness or itching?
3. Any lesions or warts on or around the affected area?
4. Any fever?
5. Any urinary symptoms?

* *Disrobing Instructions:* Remove clothing from waist down.
* *Vital Signs:* T and BP

Provider's Call: *Tray Setups and Possible Diagnostic Testing*

Female: Pelvic tray with appropriate cultures.

* If yeast or trichimonas is suspected, set up a (KOH) and Wet Prep.

(continues)

(continued)

Related Symptoms or Questions	Anticipatory Guidance
Complaint: Vaginal or Penile Discharge	
6. Any abdominal or back pain? 7. Any nausea or vomiting? (List how many episodes.) 8. List number of sexual partners. (Provider may want to ask this question.) 9. List LMP.	*Male patient:* Appropriate cultures Females with vaginal symptoms should be placed in the dorsal lithotomy position.
Complaint: Wounds	
1. Give location and a brief description of how wound occurred. 2. Is wound gaping? 3. Is there any drainage coming from the wound? (Describe appearance.) 4. Is area reddened or bruised? 5. Is any swelling present? 6. Any red streaks on or around the wound? 7. Is there any possibility of a foreign body in the wound, such as gravel, nails, pins, etc.? 8. Does patient have a fever? 9. When was last tetanus shot?	• *Disrobing Instructions:* Expose affected area. • *Vital Signs:* TPR and BP **Provider's Call:** • *Tray Setup and Possible Diagnostic Testing:* Laceration tray for open wound. (Wound should be less than 8 hours old. This may vary, so check with provider for specifics.) • *Wound Culture:* Set up for a wound culture if wound is >24 hours old and looks infected. Do not perform without a specific order from provider. • *Tetanus Shot:* If last shot was greater than 10 years ago, patient will most likely need a tetanus shot. Wait for a direct order from the provider.

Section 2-2

FOLLOW-UP APPOINTMENTS/PROGRESS NOTES

Patients will often be asked to return for a follow-up appointment after an initial visit. This can be a one-time follow-up or a series of follow-up appointments. Listening skills are critical during these visits. Patients may intentionally, or inadvertently, say things that can be significant for both their medical progress and future legal purposes. Table 2-4 lists important information that should be included in a progress note.

Table 2-4

INFORMATION THAT SHOULD BE RECORDED FOR FOLLOW-UP VISITS

Parts of the Progress Note	Description or Facts
1. Today's date and time	Determine if facility wants you to use standard or military time.
2. Indicate that this is a follow-up from the last visit. (Refer to last visit.)	If patient had diagnostic testing or other laboratory work performed, attach results to the front of the chart. *EMR Application:* When using an EMR, check to make certain that the laboratory results have been uploaded in the EMR; if not, contact the laboratory to see if they can send results before the appointment time.
3. Current symptoms	How does the patient feel now? Are symptoms better or worse? Be specific!
4. Were home care instructions followed? (If not, why?)	Did patient take all prescribed medication? Did patient change the dressing as directed? Did patient follow up with the specialist, etc.? This illustrates patient's compliance or noncompliance.
5. Observations made by the assistant	The provider will document objective findings, but the assistant should document signs that the provider may not have observed (e.g., how the dressing looked before and after removal, etc.)
6. Closing signature	First initial, last name, and credential

CHARTING EXAMPLE 1

04/15/XXXX 8:25 a.m.	Follow-up from last visit regarding UTI. "I feel much better! All symptoms are gone." Pt. states that she took of all of her antibiotic. No other concerns. J. Pugh, CMA (AAMA)

CHARTING EXAMPLE 2

| 02/17/XXXX 11:30 a.m. | *Follow-up from last visit regarding laceration to left foot. Sutures to be removed today. Dressing was soiled with dirt. Pt. states that she only changed her dressing 3 × since prior visit because she didn't have enough money to buy new bandage material. ⊕ edema and erythema around the wound. ⊕ drainage (light yellow) coming from the wound. ⊖ odor. Pt. states that she finished her antibiotic. "Foot is still very sore and I cannot wear a shoe yet." M. Baily, RN* |

CHARTING EXAMPLE 3

| 01/23/XXXX 1:30 p.m. | *Follow-up from last visit regarding hypertension and new BP med (atenolol). Pt states that she is taking the medication as directed. "The atenolol causes me to urinate all the time." Pt has not been taking home readings. "Granddaughter too busy to come over and take my BP." Pt states that she is going to buy an au- tomated BP cuff at the pharmacy so that she does not have to rely on her granddaughter. S. Amimoto, RMA* |

Section 2-3

DOCUMENTING MEDICATIONS

The administration of medication is an important task routinely performed in the medical office. Equally important is the documentation
of this medication. To understand how to properly document these procedures, you must first learn a very important rule. **NEVER DOCU-
MENT A MEDICATION THAT YOU DID NOT PREPARE AND/OR
ADMINISTER!** The person who documents the medication is the
one held accountable should a lawsuit arise. Table 2-5 lists the information that should be included when documenting medications.

Table 2-5
INFORMATION THAT SHOULD BE INCLUDED WHEN DOCUMENTING MEDICATIONS

Information to Be Documented	Description or Facts
1. Today's date and time of administration	Check to determine whether standard or military time is used.
2. Name of medication	Write out the entire name so that there are no misunderstandings.

3. Strength of medication (dose given)	The amount you draw up will vary depending on the dose that is ordered and what is available. It should be recorded the way the provider ordered it (e.g., Toradol, 200 mg, not 1 mL of Toradol). Immunizations are usually recorded in milliliters (mL): 0.5 mL of adult tetanus toxoid. Allergy medications are usually recorded in mL: 0.1 mL of allergy serum.
4. Route of administration	Was medication given IM, Subcut, ID, PO or another route?
5. Site of administration	Where was it given? Be specific (e.g., R. deltoid, L. ventrogluteal, etc.)
6. Name of provider who ordered the medication. (Medical assistants usually work under the license of a provider. Always check state delegation rules to see who is able to delegate medication tasks to medical assistants.)	Who ordered the medication? If ordered by someone outside the facility, be sure to attach the written order to the progress note.
7. Some practices want all administered medications to show the following: • **Manufacturer's Name** • **Lot Number** • **Expiration Date** (Many medical offices have medication logs in which this information can be entered. If so, you usually do not need to document this particular information in the chart.)	Many manufacturers make the same drug—be specific. If there is a problem with the medication, it is important to know the lot number so that you can inform the manufacturer. The opposite also holds true: *Never give a medication that has reached or passed its expiration date.*
8. Any problems encountered	Some offices have patients wait for 15–30 minutes following all injections. Other offices have patients wait only after administering allergy serum and antibiotics. You should report and document any local or systemic reactions, (e.g., edema, erythema, or breathing difficulties, etc.).
9. Any educational material distributed	Material that may tell the patient what to expect, such as side effects, etc. (Be certain to include the VIS date when documenting vaccines.)
10. Closing signature	First initial, last name, and credential

Immunizations will need to be documented in the chart on the progress note and on the immunization log within the chart. Immunizations are frequently documented outside the chart onto a special immunization log and are also documented into the caregiver's health record. Narcotics should be documented in the chart on the progress note and outside the chart on a special narcotics log form.

EMR Application

Most EMR programs have a medication section in which all medications are recorded. Reports can be generated from the global EMR that illustrate which patients received drugs from a particular lot number; thus separate medication logs are often not necessary when using EMR.

CHARTING EXAMPLE 1

| 02/15/XXXX 2:35 p.m. | Adult Td, 0.5 mL, IM, R. deltoid, per Dr. Smith. Manufacturer: Sanofi Pasteur, Lot #:246098, Exp Date: 2/XXXX, Gave pt. tetanus information sheet (May XXXX). No complications. M.Richwalsky, CMA(AAMA) |

CHARTING EXAMPLE 2

| 04/02/XXXX 10:00 a.m. | Allergy serum, 0.5 mL, Subcut, Right arm, per Dr. Kim. Observed small wheal about the size of a quarter at injection site during the post-injection follow-up. ⊕ erythema, ⊕ edema, ⊖ resp sx. Applied ice to area. Informed doctor of reaction. Gave pt. 1 Benadryl cap, 50 mg, PO, per Dr. Kim. The doctor would like the dose of allergy serum to be reduced to 0.1 mL next visit. J. Nutter, CMA (AAMA) |

CHARTING EXAMPLE 3

| 10/22/XXXX 3:00 p.m. | Ketorolac, 30 mg, IM, Right dorsogluteal muscle, per Dr. Jones. No local or systemic reaction during 15-minute check. Manufacturer: Vesta, Lot #:11112ADW, Exp Date: 07/XXXX, N. Ahknatova, LPN |

Section 2-4

DOCUMENTING PRESCRIPTIONS

Writing and documenting prescriptions are very important tasks in the provider's office. This section will address documentation of prescriptions. To review how to write prescriptions, turn to Section 7, in the discussion of parts of a prescription.

Every prescription must be double-checked with the provider before calling it in to the pharmacy and double-checked again with the pharmacist. The information in Table 2-6 is useful for documenting prescriptions.

EMR Application

With E-prescribing, prescriptions are a cinch. Prescriptions can be created and printed, faxed, or sent electronically using e-script software. Many providers using e-scripts create and send prescriptions on their own, so this task may not be performed by ancillary staff members in some offices. Office personnel may need to send the provider an electronic task when patients call requesting a prescription refill. Always check office protocol!

Table 2-6

INFORMATION THAT SHOULD BE INCLUDED WHEN DOCUMENTING PRESCRIPTIONS

Information to Be Documented	Description or Facts
1. Today's date and time	Check to determine whether standard or military time is used.
2. Pharmacy's name, location, phone number, and pharmacist's name	This will help to alleviate any misunderstandings as to which pharmacy was called.
3. Name of medication	Write out the entire name so there is no misunderstanding.
4. Strength of medication	Many medications come in different strengths. Be specific!
5. Amount to be dispensed	In cases in which it applies. When R is a controlled substance, the amount to be dispensed should be written out so no one can tamper with the prescription.

(continues)

(continued)

Information to Be Documented	Description or Facts
6. Special instructions	This lists how much is to be taken, how often, and how to take it (i.e., before or after meals, at bedtime, when symptoms occur), and how long to take it.
7. Any refills	List number of refills designated by the provider.
8. Who ordered the prescription	It is important to show that there was an actual order.
9. Closing signature	First initial, last name, and credential

Field Tip

It is important for all health care professionals to know the laws in their states regarding the writing and calling-in of prescriptions. Be familiar with those laws and know what schedules you are capable of handling.

CHARTING EXAMPLE 1 USING ACCEPTABLE ABBREVIATIONS

| 06/09/XXXX 2:45 p.m. | Called in prescription to Howell's Pharmacy, S. High Street, 555-0234. Spoke w/ pharmacist Bob Tucker: Amoxicillin, 250 mg, #30, Sig 1 cap tid × 10 days, No Refills per Dr. Chan. M. Baker, RMA |

CHARTING EXAMPLE 2 NOT USING ABBREVIATIONS

| 05/18/XXXX 3:15 p.m. | Called in prescription to XYZ Pharmacy, Weber Street, 297-2255. Spoke to pharmacist Chantel Allen: Atenolol, 100 milligrams, Number: 30, Take 1 capsule every day for thirty days, No Refills per Dr. Heller. E. Speck, RN |

CHARTING EXAMPLE 3 WITH ACCEPTABLE ABBREVIATIONS

| 11/19/XXXX 10:30 a.m. | Gave pt. written prescription for Ery-Tab, 250 mg, #120. Sig 1 tab bid × 10 days, No Refills per Dr. Singh. S. Green, MA |

Section 2-5

CHARTING IN-HOUSE PROCEDURES

Many procedures are performed in the ambulatory office setting. Documentation of those procedures should illustrate the following: What procedure was ordered, who ordered the procedure, whether the procedure was completed, and who performed the procedure. A good rule to apply here is: "If it is not documented, you didn't do it." Professional liability cases have been lost because of poor or missing documentation. Avoid procrastination!

Table 2-7

INFORMATION THAT SHOULD BE DOCUMENTED FOR A PROCEDURE

Information to Be Documented	Description or Facts
1. Today's date and time of procedure	Determine whether to use standard or military time.
2. List name or names of procedures.	ECG, UA, C&S, complete blood count (CBC), etc.
3. Name of provider ordering the procedure	You must always show an order when documenting a procedure. If the procedure was ordered by an outside provider, attach a copy of the order to the progress note. This will help to comply with the Clinical Laboratories Improvement Act (CLIA) and COLA guidelines.
4. If procedure is a blood draw, list this information.	• The method used to collect the blood (i.e., evacuated tube, syringe, or butterfly) • Location of blood draw • Color and number of tubes drawn • Tests ordered • Who ordered the tests and where they were sent • Acquisition number when it applies
5. List anatomical locations when referring to other types of procedures.	Examples: Sutures removed from L. foot, finger puncture, R. 3rd digit, etc.

(continues)

(continued)

Information to Be Documented	Description or Facts
6. Did patient experience any problems during or following the procedure? Record "no complications" or "patient tolerated procedure well" when no complications result.	Examples: Tingling sensation, lightheadedness, fainting, nausea or vomiting, etc.
7. Did patient receive any educational material or home care instructions?	Shows that patient was instructed on proper home care procedures. Could be important in a legal dispute.
8. Closing signature	First initial, last name, and credential.

Field Tip

Some procedures not only must be documented on the progress note but also in a special laboratory log. Examples of procedures that should have logs include specimens that are sent out of the office, In-House Testing such as rapid strep results, pregnancy results, erythrocyte sedimentation rates (ESRs), and blood glucose results.

EMR Application

Procedures may be documented in a special "Procedures" section of the EMR or directly on a progress note. Make certain that you familiarize yourself with the program's software so that you are documenting procedures in the correct location.

CHARTING EXAMPLE 1

| 02/12/XXXX 8:45 a.m. | Physical & chemical UA, per Dr. Gogotya. Results: Volume: 125 mL, Color: Yellow, Clarity: Cloudy, ⊖ Odor, SG 1.025, pH 7.0, Pr. 1+, Leuk. 2+, all other tests Norm. C. Jones, CMA (AAMA) |

CHARTING EXAMPLE 2

| 03/15/XXXX 10:30 a.m. | Venipuncture (evacuated tube method), L. cephalic vein for a CBC and amenorrhea profile per Dr. Phillips. 2 red-top tubes and 1 lavender-top tube sent to ABC Labs. Acquist # 897FT Neg complications. C. Nrare, MLT |

CHARTING EXAMPLE 3

07/11/XXXX 2:15 p.m.	Finger puncture, L 4th digit for a BS & HCT per Dr. Mendez, Results: BS 110 mg/dL and HCT 48%. S. Nelson, RMA

Section 2-6
COMPLETING AND DOCUMENTING REFERRALS

Some insurance plans require that the primary care provider (PCP) act as a "gatekeeper" for the patient. This means that the patient must contact the PCP before scheduling appointments with a specialist. The PCP must then put a referral in place for that patient.

Referrals may be performed over the telephone, by fax machine, or electronically by computer. Phone referrals use a menu selection system. Special forms can be faxed to the appropriate carrier and then sent to the referral provider. Some carriers supply the PCPs with a triplicate form that can be filled out and mailed in. One copy is sent to the carrier, one copy is sent to the referral provider, and one copy is placed in the patient's chart. Most referrals are now done online. Follow-up should be done on all referrals to ensure they were received by the insurance company. The company will usually issue a number upon receiving the referral. This number should be used any time there is correspondence regarding a claim relating to that specific referral.

Regardless of the manner in which a referral is initiated, the items listed in Table 2-8 must be included.

Table 2-8
ITEMS THAT MUST BE INCLUDED IN A REFERRAL

1. Patient's name and date of birth
2. Subscriber's insurance number and group number or name
3. ICD-9 or 10 diagnosis code(s)
4. Referring provider's name, address, and NPI number
5. Provider's name, address, and NPI number of the provider to whom the patient is being referred
6. CPT-IV codes for any procedures being requested. Check with the referral provider to determine what is necessary.

Field Tip

The appointment may be scheduled before approval; however, the patient should not be seen until authorization is obtained. Table 2-9 lists what items need to be listed when documenting a referral.

Table 2-9

ITEMS THAT MUST BE LISTED WHEN DOCUMENTING A REFERRAL

1. Today's date and time

2. Method used to obtain referral (fax, telephone, mail, etc.)

3. Name of referral provider

4. Name of referring provider (Who requested the referral?)

5. Reason for referral or diagnosis

6. Representative who authorized the referral

7. Authorization number

8. Appointment date and time with the provider to whom the patient is being referred

9. Confirmation to the patient if applicable

10. Closing signature

CHARTING EXAMPLE 1

10/08/XXXX 9:15 a.m.	Telephone referral: Obtained referral with Citizen Health for pt. to see Dr. Keith Fein for heart arrhythmia per Dr. Elonge. Spoke with Rep. Tim Andrews: Authorization #99876. Scheduled pt. to see Dr. Fein on 10/10/XXXX at 2:00 p.m. Confirmed info with pt. M. Holtsberry, CMA (AAMA)

CHARTING EXAMPLE 2

04/13/XXXX 8:45 a.m.	Faxed referral to BHC for pt. to see Dr. Chris Allen re: COPD condition per Dr. Ebihara. Stella from BHC faxed back authorization code #45789. Scheduled pt. to see Dr. Allen on 4/24/XXXX at 3:00 p.m. Called and verified this information w/ the pt. K. Economikous, LPN

CHARTING EXAMPLE 3

02/19/XXXX 9:15 a.m.	E-mailed referral request to Glen-Care for pt. to see Dr. Trey Smith regarding enlarged prostate per Dr. Hower. Awaiting approval. F. Stout, CMA (AAMA)

Section 2-7

DOCUMENTING PRE-CERTIFICATIONS AND OUTSIDE PROCEDURES

Pre-certifications are also known as pre-authorizations or "pre-certs." Pre-certifications are required by most insurance plans as well as governmental plans when a procedure is particularly expensive.

A pre-cert differs from a referral because it is specific to the procedure to be performed. It is usually, but not always, initiated by the specialist's office, unlike a referral, which is initiated by the primary care provider.

Plans differ as to what procedures need to be pre-certified. Contact the insurance company or governmental agency for specifics or refer to the manual. The reverse side of the patient's insurance card usually has a toll-free number to call for pre-certifications.

Failure to obtain a pre-certification in circumstances mandated by the insurance carrier may result in large financial losses to the patient or the clinic ordering the testing.

Table 2-10 lists the information necessary for obtaining pre-certification.

Table 2-10
PRE-CERTIFICATION INFORMATION

1. Patient's name and date of birth
2. Primary care provider's name and identification number if relevant
3. Specialist's name and identification number if relevant
4. CPT-IV codes for all procedures to be done
5. Corresponding ICD-9 or -10 codes for each procedure

The carrier's representative will either assign you a pre-certification number or tell you that the request must be forwarded for further evaluation. Hence, it is not a good idea to wait until the last minute to obtain a pre-certification. There is no guarantee of payment until the pre-certification number is assigned. Even then, the procedure may not be fully covered. Having the patient sign a disclaimer that states that payment will be made according to the individual's insurance plan will release the office from liability in cases in which the insurance company pays only a fraction of the procedure's actual cost.

Table 2-11 lists items that must be documented for a pre-certification.

Table 2-11
ITEMS THAT MUST BE DOCUMENTED FOR A PRE-CERTIFICATION

1. Today's date and time

2. Name of carrier's representative

3. Name of insurance company

4. Name of procedure and where performed (must be within network)

5. Pre-certification number

6. If pre-certification is denied or detained, list reasons and options

7. Closing signature

CHARTING EXAMPLE 1

02/22/XXXX 2:30 p.m.	Obtained pre-approval from Sandy Moomia at JTH Health to schedule pt. for a uterine ultrasound at Hardy Memorial, per Dr. Dilullo. Certification #55678F. J. Thomas, NCMA

CHARTING EXAMPLE 2

04/18/XXXX 10:00 a.m.	Spoke with Rhonda Llewellyn from Premium Health regarding permission for pt. to have an MRI of the head and neck per Dr. Aurand. Rhonda stated that the initial request was denied. She is sending the request on to be reviewed. Will call back once request has been reviewed. M. Wu, RN

CHARTING EXAMPLE 3

08/08/XXXX 11:15 a.m.	Obtained approval from Julie Santiago at AHC today for pt. to have a TURP at St. Catherine's Memorial. Authorization code #43210. Approval good for 3 months. P. Lofquist, RMA

Once authorization is granted, the medical assistant will need to call the facility where the procedure is to be performed and set up an appointment for the patient. The information listed in Table 2-12 will need to be documented when setting up an outside procedure.

Table 2-12
INFORMATION THAT MUST BE DOCUMENTED FOR OUTSIDE PROCEDURES

1. Today's date and time

2. Name of procedure or test to be performed

3. Name of facility performing the procedure and location within the facility where patient is to report

4. Name of the person you spoke with at the facility

5. Date and time of procedure

6. Name of clinician ordering the procedure

7. Any special instructions that must be given to the patient

8. Confirmation to the patient

9. Closing signature

EMR Application

The majority of EMR programs have an "orders management" section in which orders for outside procedures can be sent electronically. This works only if the diagnostic center or laboratory is electronically linked with the system being used by your health care facility. Many EMR software programs also track the patient's insurance, and thus will alert you if you try to set up a procedure at a non-participating center.

CHARTING EXAMPLE 1

| 02/23/XXXX
2:20 p.m. | Scheduled pt. for uterine ultrasound per Dr. Stein. Procedure set up at Washington Hospital on Tuesday, 2/24/XXXX at 10:00 a.m. Spoke with Judy Allen, "Pt. is to take elevator to the 2nd floor of hospital and report to the ultrasound lab. Bladder should be full. Instruct pt to drink 4–6 (8-oz) glasses of water before arriving for the test." Called and confirmed this info. w/ the pt. J. Holtsberry, MOA |

CHARTING EXAMPLE 2

11/18/XXXX 8:45 a.m.	Scheduled pt. for a PA & Lat CXR, per Dr. Sanchez. Spoke w/ Susan Fitzgerald at Davis Radiology. Appointment set for today at 10:30 a.m. Confirmed this info w/ pt. J. Beaver, RMA

CHARTING EXAMPLE 3

07/22/XXXX 9:30 a.m.	Scheduled pt. for a mammogram per Dr. Kennedy. Spoke w/ Spencer Moses at Women's Health Center. Appointment set for Thursday 07/25/XXXX for 8:00 a.m. "Instruct pt. not to wear any deodorant to the exam." Called and confirmed this info w/ pt. C. Lupinski, RMA

Section 2-8

DOCUMENTING TELEPHONE SCREENINGS

Screening of phone calls is a difficult task because of the fine-line issue. The person doing the screening not only has to determine what might be wrong with the patient, but also may have to give the patient instructions based on the nature of the complaint. This is challenging because it places the medical assistant in a role that is very similar to diagnosing or prescribing.

The authors of this handbook prefer to use the term *telephone screening* rather than *telephone triage*. Screening phone calls is different from triaging calls. Triaging calls usually involves much more responsibility than what the medical assistant or medical office assistant is legally capable of performing. The person screening the call must use a triage or screening manual that has been approved by the practice. This manual should prompt the medical assistant to ask a series of general questions. Based on the responses to those questions, the screener will follow a decision tree or algorithm that provides specific protocols to follow when the patient answers yes to certain questions. Table 2-13 lists the information that should be included in a phone call. To learn more about the screening of phone calls, refer to Section 3.

Table 2-13

INFORMATION THAT SHOULD BE INCLUDED
IN DOCUMENTATION OF A PHONE CALL

Information to Be Documented	Description or Facts
1. Today's date and time of call	Timing is especially important in possible legal cases such as accidents and work injuries. Determine whether to use standard or military time.
2. General complaint	Brief description of why the patient called
3. Date or time of onset of symptoms or the date and time of the injury	This is important for both assessment and legal purposes.
4. History of the present illness	These questions can be found in Section 3 of this handbook, in the tables corresponding to the complaint and relevant symptoms. Instructions for handling the symptoms can also be found in each chart.
5. Any self-treatment	Has the patient taken any medications or administered any treatment to alleviate symptoms?
6. If relevant, update the patient's medication information.	Do not have to list if patient is instructed to come into the office or to go to the emergency room (ER).
7. Update any drug allergies.	This is only if the call is in relation to a prescription.
8. List instructions given to the patient and the source of the instructions.	Was the patient directed to call the emergency medical services (EMS) or set an appointment, or was the patient given home care instructions?
9. Document patient's compliance or refusal to follow instructions.	This could be very important in a legal dispute.
10. Closing signature	Give first initial and last name of the individual taking the call, followed by credential.

The documentation of phone calls will usually be lengthier than
in-office entries. This is largely due to the increased legal responsibility
of the person performing the screening, as well as the additional information that must be recorded for a phone call.

CHARTING EXAMPLE 1

10/25/XXXX 2:15 p.m.	TC: Pt. c/o chest pain x 30 minutes. Pain is a "10" (1–10 Scale). "Pain starts in the center of my chest and radiates to my left side. It feels like a truck is sitting on top of my chest." ⊕ Shortness of breath, ⊕ left arm pain, ⊖ N/V, ⊖ dizziness, ⊖ Hx of heart disease. Pt. took 2 aspirin 20 minutes ago, ⊖ relief. Instructed pt. to call the EMS per pg 23 of Screening Manual. Pt. refused. Said husband would drive her to the ER. Asked to speak to husband. Informed husband of possible consequences of transporting pt. by himself. Husband agreed to call the EMS. M. Khan, R.N——————

CHARTING EXAMPLE 2

12/12/XXXX 1:40 p.m.	TC: Pt.'s mother called to say that pt. cut R. lower leg on the monkey bars while at school. Injury happened at approx. 1:00 p.m. "Cut is about 1½" long and is gaping." Bleeding is controlled. Mother washed the area and applied antiseptic ointment and a bandage to the area. Last tetanus approx. 2 years ago. Scheduled the pt. for an appointment at 3:00 today per page 45 of Screening Manual. S. Pucel, RMA ——————

CHARTING EXAMPLE 3

05/16/XXXX 9:15 a.m.	TC: Pt. c/o a possible "sinus infection" × 4 days. ⊕ Thick green nasal drainage, ⊕ HA/pressure in temple region, ⊕ Cough (nonproductive), ⊕ Fever (101°F), ⊖ Sore throat, or ear pain. Therapeutic Measures: 2 Sinaway tabs every 12 hours ("little to no relief"). Scheduled pt. to come in for an 11:00 appointment today per page 33 of Screening Manual. T. Wong, RN——————

Section 2-9

DOCUMENTING PATIENT EDUCATION SESSIONS

Patient education is vital in today's health care setting. Health care reform places greater emphasis on prevention and disease management than ever before. Types of education performed in the medical office include diabetes education, breast health, cholesterol management, testicular examinations, and medication education.

The medical office should stock pamphlets approved by the provider that can be used to enhance what is being stated during the educational session. The type of education presented in a medical office is usually considered basic and preliminary. Providers may want to send patients outside the office for more comprehensive education from certified specialists. Refer to Table 2-14 for documentation specifics.

EMR Application

Many EMR programs have health maintenance registries that alert medical personnel when a patient is due for preventative screenings and immunizations. The alert can be adjusted as a window that pops up when the chart is opened or as a soft alert that appears on a toolbar or within a particular tab. Global reports can be generated that identify all patients who are due for particular screenings or exams, so that reminders can be sent out to those patients who do not frequent the office.

Table 2-14

INFORMATION RECORDED FROM A PATIENT EDUCATION SESSION

Information to Be Documented	Description or Fact
1. Today's date and time of education	Determine if military or standard time is to be used.
2. List the topic and purpose of the education.	Examples: Smoking cessation, diabetes education, medication management
3. Document who ordered the session.	This is important when the patient is being charged for the education. Insurance companies will want to see an order from the provider.

(continues)

(continued)

Information to Be Documented	Description or Fact
4. Document who was present for the session.	Many family members assist with home care. List any additional members of the family who were present for the educational session.
5. List patient's comprehension and response to session.	It is important to note if the patient was able to understand the purpose of the session as well as what was being presented. Patient's refusal to participate in the session or negative comments made by the patient during the session also need to be noted.
6. List any educational materials that were distributed to the patient.	These may be brochures or home care instruction forms.
7. Document any special instructions that were given to the patient that were not listed in the brochures or on the home care instruction forms.	Information such as where the patient can get additional information, referral information, and under what circumstances the patient should call the office.
8. Closing signature	First initial, last name, and credential

CHARTING EXAMPLE 1

| 03/12/XXXX 4:30 p.m. | Cholesterol management education session per Dr. Legg regarding last cholesterol level of 256. Pt. appeared to understand the importance of lowering blood cholesterol and was able to repeat back the information correctly. Gave pt. home care sheet and told her to follow-up in 3 months for another cholesterol level per Dr. Legg. J. Schmidt, LPN |

CHARTING EXAMPLE 2

02/18/XXXX 2:30 p.m.	Breast health education session per Dr. Gutierrez. Demonstrated how to perform monthly self-breast exams and instructed pt. on the importance of yearly mammograms.Instructed pt. to set up a baseline mammogram. Pt. said she would call Blackwell Radiology today to schedule a mammogram. N. Cruiz, CMA (AAMA) ————————————

CHARTING EXAMPLE 3

05/12/XXXX 3:30 p.m.	Cast care management for Fx of left leg per Dr. di Napoli. Both pt. and mother of pt. were present for the session. Pt. repeated steps back and appeared to have a good understanding. Instructed pt. to call office with any signs of impaired circulation. Pt. scheduled to re-turn 6/14/XXXX for an AP and Lat X ray of the left leg per Dr. di Napoli. Gave pt. home care instructions. S. Norton, RN ————————————

Section Three
TELEPHONE SCREENINGS

INTRODUCTION

Assessment in an ambulatory care office is uniquely different from the assessment that occurs in a hospital setting or an extended care facility. Patients scheduled for an appointment in the medical office will initially be seen by a medical assistant or nurse with an evaluation by the provider.

Health care personnel employed in an office are involved in the assessment procedure. The detail of the assessment is determined by the training of the individual doing the assessment and the office protocol.

The term *assessment* usually entails screening, examining, and formulating a tentative diagnosis. Medical assistants are not trained or licensed to examine or diagnose, but should, however, have good screening capabilities. Two types of screenings take place in the medical office: office screenings and telephone screenings.

Office screening consists of asking the patient about the chief complaint and related symptoms or a history of the present illness. This provides the health care worker with information for setting up the room and having the patient disrobe appropriately.

Telephone screenings involve more than just asking questions. The medical assistant must have the ability to ask the appropriate questions based on the patient's symptoms. It is important to incorporate a telephone screening manual that represents the philosophies of all providers in the office. Using a screening manual takes the decision making out of the hands of the screener and puts it into the hands of the providers who approved the manual. The screener must be careful not to deviate from the manual. If the patient has a condition not listed on the chart or the medical assistant is unable to schedule the patient within the time limits suggested, the medical assistant will need clarification from the provider about how to handle the call.

Field Tip

Some states are very specific about who can give out telephone directives regarding patient care, so check the laws of your state before instituting a telephone screening program in your office.

The following section offers general assessment questions that can be used for telephone screenings. These tables are especially helpful for students learning assessment or screenings and are a valuable reference for medical assistants already in the workplace.

HOW TO USE THE TABLES

Each assessment table starts out with an introduction that explains some important facts about the general complaint listed at the top of the page. The tables are divided into three columns:

The **first column**, titled "Task or Question," lists either a task such as recording the date and time or a question that should be addressed to the patient.

The **second column**, titled "Response," lists responses from the patient that require the screener to take further action. **Note: If a response from the patient does not require the screener to take action beyond recording the patient's answers on the table, the "Response" column will be shaded pink.**

The **third column**, titled "Action," lists action(s) the screener should take based on the response from the patient. For example, in the Abdominal Pain/Stomach Pain table, based on the patient's response of "Yes" (in the "Response" column) to question 5 (in the "Question" column), the screener's next action (listed in the "Action" column) would be to direct the patient to call emergency medical services (EMS). The person performing the screening should progress down the table until all questions have been answered and all tasks completed. The screener will then choose the response that requires the most significant action. For example, if a person answers yes to a question that instructs the patient to schedule a same-day appointment, but also answers yes to a question that directs the patient to come in ASAP, the screener should choose the ASAP action. *You can always upgrade an action, but never downgrade an action.* If the patient answers yes to one of the questions that require an EMS action, the screener should stop asking questions and have the patient call 9-1-1 or the local emergency medical services.

You will find additional information at the bottom of each table. Information that may be included on various tables include:

- **Field Application Tips:** These are quick facts that may help the medical assistant with time management or serve as a reminder to do something.

- **Provider Call:** This involves two categories: *Home Care Instructions and Over-the-Counter Information.* These categories are listed under Provider Call because the provider is part of the

decision-making process. Many factors can alter what the patient
should do. The patient's general overall health, as well as the prescribed and over-the-counter (OTC) medications the patient is currently taking, can have a direct bearing on what the patient should
do. **Always check with the provider before giving any home
care instructions.**

- **Charting Example:** These reflect what should be documented
when the patient calls complaining of specific symptoms.

The following is a complete listing of the abbreviations that are used
in the "Action" column in the tables.

Section 3-1

ACTION ABBREVIATION AND CODE KEY

Table 3-1 lists abbreviations used in the "Action" column of the assessment tables. Each abbreviation encourages the user to direct the patient
to take a certain action when the patient answers the questions with a
particular response.

Table 3-1
ABBREVIATION AND CODE KEY

Abbreviation or Code	Description
1. **EMS** Note: Whenever "EMS" appears in the Action column of the charts in this section, it will be in red to remind the screener that this action is respond-ing to a possible life-threatening emergency.	Patient should hang up and dial 9-1-1 or the local EMS.
2. **STAT**	Patient should come in immediately. If unable to work the patient in immediately, consult provider for other options.
3. ASAP	Patient should be seen within 1–2 hours if at all possible. Consult with provider if unable to work patient in within that time frame.

(continues)

(continued)

Abbreviation or Code	Description
4. SDA	Same-day appointment. Try to work the patient in that day. If unable to work patient in that same day, consult physician for other options.
5. (24–48)	Patient should be seen sometime in the next 2 days. If unable to work patient in that time constraint, consult provider for other options.
6. PC (Provider Call)	The Provider Call section lists possible home care instructions that can be given to the patient when symptoms are mild and nonthreatening. It also lists some common OTC categories that can be suggested when the patient exhibits particular symptoms. The term *Provider Call* literally means that a provider should approve these actions before directing the patient to take them.

Section 3-2

ABDOMINAL PAIN/STOMACH PAIN

Abdominal pain can be caused by a wide assortment of problems. The abdominal region contains several organs and some abdominal pain may be referred from other sources or organs outside the abdominal region.

Abdominal pain may be very severe or even life threatening, such as a ruptured appendix or abdominal aortic aneurysm, or it may be associated with something more simplistic, such as a stomach virus. You must obtain a good history of the present illness because this will help determine if and how soon the patient should be seen. In most cases, patients with abdominal pain should be seen by the provider. Acute episodes of pain are usually more cause for alarm than chronic pain. When in doubt, always check with the provider. Table 3-2 lists the tasks, questions, responses, and actions for abdominal and stomach pain screenings.

Table 3-2

ABDOMINAL AND STOMACH PAIN SCREENINGS

Task or Question	Response	Action
1. Record today's date and the time of the call along with a brief description of the patient's concern.		
2. Record when symptoms began. Acute or sudden onset of pain is always more of a concern than chronic pain.		
3. Rate the pain on a scale of 1–10.		
4. Give location of pain. Is the pain intermittent or constant? What makes pain better or worse? Is pain acute and severe, located in the abdomen, testicle, or groin region, with an inability to walk?	Yes	EMS
5. Is there any shortness of breath or chest pain?	Yes	EMS
6. Is the patient pregnant? (females only)	Yes	EMS
7. Is pain associated with an injury or trauma?	Yes	EMS
8. Does patient have a fever? (List current temperature) Is temperature >101° F?	Yes	ASAP
9. Is pain associated with vaginal bleeding, discharge, or a missed period?	Yes	ASAP
10. Is pain associated with urinary tract symptoms or back pain?	Yes	ASAP
11. Is pain in the testes or is there swelling? (if male)	Yes	ASAP
12. Is there severe vomiting and diarrhea lasting for more than 1 day? (Record how many episodes.) Was last urination more than 8–10 hours ago? Does patient have a dry tongue and mucous membranes? *(If vomiting and diarrhea are not severe and patient does not appear dehydrated, pain is intermittent, or other family members or friends have had similar symptoms, give patient home care instructions that can be found at the bottom of the chart.)*	Yes	ASAP PC

(continues)

(continued)

Task or Question	Response	Action
13. Does pain radiate across the abdomen or is it contained within a particular location?	**Yes**	ASAP
14. Is the color of the stool black or tarry, or does it contain visible blood?	**Yes**	ASAP
15. Are there any chronic illnesses such as diabetes, atherosclerosis, coronary artery disease, chronic obstructive pulmonary disease, or any other immunosuppressive disorders?	**Yes**	ASAP
16. Is pain mild to moderate and in combination with constipation? (List last bowel movement and texture.)	**Yes**	(24–48)
17. List prescribed and OTC medications currently being taken by patient.		
18. List any drug allergies.		
19. List instructions given to patient and state where they came from (e.g., screening manual or provider, physician).		
20. Record closing signature.		

Field Tip

Certain medications such as aspirin, corticosteroids, and nonsteroidal anti-inflammatory drugs (NSAIDs) may cause abdominal pain or stomach pain. Alert the provider when pain may be related to a medication.

Provider's Call

Home Care Instructions

1. Stop eating solids; this will only worsen symptoms.
2. Sip clear liquids such as water, clear juice, and broth until pain has subsided. If unable to keep liquids down, suck on some ice chips.
3. May add dry toast, soda crackers, soups, applesauce, and gelatin as pain subsides.
4. Avoid dairy products, caffeine, alcohol, and spicy foods.
5. Notify office or seek medication attention if pain changes in frequency, intensity, or location.

6. Heat therapy may be beneficial in minimizing pain. Examples of heat therapy include taking a warm bath or applying a heat pack to the affected area.

Do not use heat in cases of possible appendicitis, excessive menstrual bleeding, or possible pregnancy.

OTC—Over-the-Counter Medications

If the patient's symptoms appear to be related to indigestion, the provider may want you to suggest the use of an over-the-counter antacid. Instruct the patient to stay away from foods that aggravate the indigestion such as: caffeine, alcohol, spicy foods, colas, etc. If symptoms are more gastrointestinal and involve diarrhea, the physician may encourage the use of a common OTC antidiarrheal medication. Always check with the physician before suggesting any OTC meds.

CHARTING EXAMPLE

03/22/XXXX 2:00 p.m.	TC: Pt. c/o continuous lower abdominal pain, pain scale level ("8") × 3 hours. Pain radiates from naval area to the R. side. Fever (101°F). Last bowel movement was 8 hours ago (normal color and texture). "I feel constipated right Now." ⊕ Indigestion, ⊖ urinary symptoms (last urination 6 hours ago) ⊕ dry mouth, ⊕ sunken eyeballs, LMP 3/15/XX, ⊖ vaginal. Sx, ⊖ ℞ drugs, ⊖ OTC drugs, NKDA. Instructed pt. to come for a 3:00 appointment per screening manual, page 66. J. Garrett, CMA(AAMA) ————————

Section 3-3

ALLERGIC REACTION/ANAPHYLAXIS

Allergic reactions may occur immediately or up to 24 hours following exposure to the offending agent. Offensive agents include medications, insect stings or bites, foods, laundry detergents, and soaps. Reactions may be mild, such as a local rash, redness, or swelling, but may progress to a more severe reaction known as anaphylaxis.

Symptoms of anaphylaxis include constriction of the throat, tongue, or bronchial tubes, difficult or labored breathing, and unconsciousness. If the patient does not receive immediate medical attention, the patient may die. Good assessment skills are critical when developing any complaint that could be life threatening. Table 3-3 lists the tasks, questions, responses, and actions for allergic reaction and anaphylaxis screenings.

Table 3-3

ALLERGIC REACTION AND ANAPHYLAXIS SCREENINGS

Task or Question	Response	Action
1. Record today's date and the time of the call along with a brief description of the patient's concern.		
2. Record when symptoms began.		
3. What does the patient think caused this attack?		
4. Does the patient have a history of anaphylaxis?	Yes	EMS
Does the patient have an EpiPen or equivalent that has been prescribed by the provider?	Yes	Administer medication following directions on package insert.
5. Does the patient have any shortness of breath or respiratory distress?	Yes	EMS
6. Does the patient have swelling of the tongue, lips, or throat or difficulty in swallowing?	Yes	EMS
7. Does the patient have any chest pain?	Yes	EMS
8. Does the patient feel dizzy or faint?	Yes	EMS
9. Does the patient have a rash, itching, or hives?		
If onset is new and the rash is red, hives are present or there is intense itching?	Yes	EMS
For mild symptoms of itching, rash, swelling, or hives with no breathing problem		PC
10. Does the patient have nausea, vomiting, or diarrhea?	Yes	EMS
11. Does the patient have a severe headache?	Yes	EMS

12. Does the patient have a history of seasonal allergies and want some comfort advice?	**Yes**	Should try what has worked well in the past. If symptoms are worse than usual, ASAP.
13. List any self-treatment. Has it helped?		
14. List current prescribed and OTC medications.		
15. List any drug allergies.		
16. List instructions given to patient and state where they came from (e.g., screening manual, provider).		
17. Record closing signature.		

Provider's Call

Home Care Instructions

1. Identify and eliminate the offensive agent (detergents, medications, etc.).
2. If offensive agent appears to be a medication, alert physician to determine what the patient can take in its place.
3. Try soaking in a cool bath. (May add 1 cup of baking soda to water.) Do not rub area with a towel; pat dry.
4. Warm baths and heat should be avoided.
5. Have patient start a diary and list what foods, detergents, etc., make them worse.

OTC—Over-the-Counter Medication

Some providers may suggest the use of an antihistamine such as Benadryl. Always check with the provider before suggesting any medications.

CHARTING EXAMPLE

10/21/XXXX 2:00 p.m.	TC: Pt. c/o rash on arms and legs × 2 days. ⊕ Itching, ⊖ hives, ⊖ HA, ⊖ SOB or swelling of throat, ⊖ chest pain, ⊖ N/V or stomach discomfort. Pt. just started using a new laundry detergent. No current or prescribed drugs, NKDA. Pt. instructed to stop using current laundry detergent. Start Benadryl, 50 mg q 6–8 hrs, per Dr. Kryszczuk. Pt. to call if sx do not get better. S. Esposito, RN ————

Section 3-4

ANXIETY AND STRESS SCREENINGS

Everyone suffers from anxiety and stress at some point. Stress is a normal part of life. "Healthy" stress or good stress can actually motivate behavior, whereas "unhealthy" stress or bad stress interferes with normal daily activities. A person who suffers from unhealthy stress is unable to handle ordinary situations such as constructive criticism from the boss, overcooking a casserole, etc. Chronic stress can lead to diseases such as heart disease and cancer. Stress that becomes progressive can lead to severe panic attacks, which may result in breathing disorders and heart irregularities. It is important to be calm and supportive when dealing with an anxious patient. Avoid comments that could be misconstrued or those comments that could make the patient feel even more anxious. Table 3-4 lists the tasks, questions, responses, and actions for anxiety and stress screenings.

Table 3-4

ANXIETY AND STRESS SCREENINGS

Task or Question	Response	Action
1. Record today's date and the time of the call.		
2. Give a brief description of the patient's complaint, using the patient's own words.		
3. Record when symptoms began.		
4. Does the patient have a history of anxiety or stress?		
5. Does the patient have breathing problems?	Yes	EMS
6. Does the patient have any heart irregularities?	Yes	EMS
7. Does the patient's behavior appear to be psychotic or delusional?	Yes	EMS
8. Is this the patient's first anxiety attack?	Yes	ASAP
9. Does the patient have visual or auditory hallucinations?	Yes	ASAP
10. Does the patient have excessive sweating, trembling or shaking, or crying?	Yes	ASAP
11. Does patient have recent weight loss?	Yes	(24–48)

12. Is patient unable to concentrate?	**Yes**	**(24–48)**
13. Is this a chronic condition?	**Yes**	**(24–48)**
14. List current prescribed and OTC medications taken by patient.		
15. List any drug allergies.		
16. List instructions given to patient and state where they came from (e.g., screening manual, provider).		
17. Record closing signature.		

CHARTING EXAMPLE

02/12/XXXX	TC: Pt. c/o "anxiety attack" × 3 hours. ⊕ shortness
3:15 p.m.	of breath at rest earlier today (normal now). ⊖ Heart
	related sx, ⊖ visual or auditory hallucinations, ⊖ ex-
	cessive sweating, ⊕ trembling and crying, ⊕ inability
	to concentrate, ⊖ weight loss. ℞ Prozac, ⊖ OTCs, NKDA.
	Instructed pt. to come in for 4:00 appointment per
	screening manual, Page 86. J Pugh, CMA (AAMA)

Section 3-5

BACK PAIN

Back pain can be caused by a host of different problems. Diseases such as urinary tract infections and osteoporosis are just a couple of diseases that may present with back pain. Severe lower back or lumbar pain that is unaffected by activity and may include symptoms of shock could involve a life-threatening aneurysm. The majority of back pain is caused by muscle, ligament, or disc pain. Movement will usually aggravate this kind of pain. Slipped or ruptured discs are also the cause of many lower back pain episodes. A slipped disc may lead to entrapment of the nerves, which may cause a condition known as sciatica. Sciatica usually starts in the lower back and may extend down the affected leg and foot. Tingling and numbness may also be associated with this pain.

All acute episodes of back pain should be evaluated. Asking appropriate questions will help the screener prioritize how quickly the patient should be seen. Chronic pain that recurs should also be evaluated, but will usually not take precedence over acute attacks unless patient is in excruciating pain. Table 3-5 lists the tasks, questions, responses, and actions for back pain screenings.

Table 3-5
BACK PAIN SCREENINGS

Task or Question	Response	Action
1. Record today's date and the time of the call.		
2. Give brief description of the patient's complaint, using the patient's own words.		
3. Record when symptoms began.		
4. Was pain caused by a traumatic episode followed by an inability to move or walk?	Yes	EMS
5. Does patient have loss of bladder or bowel control in association with the pain?	Yes	EMS
6. Is pain sudden and severe and unchanged by movement?	Yes	EMS
7. Rate pain on a scale from 1 to 10. Is pain rating a 5 or higher?	Yes	SDA
8. Is pain in conjunction with urinary symptoms?	Yes	SDA
9. Is pain in combination with a fever?	Yes	SDA
10. Is back pain in conjunction with abdominal pain?	Yes	SDA
11. Does pain radiate down the leg or combine with numbness or tingling?	Yes	(24–48)
12. List current prescribed and OTC medications.		
13. List home care treatment. Does it work?		
14. List any drug allergies.		
15. List instructions given to patient and state where they came from (e.g., screening manual, provider).		
16. Record closing signature.		

Provider's Call

Home Care Instructions

The majority of patients with back pain will be seen, but the following are some comfort measures that the patient can implement in the meantime. Patients in acute pain can apply ice bags wrapped in a towel every 2–4 hours for the first 48 hours. This will help reduce swelling and inflammation. After 48 hours, treatment may be alternated with heat therapy. Sleeping on a firm mattress with a flat pillow may help relieve pain. Placing a pillow between the patient's legs while lying on the side may also help to alleviate pain.

OTC—Over-the-Counter Medication

Using aspirin products and ibuprofen may also be helpful. Check the patient's drug allergy status and as always, check with the provider before suggesting any OTC medications.

CHARTING EXAMPLE

08/08/XXXX 11:15 a.m.	TC: Pt. c/o lower back pain, pain scale level ("6") × 2 days ⊖ Injury or radiation of pain, ⊕ urinary sx that include frequency, burning, and pain on urina- tion. ⊖ Abd pain or loss of bladder or bowel control. ⊕ Fever ("99–100° F") ℞: Temazepam, 15 mg. Self- treatment: Motrin 400 mg q 4–6 hours × 2 days. Little relief, no other OTCs, NKDA. Instructed pt. to come in for a 2:00 appt, per screening manual page 64. K. Durr, LPN

Section 3-6

BURNS

Before assessing a burn, one must understand how to classify burns. Table 3-6A defines burns by type and degree. It also lists basic first aid for different types of burns. To determine the extent of burns, see Figure 3-1. Table 3-6B lists the tasks, questions, responses, and actions for burn screenings.

Table 3-6A
BURN DESCRIPTIONS

Type	Degree
Thermal Burn: Caused by heat, such as a hot surface or flames **First Aid:** Follow the first-, second-, and third-degree first-aid tips in the degree column.	**First-Degree Burn:** A superficial burn involving the first layer of skin **Symptoms:** Reddening of the skin, warmth, and pain. Skin remains intact. **First Aid:** Applying cold water to the area should stop the burning. An appointment is usually not necessary.
Chemical Burn: Caused by contact with acids or alkalis **First Aid:** Clothes should be removed and the area flooded with water for a minimum of 15 minutes. Dry chemicals should be brushed off before flushing the patient's skin (some dry chemicals are activated by water). Cover with a sterile dressing. Should be assessed by a provider.	**Second-Degree Burn:** These burns extend into the dermis or second layer of skin. Also referred to as a partial-thickness burn. **Symptoms:** Skin may appear white to pink. May have some fluid loss and blisters. Mild to moderate pain. **First Aid:** Wash with antibacterial soap. Cover with a nonstick sterile dressing. Second-degree burns should be assessed by the provider.
Electrical Burn: Occurs after contact with electrical wiring. An electrical burn can be caused by a lightning strike. Hard to assess outwardly. Internal injuries not visible to the naked eye could be present. **First Aid:** Make sure electrical source has been shut down before applying first aid. Administer cardiopulmonary resuscitation (CPR) if necessary, and call the EMS.	**Third-Degree Burn:** Involves all three layers of the skin and is also referred to as a full-thickness burn. **Symptoms:** No blisters. Skin may appear white and leathery. Usually no pain. Thrombosed vessels may be present. **First Aid:** Should be treated by a provider. May require hospitalization.

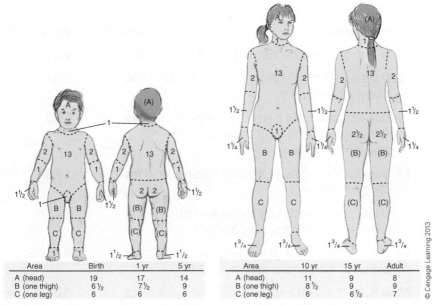

Figure 3-1: The Lund and Browder chart is used for estimating the extent burns in infants and children.

Table 3-6B
BURN SCREENINGS

Task or Question	Response	Action
1. Record today's date and the time of the call.		
2. Record the nature of the complaint in patient's own words. A complete description of the burn is necessary for the screener to answer questions 8–11. Patient will not know what degree burn they have; thus the burden is on the screener to assess the degree of the burn. Use Table 3-6A to guide you.		
3. Record date and time of onset of the burn.		
4. Does the patient have any respiratory problems?	**Yes**	**EMS**
5. Does patient have any heart palpitations?	**Yes**	**EMS**
6. Is skin clammy or does patient appear to be confused?	**Yes**	**EMS**

(continues)

(continued)

Task or Question	Response	Action
7. Is burn a chemical or electrical burn?	Yes	EMS
8. Does burn cover a large surface area larger than the size of a first?	Yes	EMS
9. Does the burn cover a large surface area? (anything greater than 18% or involves the face, hands, feet or genitals.)	Yes	EMS
10. Does burn wrap around the circumference of any body part?	Yes	EMS
11. Does burn appear to only involve the first layer of skin and is small in diameter?	Yes	PC
12. Does patient have a chronic illness or a disease that compromises immunity?	Yes	ASAP
13. Is burn more than 1–2 days old? Does it have a colored drainage seeping from the area or a foul odor or is it very painful?	Yes	SDA
14. When was last tetanus shot?	If >10 years	SDA
15. Was any home care treatment applied?		
16. List any OTC medications.		
17. List any prescribed medications the patient is currently taking.		
18. List any drug allergies.		
19. List instructions given to patient and state where they came from (e.g., screening manual, provider).		
20. Record closing signature.		

Provider's Call

Home Care Treatment

Submerge burn in cool water to help reduce pain. Increase fluid intake by at least 30%; encourage the patient to force fluids such as water. Patients should not break blisters. Popping blisters allows bacteria to enter into the burn area. If fluid from blisters is cloudy or milky in appearance or odiferous, patient should be instructed to come into the office.

OTC—Over-the-Counter Medication

Provider may suggest the use of OTC pain relievers such as acetaminophen or ibuprofen. A current medication list should be obtained before checking with provider on the use of OTC meds. As always, never suggest any OTC medications without a direct order from the provider.

Sunburn Prevention

The best defense against sunburn is prevention. Encourage patients to use a sunscreen with a protection factor of 15 or above. Limit sun exposure time and wear proper clothing. A sunburn is usually a first-degree burn unless blisters are present. If patient gets a sunburn, immerse area in cold water or place cool compresses on the area. Do not break blisters. Patient should be seen if blisters appear, because this indicates there is a second-degree burn.

CHARTING EXAMPLE

02/15/XXXX 2:30 p.m.	TC: Pt. states that she burned her ® arm on curling iron approximately 2 hours ago. Area is red and warm to the touch. Clear exudate is seeping from the area. ⊖ Blisters, ⊖ resp. problems, ⊖ chronic illness, ⊕ intense pain, pain scale ("10"). Pt. Applied cold water to area, but pain is getting worse. ⊖ OTC, ⊖ ℞, NKDA. Set pt. for a 3:30 appointment today per screening manual, page 32. M. Paker, CMA (AAMA)

Section 3-7

CHEST PAIN

Chest pain can be a symptom of many different conditions ranging from life-threatening emergencies such as a myocardial infarction to something much less threatening such as gastrointestinal disturbances or muscle pain. Conditions that cause chest pain have similar symptoms and it is difficult to distinguish one from another.

An important rule to remember when screening chest pain is: **Treat all chest pain as though it is a potential emergency.** It is important to realize that patients do not have to complain of chest pain to be in the middle of a myocardial event. The patient may only have one related symptom such as neck or jaw pain, sweating, shortness of breath (SOB), nausea and vomiting (N/V), or dizziness. The history is more important than symptoms when assessing chest pain. A caller who has a history of heart problems needs to be evaluated immediately. Table 3-7 lists the tasks, questions, responses, and actions for chest pain screening.

Expect denial! Many patients having chest pain attribute the pain to something other than heart ailments.

Table 3-7

CHEST PAIN SCREENINGS

Task or Question	Response	Action
1. Record today's date and the time of the call.		
2. Record the nature of the complaint in the patient's own words. Patient may not use the word *pain* in the complaint. Many patients describe it as chest pressure.		
3. Record when symptoms began.		
4. Did the patient lose consciousness?	**Yes**	**EMS**
5. Is pain going on now and does pain stay when patient is resting? If pain has subsided and no other symptoms currently exist, advance to question 13.	**Yes**	**EMS**
6. Does patient have continuous hiccoughs in conjunction with the chest pain?	**Yes**	**EMS**
7. Does patient have a history of heart ailments?	**Yes**	**EMS**
8. If patient has a history of angina, has the pattern changed?	**Yes**	**EMS**
9. Does the pain radiate to arm, neck, or jaw?	**Yes**	**EMS**
10. Does patient have any breathing problems?	**Yes**	**EMS**
11. Is patient experiencing any sweating?	**Yes**	**EMS**
12. Is pain in combination with nausea and vomiting?	**Yes**	**EMS**
13. If pain is not in conjunction with any other symptoms, and it worsens with movement.		**SDA**
14. If patient is not in acute pain at this time, and there are no other symptoms.		**(24–48)**
15. List any home treatment that the patient has tried. Does treatment help relieve symptoms?		
16. List any OTC medications the patient is currently taking.		
17. List any prescribed medications the patient is currently taking.		

18. List any drug allergies.		
19. List instructions given to patient and state where they came from (e.g., screening manual, provider).		
20. Record closing signature.		

Provider's Call

If patient takes nitroglycerin, discuss with the provider for immediate recommendations. Patients who do not have a history of angina may be encouraged to take an aspirin while waiting for EMS.

CHARTING EXAMPLE

06/11/XXXX 4:30 p.m.	TC: Pt. states: "I have had chest pain for the past 1/2 hour. It feels like someone is sitting on my chest." Pain level ("10"). ⊕ shortness of breath, ⊕ radiation to the left arm and jaw, ⊖ N/V, ⊖ Hx of heart disease. Instructed pt. to take one ASA, per Dr. Epstein and to call the EMS. Pt.'s husband took phone and said that he would call EMS. He will call later to let us know what happens. C. Spangler, RMA ————

Section 3-8

COLD, COUGH, AND INFLUENZA (FLU)

Cold and flu season is typically during the winter months but can occur during any season. Colds or upper respiratory infections (URIs) are caused by viruses. Many URIs start out with a runny or stuffy nose, sneezing, slight fever, and sore throat. If symptoms progress and patient complains of pressure or pain in the sinuses, there may be an infection that will need to be treated. The duration of the symptoms is an important piece of information to relay to the provider. A productive cough may indicate that the infection is no longer a URI but has progressed to the lower respiratory tract (bronchi and lungs).

Influenza usually starts out with fever greater than 101° F degrees with body aches in the beginning stages and may progress into a productive cough. In some patients, it may progress to pneumonia. Patients at greatest risk are those with compromised immune systems, the elderly, and the very young. All persons, regardless of risk, should be encouraged to have a flu shot every year. This will decrease the overall influenza risk to everyone. Table 3-8 lists the tasks, questions, responses, and actions for cold, cough, and influenza screenings.

Table 3-8

COLD, COUGH, AND INFLUENZA SCREENINGS

Task or Question	Response	Action
1. Record today's date and the time of the call.		
2. Give a brief description of complaint in patient's own words.		
3. Record when symptoms began.		
4. Does patient have runny or stuffy nose?	Yes	(24–48)
5. Does patient have a sore throat? (If throat has been sore more than 3 days or patient has white patches on back of throat)	Yes	SDA
6. Does patient have a productive cough? List color of phlegm or sputum.	Yes	SDA
7. Does patient have a nonproductive cough that has lasted for more than a week?	Yes	(24–48)
8. Does patient have SOB? Does the patient have shortness of breath?	Yes	ASAP
9. Does patient have sinus pressure or pain?	Yes	SDA
10. Does patient have any light sensitivity?	Yes	SDA
11. Does patient have a fever of 101° F or higher?	Yes	SDA
12. Does patient have any ear pain or pressure?	Yes	SDA

13. What home care treatment has the patient tried? Has it helped?		
14. List all OTC medications and prescribed medications that the patient is taking.		
15. List any drug allergies.		
16. List instructions given to patient and state where they came from (e.g., screening manual, provider).		
17. Record closing signature.		

Provider's Call

OTC—Over-the-Counter Medication

Patients who do not require a visit with a provider may take OTC medications such as decongestants, antihistamines, and cold or flu remedies. Check with provider before recommending any medications. Have current OTC and prescribed list ready when consulting with physician about OTC medications.

CHARTING EXAMPLE

09/12/XXXX 10:30 a.m.	TC: Pt. c/o "cold sx" × 2 weeks. ⊕ nasal drainage ("Green and thick"), ⊕ sinus pressure behind eyes, ⊕ light sensitivity, ⊖ sore throat, ⊖ ear pain, ⊖ cough, ⊕ Fever (103° F). Pt. has been taking Extra Strength Sudafed with little to no relief. ⊖ ℞, NKDA. Instructed pt. to come in for SDA per screening manual, page 35. M Heller, EMT

Section 3-9

CONSTIPATION

Constipation can be described as the inability to pass stool, the passing of hard stools, or straining during bowel movements. Normal frequency of bowel movements can range anywhere from 1–3 times per day to 3 times per week. Always get a history of patient's "usual" bowel habits. Constipation can and usually does increase with age. Seldom is constipation an emergency unless the patient has a bowel obstruction.

Symptoms of a bowel obstruction include the inability to pass gas or stool by way of the rectum, N/V, and severe abdominal cramping. Patients who are elderly or who have debilitating disease may be prone to fecal impaction. This may require a manual disimpaction. The call should be forwarded to the provider in cases in which obstruction or impaction is suspected or the patient should be directed to come in right away. Table 3-9 lists the tasks, questions, responses, and actions for constipation screening.

Table 3-9
CONSTIPATION SCREENINGS

Task or Question	Response	Action
1. Record date and the time of the call.		
2. Give a brief description of complaint in patient's own words. Does patient have a history of constipation?		
3. Record date of last bowel movement and texture.		
4. Does patient have abdominal pain? Is pain severe or in combination with an inability to walk?	Yes	EMS
5. Has patient had a history of grossly bloody stools or black, tarry stools?	Yes	ASAP
6. Is patient unable to pass gas or stool?	Yes	ASAP
Does patient have severe nausea and vomiting in combination with constipation?	Yes	EMS
7. Does patient have a fever? (List temperature and route.) Is temperature >101° F?	Yes	ASAP
8. Does patient have a debilitating disorder or neurological impairment?	Yes	ASAP
9. What self-treatments has the patient tried? Has patient obtained any relief?		
10. List all OTC and prescribed medications that the patient is currently taking.		
11. List any drug allergies.		
12. List instructions given to patient and state where they came from (e.g., screening manual, provider).		
13. Record closing signature.		

Provider's Call

Home Care Instructions

Go to the bathroom as soon as you have the urge. Waiting can lead to constipation. Try soaking in a tub of warm water or applying warm compresses to the anal sphincter. An increase in fiber, bran, water, raw vegetables, and fruits will help with regularity. Eliminate fats and sugars from the diet. Exercise will also assist with bowel elimination. Patients should call if symptoms worsen or do not improve.

OTC—Over-the-Counter Medication

Many medications can assist with bowel elimination, such as osmotic agents, laxatives, and suppositories or enemas. Check with provider before recommending any medication.

CHARTING EXAMPLE

| 06/26/XXXX
3:20 p.m. | TC: Pt. c/o "constipation" × 3 days. Last bowel movement on 6/24/XXXX ("normal texture") Usual bowel habits: 1 BM every 1–2 days. ⊕ rectal gas, ⊕ abd. "pressure" (⊖ pain), ⊖ N/V, ⊖ bloody or tarry stools, ⊖ fever, ⊖ debilitating or neurological impairment, Self-treatment: Prunes (⊖ relief), ⊖ OTCs, ⊖ Rx, and NKDA. Gave pt. home care instructions per page 36 of screening manual. Instructed pt. to take 2 (5-mg tablets) of Dulcolax at bedtime per Dr. Jones. Pt. to call back if sx. worsen or if patient gets no relief by tomorrow. G. Costanza, CMA (AAMA) ——————— |

Section 3-10

DEPRESSION

All of us have or will struggle with depression during this journey we call life. Several contributing factors may lead to depression. Situational circumstances, such as the loss of a loved one or the loss of a job, may lead to acute episodes of depression. Chronic depression may be related to a chemical imbalance and these patients will usually be on antidepressant therapy. Any patients who display signs of possible harm to themselves or someone else must be evaluated right away. Some providers do not feel adequate to handling these types of problems. Check with the providers in your practice to see if they have a referral list of mental health centers that specialize in dealing with these disorders. Check patient's insurance coverage for participating providers before making a referral. Table 3-10 lists the tasks, questions, responses, and actions for a depression screening.

Table 3-10
DEPRESSION SCREENINGS

Task or Question	Response	Action
1. Record today's date and time.		
2. Describe symptoms in patient's own words.		
3. Record when symptoms began.		
4. Does patient have a history of depression? Does patient take medication for depression? (Record name and type.) Does patient take the medication as prescribed?		
5. Does patient know of any factors that may have contributed to this episode?		
6. Has patient attempted suicide with this current bout of depression?	Yes	EMS
Has the patient attempted suicide in the past?	Yes	EMS
7. Has patient had any auditory or visual hallucinations?	Yes	EMS
8. Does patient have a substance abuse or alcohol problem?	Yes	ASAP
9. Has the patient had a baby in the last 6 months?	Yes	ASAP
10. Has patient had a decrease or increase in appetite lately?	Yes	(1 week)
Has patient lost or gained more than 5 lbs in the last week?	Yes	ASAP
11. Does patient feel hopeless?	Yes	ASAP
12. Does patient have a hard time concentrating?	Yes	(1 week)
13. Does patient notice an increase in fatigue?	Yes	(1 week)
14. Has there been a change in sleeping habits?	Yes	(1 week)
15. Does patient have a counselor or practitioner other than the physician who has treated this disorder in the past? When was the last visit?		

16. List any current OTC or prescribed medications that the patient is taking that are not listed above.		
17. Does patient have any known drug allergies?		
18. List instructions given to patient and state where they came from (e.g., screening manual, provider).		
19. Record closing signature.		

Field Tip

When possible, patients who appear to be in acute distress should be assessed by the provider at the time of the call. The provider may determine that the patient needs to be referred to a mental health specialist, clinic, or hospital.

CHARTING EXAMPLE

01/23/XXXX 8:30 a.m.	TC: Pt. c/o "severe depression" × 1 week. ⊕ hx. of depression, currently taking Prozac, 20-mg daily. ("taking as directed"). "My girlfriend broke up with me and I just want to die," ⊕ loss of appetite, ⊕ weight loss (5 lbs in last week), ⊕ fatigue ("cannot sleep"), ⊖ substance or alcohol abuse, inability to concentrate in school, "I can't do anything but cry." Has seen counselors at South West Mental Health Center in the past but does not remember who. ⊖ ℞, ⊖ OTC, NKDA. Instructed pt. to come in for a 9:30 appt. per Dr. Patel. J. Harnett, RN ————

Section 3-11
DIARRHEA

Bowel habits will vary from person to person. Some individuals may have as many as 2–3 bowel movements per day, whereas others might have 2–3 bowel movements per week. Some patients misinterpret what diarrhea actually is. Patients may describe soft bowel movements as diarrhea. Diarrhea is usually described as an increase in the frequency or water content of bowel movements. Significant diarrhea may result in liquid stools that occur at least 3–4 times a day. It may be acute (sudden onset, short duration) or chronic (recurring, long duration). Acute episodes of diarrhea are usually caused by infectious organisms such as bacteria, viruses, and parasites. Another common cause of diarrhea is food poisoning. Symptoms of food poisoning usually occur 6–12 hours after ingestion of the contaminated food. Food poisoning is often accompanied with vomiting. Certain drugs such as antibiotics, antacids, and quinidines taken within a 3-month period can result in diarrhea. A history of recent travel, as well as recent exposure to others with similar symptoms, may be helpful in identifying the causative organism. Table 3-11 lists the tasks, questions, responses, and actions for diarrhea screening.

Table 3-11
DIARRHEA SCREENINGS

Task or Question	Response	Action
1. Record today's date and the time of the call.		
2. Give a brief description of the patient's complaint in the patient's own words.		
3. Record when symptoms began.		
Has diarrhea been present for more than 1–2 weeks and appears to be getting worse?	Yes	(24–48)
4. Describe texture and frequency of bowel movements.		
5. Does patient have abdominal pain?		
Is pain constant and severe?	Yes	EMS
Is pain intermittent but not severe?	Yes	(24–28)
6. Is abdomen tender or swollen?	Yes	EMS
7. Has there been a change in skin color (blue-gray) or are there any breathing problems?	Yes	EMS
8. Has patient fainted in association with the diarrhea?	Yes	EMS
Does patient feel lightheaded on movement or likely to faint now?	Yes	EMS
9. Are stools bloody? Is toilet covered with blood?	Yes	EMS

10. Does patient have any vomiting? List frequency and appearance. Does patient appear to be dehydrated? (Look for symptoms of dehydration on the last page of this chart.)	**Yes**	ASAP
11. Has patient taken antibiotics, antacids, or quinidines in the past 3 months?	**Yes**	ASAP
Is patient taking any immunosuppressive drugs?	**Yes**	ASAP
Is patient taking any other medications that may cause diarrhea?	**Yes**	**(24–48)**
12. Does patient have a fever? Is fever >101° F?	**Yes**	ASAP
13. Are bowel movements mixed with blood or do they appear tarry?	**Yes**	ASAP
14. Does the patient have insulin-dependent diabetes?	**Yes**	ASAP
15. Has patient been exposed to anyone with similar symptoms or recently traveled to a different country?	**Yes**	**(24–48)**
16. Are symptoms mild to moderate and have not lasted more than a few days?	**Yes**	PC
17. What has patient taken for symptoms? Was there any relief?		
18. List all prescribed medications and any OTCs the patient is currently taking that were not listed above.		
19. List any drug allergies.		
20. List instructions given to patient and state where they came from (e.g., screening manual, provider).		
21. Record closing signature.		

Field Tip

Infants, young children, and the elderly can become dehydrated quickly and should be assessed by a provider promptly for symptoms of dehydration.

Dehydration Symptoms

Reduced or no urine output for past 8–10 hours, dry mucous membranes, or a decrease in skin turgor.

Provider's Call

Home Care Instructions

Patients who have mild to moderate symptoms that appear to be viral may try the following: Sip clear liquids for 2 days (flat sodas, broth, gelatin, dilute clear juices; no fruit juices that are colored). Patient may add rice, applesauce, toast, crackers, and bananas after 48 hours. Eat several small portions throughout the day until symptoms have subsided. Avoid all dairy products.

OTC—Over-the-Counter Medications

The provider may want to instruct patient to take an antidiarrheal medication (e.g., Kaopectate, Imodium). As always, double-check with provider before giving any medication suggestions.

CHARTING EXAMPLE

08/12/XXXX 10:15 a.m.	TC: Pt. c/o "diarrhea" × 2 days. (1–2 episodes per day, loose and watery) ⊖ blood or pus, ⊕ abd. cramping (↑ pc) ⊖ fever, ⊕ N/⊖ V, not outside the country recently, ⊕ family history of symptoms. (husband and daughter have similar sx.) ⊖ dehydration sx, ⊖ chronic illnesses, OTC: 3 doses of Imodium over past 2 days (little relief). ⊖ Other OTCs, ⊖ ℞, Drug Allergy: Penicillin. Instructed patient to follow home care instructions per screening manual, page 64. Pt. to call if sx do not improve or worsen. J. Allen, CMA (AAMA) ——————————————————————

Section 3-12

EAR PAIN

Table 3-12A summarizes three types of ear infection. This table is not to be used for diagnosing but rather to help identify the different types of ear infections.

Table 3-12A
TYPES OF EAR INFECTIONS

Otitis Externa or "Swimmer's Ear"	Otitis Media	Otitis Interna
Definition: Inflammation of the outer ear	**Definition:** Inflammation of the middle ear space	**Definition:** Inflammation of the inner ear; also known as labyrinthitis
Cause: Usually caused by frequent water in the ear. This makes the environment more susceptible to bacterial and fungal growth.	**Causes:** Fluid accumulation in the middle ear space (called the eustachian tube) leads to a middle ear infection, either an acute or chronic otitis media. Bacteria or viruses from the upper respiratory tract proliferate into the trapped fluid, setting up an environment for a bacterial infection.	**Possible Causes:** May be due to a bacterial or viral infection May also occur as a result of head trauma
Symptoms: Moderate pain. Pain usually worsens when the earlobe is pulled. Patient may have an odiferous yellow drainage coming from the ear.	**Symptoms:** Patients may describe symptoms of ear popping, pressure, or a stabbing pain. Short-term hearing loss may occur. Pain usually increases with swallowing or chewing or in a supine position.	**Symptoms:** Patient may complain of vertigo and vomiting.
Treatment: Antibiotic eardrops	**Treatment:** Systemic antibiotics	**Treatment:** Systemic antibiotics and anti-vertigo medication

Same-day appointments should be given to patients with possible ear infections. Table 3-12B lists the tasks, questions, responses, and actions for ear pain screenings.

Table 3-12B
EAR PAIN SCREENINGS

Task or Question	Response	Action
1. Record today's date and the time of the call.		
2. Give a brief description of complaint in patient's own words.		
3. Record the date of onset list.		
4. Is ear pain the result of trauma to the ear or head?	**Yes**	ASAP
5. Is there a possible foreign body in the ear?	**Yes**	ASAP
6. Is patient in significant pain? (Rate pain on a scale from 1 to 10.)	**Yes**	ASAP
7. Does patient have a colored drainage coming from the ear?	**Yes**	ASAP
8. Does patient have a fever? List temperature. Is temperature >101° F?	**Yes**	ASAP
9. Does patient have dizziness or vomiting in conjunction with the ear pain?	**Yes**	ASAP
10. Are patient's symptoms related to pressure changes as in flying or being underwater?	**Yes**	ASAP
11. Does patient have neck or facial pain or swelling in relation to ear pain?	**Yes**	ASAP
12. Is there any visible swelling in the canal?	**Yes**	ASAP
13. Has patient had any cold symptoms such as a runny nose, sore throat, or sinus congestion?	**Yes**	SDA
14. Has patient tried any self-treatment? Has patient obtained any relief?		
15. List all OTC and prescribed medications being taken by the patient.		
16. List any drug allergies.		
17. List instructions given to patient and state where they came from (e.g., screening manual, provider).		
18. Record closing signature.		

Field Tip

Patients should avoid putting anything into their ears such as Q-tips, bobby pins, or keys. To relieve pain, patient may try applying warm compresses or heating pad to affected ear. Lie with the affected ear down.

Provider's Call

OTC—Over-the-Counter Medications

The use of decongestants may be indicated for patients with blocked eustachian tubes. Check with provider before giving out OTC advice.

CHARTING EXAMPLE

02/17/XXXX 2:30 p.m.	TC: Pt. c/o R. ear pain ("10") × 2 days. ⊖ foreign body, ⊖ drainage, ⊕ fever (102° F) ⊖ dizziness, ⊖ N/V, ⊕ nasal drainage (clear), ⊖ sore throat, ⊖ sinus pressure, ⊖ neck or facial pain, ⊖ pressure changes. OTC: Sudafed ("little relief"). No other OTCs, ℞: None, NKDA. Scheduled pt. for a 3:15 appointment today per screening manual, page 44. N. Slavomir, RMA

Section 3-13

EYE DISORDERS

There are many causes of eye pain and visual disturbances. These causes may be associated with an injury or brought on by a pathological process. Eye injuries and foreign bodies in the eye should be evaluated as soon as possible to determine the extent of their severity. Eye injuries accompanied by a loss of vision, photophobia, or excessive tearing are definite concerns for immediate action.

A sudden onset of pain or visual impairment may be symptomatic of something that is more sight-threatening than chronic symptoms. Tunnel vision, floaters, or flashes of light may be indicative of a serious pathological condition.

One important point to remember when screening eye injuries is that a delay in diagnosis may result in serious consequences that can lead to a permanent loss of vision. Table 3-13 lists the tasks, questions, responses, and actions for eye screenings.

Table 3-13

EYE SCREENINGS

Task or Question	Response	Action
1. Record today's date and the time of the call.		
2. Give a brief description of patient's complaint using the patient's own words.		

(continues)

(continued)

Task or Question	Response	Action
3. Record date and time of onset of injury or symptoms.		
4. Does patient have a complete loss of vision?	**Yes**	**EMS**
5. Did a chemical get into the patient's eye?	**Yes**	**EMS** Flush with water until EMS arrives.
6. If pain is involved, rate on a scale from 1 to 10. Was pain sudden or severe?	**Yes**	**STAT**
7. Was eye condition related to a traumatic injury?	**Yes**	**EMS**
8. Does patient have a foreign body in the eye?	**Yes**	**EMS**
9. Does patient have any changes in vision such as blurring, flashes of light, or floating objects?	**Yes**	**STAT**
10. Does patient have uncontrollable tearing in association with an injury?	**Yes**	**STAT**
11. Does patient have any medical history that may have contributed to the symptoms (e.g., diabetes, glaucoma, etc.)?	**Yes**	ASAP
12. Any new photophobia or light sensitivity?	**Yes**	**SDA**
13. Does patient have red eyes with a purulent discharge?	**Yes**	**SDA**
14. Does the patient have red eyes with a non-purulent discharge?	**Yes**	**PC**
15. Does the patient have a sty?	**Yes**	**PC**
16. What has patient done for the symptoms?		
17. List current OTC and prescribed medications that the patient is taking.		
18. List any drug allergies.		
19. List instructions given to patient and state where they came from (e.g., screening manual, provider.)		
20. Record closing signature.		

> **Field Tip**
>
> Some providers may want eye injuries and disorders evaluated by an eye specialist, especially in cases in which the patient is already under the care of an ophthalmologist.

Provider's Call

Home Care Instructions

If there is a foreign body or penetrating object in the eye, do not cover the eye. You may be advised to instruct the patient to cover the eye if it is light sensitive. Eyes that are matted shut may be loosened up by applying warm compresses. Styes should not be squeezed. Applying warm compresses throughout the day should help to reduce the size of a sty. Patients with several styes or a history of styes should be evaluated for etiology and prophylactic treatment.

CHARTING EXAMPLE

02/15/XXXX 11:15 a.m.	TC: Injured R. eye × 1 hour ago. "I accidentally stuck the mascara applicator in My eye while applying my makeup." ⊕ Redness, ⊕ eyelid swelling, ⊕ pain ("10"), ⊕ excessive tearing, ⊕ blurred vision. Home Treatment: Irrigated R for 10 min. w/water. "Feels like something is still in my eye." ⊖ OTCs, ⊖ ℞, NKDA. Instructed pt. to come in at ⊖ 11:45 for an appt. and to cover R. eye OD with a clean bandage per screening manual, page 67. Pt. agreed. C. Daniels, MOA

Section 3-14
FAINTING

The technical term for fainting is syncope. Syncope may be the result of something severe such as a disturbance in heart rhythm or something benign as in a sudden drop in blood pressure. Other conditions that may cause the patient to lose consciousness include seizures, hypoglycemia, and vertigo.

A common event that may occur is a vasovagal response. This might occur during or following a blood draw or after the announcement of alarming news. Postural syncope is usually the result of a sudden and severe drop of blood pressure upon standing. This occurs more often in elderly patients, diabetic patients, pregnant patients, and in patients who are dehydrated.

Fainting is generally not serious if it is an isolated event, but the screener must collect the following information: Did an injury occur when the patient fainted? Did the patient lose consciousness as in a hypoglycemic reaction or a seizure disorder, or was the syncope related to a heart disorder? Patients will usually only lose consciousness a few seconds to 1–2 minutes in true syncope episodes. Patients who lose consciousness for longer periods or who struggle to gain full faculties must be evaluated as soon as possible. Asking the appropriate questions will assist the screener in following the correct protocol. Table 3-14 lists the tasks, questions, responses, and actions for fainting screening.

Table 3-14
FAINTING SCREENINGS

Task or Question	Response	Action
1. Record today's date and time of visit or call.		
2. Give a brief description of the patient's complaint using the patient's own words.		
3. Record onset of event and list prior events and any contributory facts.		
4. Is patient unconscious now?	Yes	EMS
5. Were symptoms preceded or followed by chest pain or shortness of breath?	Yes	EMS
If no current heart symptoms, does patient have a history of heart problems or has the patient ever had a stroke?	Yes	EMS
6. How long was the patient unconscious?		
Was patient unconscious >2 minutes?	Yes	EMS
Was patient unconscious <2 minutes with no other symptoms?	Yes	SDA
7. Did the patient sustain any injuries as a result of the fall?	Yes	Response will be according to the severity of injuries received.

8. How does patient feel now?		
If patient is apprehensive with no other symptoms.		ASAP
If patients feels fine and answered "no" to any other question that required a response.		PC
9. List current OTC and prescribed medications.		
10. List any drug allergies.		
11. List instructions given to patient and state where they came from (e.g., screening manual, provider).		
12. Record closing signature.		

Provider's Call

Home Care Instructions

If patient's syncope episode did not require any action listed in the chart and patient appears to be fine now, encourage patient to rest with feet elevated. Patient should drink lots of fluids and be careful when moving from a sitting or lying position to a standing position. If patient feels that the episode might have been related to low blood sugar, encourage the patient to drink something that will get glucose into the bloodstream quickly (e.g., a fruit juice) followed by a protein snack to prevent rebound hypoglycemia. Encourage patient to call back if symptoms return.

CHARTING EXAMPLE

| 06/26/XXXX 10:35 a.m. | TC: Pt.'s husband called to say that pt. fainted approximately 15 minutes ago. Pt. was unconscious for about 2 minutes. Husband caught patient prior to hitting the ground. ⊖ injuries. Pt. c/o dizziness prior to fall but no other sx. ⊖ past hx of syncope, ⊖ hx of heart or seizure disorders. Husband says that wife is fully conscious but very fatigued. ⊖ OTC, ℞: Triphasil 21, NKDA. Husband would like for wife to be evaluated, he is very concerned about her. Instructed husband to call the EMS per Dr. Murarka. D. Bobb, RMA ——————— |

Section 3-15

FEVER

A fever is usually associated with an infectious or inflammatory response. It is the body's natural way of protecting itself against a causative organism; therefore it is not always best to reverse a fever right away. It is important for the screener to ask questions that will help in determining if the fever is the result of a more benign condition such as a mild virus or a more serious condition such as a severe bacterial infection. Adult patients who have fevers >102° F most often should be evaluated.

In the pediatric patient, the age of the child determines the concern for an elevation in the body temperature. In an infant less than 2 months of age, a temperature elevation of 100.6° F is a reason for immediate evaluation. In a child over the age of 1 year of age, a fever of 101° F will usually prompt an evaluation of the child after 48 hours of fever in the absence of severe illness. Patients who have a compromised immune system, such as patients undergoing chemotherapy and patients with human immunodeficiency virus (HIV), are more of a concern than those with a healthy immune system. The screener will need to ask appropriate questions that will help to differentiate the seriousness of the illness. Table 3-15 lists the tasks, questions, responses, and actions for fever screening.

Table 3-15
FEVER SCREENINGS

Task or Question	Response	Action
1. Record today's date and time of visit or call.		
2. Give a brief description of the patient's complaint using the patient's own words. Record patient's current temperature. If the patient has not taken temperature, have patient take it and call you back.		
Is fever >100.6° F for an infant or >101° F in a child over age 1 year?	**Yes**	**SDA**
3. Record date or time of onset.		
Has fever been present for 3 days or more?	**Yes**	**SDA**
4. Is patient currently having a seizure?	**Yes**	**EMS**
Has patient had a seizure with this course of fever?	**Yes**	**EMS**

5. Is patient hard to arouse or has the patient lost consciousness?	**Yes**	**EMS**
6. Is patient delirious?	**Yes**	**EMS**
7. Is patient unable to swallow?	**Yes**	**EMS**
8. Is patient having chest pain or shortness of breath?	**Yes**	**EMS**
9. Does patient have a stiff neck in conjunction with fever?	**Yes**	**EMS**
10. Does patient have a temperature >102° F following a surgical procedure?	**Yes**	**ASAP**
11. Does patient have signs of dehydration? (No urine output for past 10–12 hours, dry mouth, or poor skin turgor)	**Yes**	**ASAP**
12. Does patient have urinary symptoms, vaginal symptoms, or penile symptoms? (Record last monthly period for females.)	**Yes**	**SDA**

13. Does patient have abdominal pain?
  Is pain severe?
  Is pain moderate?
	
	Yes
	Yes
		
		EMS
		SDA

14. Does patient have sinus symptoms associated with a colored drainage, light sensitivity, or pain in the sinus area?	**Yes**	**SDA**
15. Does patient have a productive cough?	**Yes**	**SDA**
16. Does patient have severe throat pain or ear pain?	**Yes**	**SDA**
17. If the patient has a fever and did not answer yes to a question that required a response above.		**PC**
18. What has patient done for symptoms? Has patient obtained any relief as a result of self-treatment?		
19. List all OTC and prescribed medications that were not listed above currently being taken by the patient.		
20. List any drug allergies.		
21. List instructions given to patient and state where they came from (e.g., screening manual, provider).		
22. Record closing signature.		

Provider's Call
Home Care Instructions
Patient should increase fluid intake. Soaking in a tub of tepid water may help to reduce fever. Avoid chilling because it will increase body temperature. Dress lightly and avoid heavy covers.

OTC—Over-the-Counter Medications
Numerous OTC medications will reduce fever. Check with the provider before advising any patient to take OTC medications.

CHARTING EXAMPLE

02/11/XXXX 2:30 p.m.	Pt., age 25 female, c/o an intermittent fever ("100–103° F") × 2 days. ⊖ seizures or loss of consciousness, ⊖ delirium, throat or swallowing problems, ⊖ sinus sx, ⊖ ear pain, ⊖ abd pain, no sx of dehydration, ⊕ urinary sx that include frequency, and pain upon urination × 1 day, ⊖ blood in urine, ⊖ vag. sx, LMP 02/01/XXXX Current OTC: None, Current ℞: Atenolol, 50 mg/d, Drug Allergies: Tetracycline. Instructed pt. to come in for a 4:30 appointment/screening manual, pg 24. S. Crabtree, CMA(AAMA)

Section 3-16
HEADACHES/HEAD TRAUMA

Head pain is one of the leading types of pain expressed by patients. Many factors contribute to head pain. The majority of head pain is benign and can be relieved with OTC preparations. A small percentage of patients with benign headaches will not gain relief from OTC preparations and will require something stronger to relieve their symptoms. Examples of benign conditions that cause headaches include muscle strain, migraines, and muscle contractions.

Some headaches are caused by a buildup of fluids in the sinus cavities. Decongestants may help to relieve sinus congestion, but it is important to determine if there is the possibility of a bacterial infection. Fever and pain on palpation are signs that could signify that the infection is bacterial and that the patient needs to be evaluated.

A small percentage of headaches are considered to be malignant and could be life threatening. Meningitis, brain hemorrhage, and brain tumors are all examples of life-threatening conditions and must be evaluated immediately.

Keep in mind that only a provider can diagnose and that the role of the screener is to ask the appropriate questions that help with prioritization. Symptoms that could signify the need for immediate care include:

- A sudden onset of excruciating pain.
- Neurological symptoms in conjunction with the headache, the inability to speak, paralysis, blurred vision, etc.
- A change or a loss of consciousness with the headache.
- Neck pain or stiffness and high fever in combination with the headache.

The screener must also keep in mind the patient's past history. If the patient has a history of headaches such as migraines or cluster headaches, it will need to be noted. If the headache has changed its pattern, it becomes more of a concern. Follow the criteria on the chart for head trauma protocol. Table 3-16 lists the tasks, questions, responses, and actions for head pain and trauma screenings.

Table 3-16
HEAD PAIN AND TRAUMA SCREENINGS

Task or Question	Response	Action
1. Record today's date and the time of the call.		
2. Give a brief description of the patient's complaint using the patient's own words. Rate the pain on a scale of 1 to 10.		
3. Record date or time of onset.		
Did pain came on suddenly and is excruciating?	**Yes**	EMS
4. Is the pain the result of a traumatic injury?	**Yes**	EMS
Is there any neck pain, tingling, or paralysis?	**Yes**	EMS
Are there any fluids coming from the patient's ears, nose, or mouth?	**Yes**	EMS
Are pupils dilated in one or both eyes?	**Yes**	EMS
Has patient developed black eyes or bruising behind the ears within 24 hours of the injury?	**Yes**	EMS
5. Does patient have any change in mental status, paralysis, vision loss, an inability to speak, hearing loss, or loss of consciousness?	**Yes**	EMS
6. Does patient have a stiff neck or high fever in combination with the headache?	**Yes**	EMS

(continues)

(continued)

Task or Question	Response	Action
7. Does patient have a history of hypertension? Is blood pressure severely elevated?	**Yes**	**EMS**
8. Is pain moderate and getting worse?	**Yes**	**STAT**
9. Does patient have nausea but no vomiting?	**Yes**	**ASAP**
10. Does patient have a colored purulent nasal drainage?	**Yes**	**STAT**
11. Does patient have a history of migraines or cluster headaches?		
Has this episode changed its pattern?	**Yes**	**ASAP**
Are prescribed medications not helping?	**Yes**	**ASAP**
12. Does patient have facial swelling?		
Is swelling mild?	**Yes**	**SDA**
Is swelling significant?	**Yes**	**STAT**
13. If patient has mild to moderate head pain and has not answered yes to a question that required a response above.		**PC**
14. What has patient taken to relieve symptoms? Has patient had any relief?		
15. What OTC and prescribed medications is patient currently taking that were not listed above?		
16. Does patient have any drug allergies?		
17. List instructions given to patient and state where they came from (e.g., screening manual, provider).		
18. Record closing signature.		

Provider's Call

Home Care Instructions

- *Headache:* If patient's pain did not require a response, the following guidelines may be given to the patient.
  1. Move to a noise-free environment.
  2. Try applying heat and cold packs to the area affected.
  3. Dim the lights or turn lights off.

4. Gently massage affected areas.

5. Stay away from odors such as perfumes and sprays that may trigger headaches.

6. Soak in a warm tub; it may offer some comfort.

7. Try lying down; adjust pillows in a way that provides the most comfort.

- **Injury:** If patient's injury did not require a response, the following guidelines may be given to the patient.

1. Observe patient for signs discussed on the chart.

2. Observe patient for alertness for the first 12 hours. Wake every 2 hours and ask questions that have easy responses (i.e., name, address, school, etc.). Continue to observe for 3 days. If symptoms worsen, patient or family member should call back.

OTC—Over-the-Counter Medication

Some patients will ask for advice concerning OTC medications. There are many OTC products that provide relief for head pain. Check with physician before suggesting any OTC medications.

CHARTING EXAMPLE

08/02/XXXX 9:45 a.m.	TC: Pt's wife called to say that husband c/o HA ("10⊕") × 2 hours. Husband states: "I have never had a HA like this before! Pain is intensifying" ⊕ N/V (3 episodes), Instructed wife to call the EMS per screening manual, pg 67. Wife will call back after EMS performs an evaluation. C. Perrino, CMA, (AAMA)

Section 3-17
INSECT BITES OR STINGS

The majority of insect bites and stings are not dangerous. Two common reactions that can occur as a result of an insect bite or sting are a local reaction and a systemic or generalized reaction. The most common reaction is a local reaction that may involve pain, redness, and swelling in the area. These symptoms will usually subside over the next several hours.

A systemic reaction is much more of a concern and usually occurs when the patient develops an allergic reaction to the venom. Swelling of the throat, tongue, or chest, wheezing, hives, and watery, itchy eyes are all symptoms of a possible anaphylactic reaction and require immediate action. A background of the patient's history can save precious moments in the screening process if the patient has had a prior allergic reaction. Table 3-17 lists the tasks, questions, responses, and actions for insect bites or stings.

Table 3-17
INSECT BITES OR STING SCREENINGS

Task or Question	Response	Action
1. Record today's date and the time of the call.		
2. Give a brief description of the patient's complaint using the patient's own words.		
3. Record date or time the bite or sting occurred.		
4. Is patient having any problems breathing? Is there swelling around the eyes, in the throat, tongue, or lip area? Does patient feel lightheaded or have a rash that is widespread?	Yes	EMS
5. Is patient allergic to what bit or stung them?	Yes	EMS
If yes, does patient have an EpiPen?	Yes	**Read and follow directions with EpiPen**
6. Did patient see what bit or stung him or her? Was patient bitten by anything that could be considered poisonous such as a scorpion or black widow spider?	Yes	EMS
7. Is stinger still inside patient?	Yes	PC
8. Does patient have swelling and redness in the local area?	Yes	PC
If bite or sting occurred >24 hours ago and swelling or redness is not subsiding or getting worse.	Yes	SDA

9. Does patient feel sick or apprehensive in conjunction with the sting or bite?	**Yes**	ASAP
Does patient have a fever, rash, or enlarged glands from bite or sting that occurred >24 hours ago?	**Yes**	ASAP
Does area look infected? (red streaks, purulent discharge, etc.)	**Yes**	ASAP
10. Was patient bitten by a tick?	**Yes**	(24–48)
11. List all OTCs and prescribed medications currently being taken by the patient.		
12. Does patient have any known drug allergies?		
13. List instructions given to patient and state where they came from (e.g., screening manual, provider).		
14. Record closing signature.		

Provider's Call
Home Care Instructions

- *Local Reaction:* Apply ice to area and elevate.
- *Tick Removal:* Grasp the body of the tick firmly with some tweezers and pull out the head.
- *Stinger Removal:* Scrape off with fingernail or the blade of a knife. Do not attempt to pull stinger out; this could release more venom under the skin.

OTC—Over-the-Counter Medication

Antihistamines can help to reverse local reactions. Check with physician before directing the patient to take any medication.

CHARTING EXAMPLE

05/16/XXXX 2:30 p.m.	TC: Pt. c/o a bee sting to R. calf muscle × 30 minutes ago. ⊖ Hx of bee sting allergies, ⊖ SOB, ⊖ swelling to throat, tongue, lips, or eyes. ⊕ swelling at the site (about the size of a quarter), ⊕ redness, "warm to the touch." Pt. does not see stinger. ⊖ OTCs, ⊖ ℞, NKDA. Instructed pt. to apply ice and elevate R. Leg per page 24 of screening manual. Pt. to call if sx worsen. T. Ausfeldt, RN

Section 3-18

NOSEBLEEDS

Many factors can contribute to nosebleeds but most often they are a result of trauma. Self-induced trauma may occur from picking, blowing, and rubbing the nose. Environmental conditions may cause the nasal passages to become dry. Patients who suffer from allergies and sinusitis are at greater risk for nosebleeds. The majority of nosebleeds occur in the anterior portion of the nose and usually only involve one nostril. Nosebleeds that occur in the posterior portion of the nose are usually more serious and much harder to control. Both nostrils are usually involved in posterior bleeds. Table 3-18 lists the tasks, questions, responses, and actions for nose bleed screenings.

Table 3-18
NOSE BLEED SCREENINGS

Task or Question	Response	Action
1. Record today's date and time of call or visit.		
2. Give a brief description of the patient's complaint, using the patient's own words.		
3. Note time of onset. If bleeding longer than 30 minutes and nose is still bleeding profusely.	Yes	EMS
4. Has patient lost consciousness or does patient appear to be confused or having difficulty seeing, speaking, or walking?	Yes	EMS
5. Does patient have a history of hypertension and is the nose bleeding profusely?	Yes	EMS
6. Is patient on blood thinner medication? If patient has been applying pressure to nostrils, does nose continue to bleed after 10 minutes?	Yes	STAT
7. Is nosebleed the result of a traumatic injury?	Yes	STAT
8. Does patient have recurring nosebleeds?	Yes	PC
9. If nosebleed is mild to moderate and patient has not answered a question that required a response.	Yes	PC
10. List all OTC and prescribed medications that are currently being taken by the patient.		
11. List any drug allergies.		

12. What has patient done to control the bleeding? Has the bleeding subsided?		
13. List instructions given to patient and state where they came from (e.g., screening manual, provider).		
14. Record closing signature.		

Provider's Call
Home Care Instructions

If bleeding appears to be coming from only one side and is minimal to moderate flow, have patient lean head forward and pinch nostrils toward the front of the nose for 10–15 minutes. Continue sitting straight up for another 20–30 minutes after initial treatment. Placing a cold pack at the bridge of the nose may help in constricting blood flow and thus minimizing blood loss. Patient should call back if bleeding does not stop within 15–30 minutes.

Lubricating the nasal passages with petroleum jelly and using a humidifier will help to keep the nasal passages moist and reduce nosebleeds.

Caution: If patient has a bleeding disorder, is on anticoagulation therapy, or bleeding is especially heavy coming from both sides of the nostrils, lean forward but do not pinch nostrils and either call the EMS or come in ASAP.

CHARTING EXAMPLE

08/12/XXXX 2:15 p.m.	TC: Pt. c/o nosebleed × 20 min. "Bleeding is coming from the right nostril and has slowed down significantly but will not completely stop." ⊖ loss of consciousness or confusion, ⊖ bleeding disorders or anticoagulation therapy, ⊖ hx of nosebleeds, ⊖ hypertension, ⊖ sinusitis, ⊖ OTC, ⊖ Rx, NKDA. Gave pt. home care instructions, on pg. 67 of screening manual. Pt. to call if sx worsen. J. Byun, LPN ————————————

Section 3-19
RASHES AND SKIN DISORDERS

Rashes are a common complaint from patients seeking medical attention. The term *rash* is ambiguous and can mean different things to different people. The screener will need to ask the patient to use specific terms to describe the rash. Obtaining a history of the present illness will be just as important as the description of the rash itself because so many rashes are similar in appearance.

Many factors can stimulate a rash. Chemicals, drugs, pets, insect bites and infestations, as well as environmental factors are just a few. Rashes are usually self-limiting and do not pose any serious health risk; however, some rashes are the proliferation of symptoms that occur in life-threatening emergencies.

The screener should know some basic information before screening these types of calls. Table 3-19A describes some typical rashes seen in the medical office and their symptoms. *The table is not to be used for diagnosing, but rather to help identify which patients need to be seen and the order in which they are to be seen.* Table 13-19B lists the tasks, questions, responses, and actions for rash screenings.

Table 3-19A
RASH CLASSIFICATION TABLE

Condition	Appearance and Duration	Action or Home Care Instructions
Chickenpox	Usually starts with a fever. Within 24 hours, red macules will appear on the trunk of the body and face, but are seldom seen on extremities. Disease progression is macules-papules-fluid-filled vesicle. Vesicles will crust over and dry out. Patient is contagious until all rash is crusted over. Whole process takes about 10 days to 2 weeks. Transmitted via skin contact and through the air. Incubation period is usually 10–21 days.	Usually manageable at home. More serious in adults. Should be seen if patient appears very ill or has a high fever >102° F or the area appears to be infected. Refer to Home Care Instructions of management of itching.
Diaper rash	Diaper rash is usually the result of excessive wet diapers. The rash might be intensified when the baby has runny stools.	Area needs to be kept clean and dry. Applying a diaper ointment with a zinc compound will help to provide a barrier. If diaper rash does not respond to this treatment, patient should be seen.

Drug rash	Can be hives or a generalized rash. Itching may be present, especially with hives, but there may be no itching at all. Rule out all other irritants that may be causing the rash or hives. Drug reactions may progress into a more serious anaphylactic reaction. Always ask about shortness of breath, throat swelling, and chest tightness.	If patient exhibits signs of anaphylaxis, have patient call the EMS. If it does appear that the causative agent is a medication, the patient needs to discontinue the medication and be given an appointment the same day.
Eczema	An itchy skin rash due to allergies; generally a food allergy.	Patient should be scheduled for an appointment for identification and treatment options.
Impetigo	A contagious bacterial infection usually caused by staphylococcus or streptococcus. Symptoms include yellow to red weeping pus-filled lesions. Commonly found on the cheeks, nose, and mouth.	Encourage patient not to scratch lesions. Patient will need to be seen for confirmation and treatment purposes.
Lyme disease	Symptoms usually occur 1–2 weeks after a tick bite. A hard lump may appear at the site of the bite encased in a red ring resembling a "bulls-eye." Other symptoms include headache, stiff neck, and joint pain.	Evaluation by a provider once a rash appears is important so that treatment can begin in the early stages of the disease.
Poison ivy, oak, and sumac	Contracted through oily plant resin that can remain on the skin for up to a week. Can also be transmitted through animals, camping equipment, and the air. Symptoms include an itchy rash that blisters.	Patients who have blisters around the eye area or genital area or the mouth should be seen. Patients who may have a secondary infection should also be seen. Shower several times within the first several hours to remove the resin from the skin. Wash clothes, animals, and any equipment that may contain the resin. Follow home care instructions on page 118 for itching.

(continues)

(continued)

Condition	Appearance and Duration	Action or Home Care Instructions
Meningitis	Inflammation of the meninges, the tissue that covers the brain and spinal cord. Symptoms include continuous headache, stiff neck, chills, fever, light sensitivity, and vomiting. A red or purple rash with or without papules may occur with some forms of meningitis. Mental confusion, seizures, and unconsciousness may be progressive signs of the disease.	Call EMS or advise the patient to be seen in an emergency department immediately. Bacterial meningitis is life threating. It is impossible to determine whether it is a viral or bacterial meningitis until a lumbar puncture and laboratory testing are completed.
Scabies	A mite that is contagious. Usually starts with an intense itchy linear rash composed of scaly papules. The mite burrows into the skin, and secondary lesions may appear between the fingers, armpits, waistline, trunk, and penis. Symptoms are worse at night.	Patient needs to be seen for diagnosis and treatment.
Scarlatina	Rash caused by streptococci bacteria. Symptoms include, fever, chills, sore throat, vomiting, malaise, and abdominal pain. Tonsils and throat are swollen and red. An exudate may be present. A red pimply rash develops within 12 hours of onset of the fever.	Patient will need to be evaluated as early as possible for diagnosis confirmation and treatment options.

Table 3-19B
RASH AND SKIN DISORDER

Task or Question	Response	Action
1. Record today's date and time of call or visit.		
2. Give a brief description of the patient's complaint using the patient's own words. (Describe the rash and give location.)		
Is rash on ears, in the eyes, or in the mouth?	**Yes**	**SDA**
Is rash in the genital region?	**Yes**	**(24–48)**
3. Record duration of rash.		
4. Has patient started a new medication recently?		
Does patient have any shortness of breath or swelling of the tongue or throat?	**Yes**	**EMS**
If patient only has rash or hives in conjunction with medication.		**SDA**
5. Does patient have a high fever, stiff neck, or headache in conjunction with the rash?	**Yes**	**EMS**
6. Does patient have symptoms on rash classification chart that suggest an office visit?		**See Rash Classification Chart**
7. Does skin around the rash appear to be infected? (purulent discharge, odiferous, or swelling?)	**Yes**	**SDA**
8. List any current OTC or prescribed medications.		
9. List any drug allergies.		
10. List instructions given to patient and state where they came from (e.g., screening manual, provider).		
11. Record closing signature.		

Field Tip

In cases in which it is apparent that a child has an identifiable rash such as chickenpox or diaper rash, stick with the related responses.

Provider's Call
Home Care Instructions for Patients with Poison Ivy, Oak, or Sumac

Apply calamine lotion or its equivalent with a cotton ball to the affected area. Taking an oatmeal or baking soda bath or adding a bath oil like Alpha Keri bath oil may give the patient some relief from the itching.

OTC—Over-the-Counter Medications

Using antihistamine OTC medications such as Benadryl may help to reduce itching. As always, check with provider before suggesting any OTC medications.

CHARTING EXAMPLE

| 12/03/XXXX 2:15 p.m. | TC: Mother states: "I think my child has chickenpox; other kids in the daycare have it." Sx include fever (101° F) and a few flat red spots on the back and neck. No other sx. ⊖ OTC, ⊖ ℞, NKDA. Gave mom home care instructions on page 28 of screening manual. Mom to call with any additional concerns. D. Hood, CMA (AAMA) |

Section 3-20
STRAINS, SPRAINS, AND FRACTURES

On occasion, patients call with an injury to their extremities. Some causes of extremity injuries are contusions, strains, sprains, dislocations, and compartment swelling. Table 3-20A will help the screener identify common symptoms for each type of injury. *This chart is not to be used for diagnosing, but rather to help identify which patients need to be seen and the order in which they are to be seen. Only a qualified provider has the authority to diagnose.* Table 3-20B lists the tasks, questions, and responses, for contusions, strains, sprains, dislocations, fractures and compartment syndrome.

Table 3-20A

STRAINS, SPRAINS, AND FRACTURE DESCRIPTIONS

Contusions	Strains	Sprains
Also referred to as a bruise. Usually occurs as the result of a traumatic episode. The skin stays intact, but the blood vessels leak underneath the skin, causing discoloration, pain, and swelling. The skin is initially red or purple and then turns green to yellow to brown. The application of ice may help to decrease swelling.	Trauma to a muscle or tendon from overuse or overextension. Patient may experience slight to moderate pain, which will intensify on movement. Little to no swelling involved. Skin color is generally normal, but may have some bruising. Common sites for strains include the calf, wrist, and shoulder. Follow home care instructions and set a same-day appointment.	A sprain is usually caused from a traumatic injury that results in a tear to the ligaments. Common sites of injury include the ankle, shoulder, wrist, and knee. Usual symptoms include localized swelling and pain. Pain will greatly intensify with movement, especially weightbearing and turning or twisting the extremity. Follow home care instructions and set a same-day appointment.
Dislocations	Fractures	Compartment Syndrome
The temporary displacement of a bone from its normal position in the joint. Usually caused by a traumatic injury. Shoulder and fingers are common sites for dislocations. Symptoms include pain, swelling, skin discoloration, numbness or tingling, and loss of mobility. Symptoms may start hours after injury has occured. Apply ice and call EMS in extreme cases, go to the emergency room, or set a same-day appointment.	Fracture is a break to the bone. There are several types of fractures. Symptoms include intense pain, particularly on movement, and swelling. Bone may look deformed. Patient should be seen ASAP and apply ice, elevate, and immobilize extremity involved before being seen. In cases in which the bone is protruding through the skin, the EMS should be called and the patient should be treated for shock.	May occur after a traumatic injury. Usually the result of increased fluid and pressure within a digit or extremity. This can impair circulation to the muscles and nerves, causing extensive damage. Symptoms include excessive swelling, intense pain, and a loss of sensation. Patient needs immediate intervention in the emergency department.

Table 3-20B
STRAINS, SPRAINS, AND FRACTURE SCREENINGS

Task or Question	Response	Action
1. List today's date and time of visit or call.		
2. Give a brief description of the complaint, using the patient's own words. Be sure to list exact location.		
3. Date or time of onset.		
4. Is a bone coming through the skin?	Yes	EMS
5. Is limb severed?	Yes	EMS
6. Has the limb lost partial or total feeling?	Yes	EMS
7. Does the limb look extremely deformed?	Yes	EMS
8. Is there uncontrollable bleeding?	Yes	EMS
9. Is patient unable to use or bear weight on extremity?	Yes	ASAP
10. Does patient have excessive swelling or decreased range of motion?	Yes	ASAP
11. Does patient have diabetes?	Yes	ASAP
12. Does patient have new tingling in the extremity or loss of sensation?	Yes	ASAP
13. Does patient have swelling or discoloration to an area that has already been splinted or casted?	Yes	ASAP
14. If patient did not answer yes to any of the questions above requiring a response.		PC
15. List any current OTCs or prescribed medications currently being taken by patient.		
16. List any drug allergies.		
17. List instructions given to patient and state where they came from (e.g., screening manual, provider).		
18. Record closing signature.		

Field Tip

Whenever an injury could potentially become a legal matter, as in the case of an automobile or industrial accident, list where the injury occurred and what the patient was doing at the time of the accident and have the patient fill out an accident report. Check office policy before scheduling a work-related injury. Some offices do not participate in such cases. Separate charts are usually made up for these types of incidents. Check the protocol in your office.

Provider's Call

Home Care Instructions

Use the RICE treatment for initial injuries: Rest, Ice, Compression, and Elevation. Wrap ice packs in a towel and apply for 15–20 minutes per treatment. Treatment may be repeated every 2–4 hours for the first 24–48 hours. Heat packs may be applied after the first 24 hours using the same technique as cold therapy after swelling has subsided.

CHARTING EXAMPLE

| 08/13/XXXX 11:15 a.m. | Pt. c/o a "twisted right ankle" approx 1 hour ago. Pt.'s shoe came off foot and ankle twisted as she got out of her car. ⊖ open injuries, ⊖ bleeding, ⊖ loss of sensation, ⊕ edema, "Ankle is twice the size it normally is" ⊕ pain ("10 ⊕".) ⊖ deformity, OTC: Cultrate, ℞: Cardura (1 mg daily). Drug Allergy: Penicillin. Instructed pt. to come in for a 12:00 appointment per screening manual, page 66. Pt. Agreed. C. Taylor, MOA ———— |

Section 3-21

URINARY TRACT SYMPTOMS

Both males and females may call the office with urinary symptoms, but the majority of calls are usually from females. Urinary symptoms may start out as minor, but can exacerbate quickly. The majority of urinary tract infections begin in the lower urinary tract (the bladder and urethra) and migrate upward toward the kidneys.

Lower urinary symptoms include dysuria (painful urination), frequency (having the urge to urinate often), and nocturia (increased urination at night). Some patients may also experience some light abdominal pressure or pain. Upper urinary tract symptoms or kidney involvement may include these symptoms plus nausea, vomiting, fever, and lower back pain.

Urinary symptoms may be related entirely to the urinary tract, but sometimes are combined with genital symptoms. The person doing the screening will need to do a history of the present illness to help identify which organs may be involved.

The majority of providers want to evaluate patients with urinary symptoms. Others want patients who are just starting to exhibit symptoms of a lower urinary tract infection to try home treatment first. Check the protocol of your office before suggesting any home care treatment. Table 3-21 lists the tasks, questions, responses, and actions for urinary tract screenings.

Table 3-21
URINARY TRACT SCREENINGS

Task or Question	Response	Action
1. List date and time of call or visit.		
2. Give a brief description of complaint, using the patient's own words.		
3. List when symptoms began.		
4. Does patient have excruciating lower back pain or abdominal pain with visible blood in urine?	Yes	EMS
Does patient have low to moderate lower back pain that is new?	Yes	SDA
5. Does patient have blood or pus in urine?	Yes	SDA
6. Does patient have a fever? If yes, is temperature >101° F?	Yes	SDA
7. Is patient unable to urinate?	Yes	ASAP
8. Does patient have nausea and vomiting in conjunction with urinary symptoms?	Yes	SDA
9. Does the patient have diabetes?	Yes	SDA
Does patient have any other chronic or debilitating diseases?	Yes	SDA
10. Does patient have a recurrent history of urinary tract infections and think this is exactly like past infections?	Yes	PC
11. Does patient have any penile or vaginal symptoms in combination with urinary symptoms? If yes, list last monthly period for female patients and list all related symptoms. (Look under Vaginal/Penile Symptoms for a complete listing of symptoms.)	Yes	SDA

12. Record all OTC and prescribed medications currently being taken by patient.		
13. Record any drug allergies.		
14. List instructions given to patient and state where they came from (e.g., screening manual, provider).		
15. Record closing signature.		

Provider's Call

Home Care Instructions

1. Increase fluid intake. Water and fruit juices high in vitamin C are good choices.
2. Caffeine products, spicy foods, and carbonated beverages usually aggravate symptoms.
3. Avoid bath gels, bubble bath, feminine hygiene products, and scented toilet paper.
4. Good hygiene before and after intercourse may help to reduce risks of infection. Couples may want to refrain from intercourse until the causative organism has been identified and all symptoms have subsided.

Special Provider's Call

Some providers may want to prescribe an antibiotic over the phone to patients who have a history of UTIs, as long as symptoms appear to be related to the lower urinary tract. *This decision can only be made by the provider.* Other providers will have the patient drop off a urine sample at the office and call the patient once the urine has been tested.

CHARTING EXAMPLE

04/14/XXXX 3:15 p.m.	TC: Pt. c/o urinary sx × 2 days. "I go to the bathroom all the time." (3–4 × /night), ⊕ pain ("6") upon urination, ⊖ nocturia blood or pus, ⊕ abd. pressure, ⊖ back pain, ⊖ fever, ⊖ OTCs, and ℞: NKDA. Set pt. up for 4:00 appt. today per screening manual, pg. 77. N. Goswami, CMA (AAMA)

Section 3-22

VAGINAL SYMPTOMS

It is normal as well as healthy for a woman to have some vaginal secretions. Amounts of secretion will vary throughout a woman's cycle and lifetime. Hormones greatly influence the amount and consistency of vaginal secretions.

A change in color or odor may point to an infectious organism. Yeast is a common type of organism found in the vaginal tract. Individuals may be more prone to yeast infections while taking certain types of antibiotics. Symptoms of yeast infections include a white discharge that is thick and may have a cottage-cheese texture. A mild odor, similar to that of baking bread, may be present but more often the secretion is odorless. The patient may experience mild to moderate itching and vaginal erythema. OTC products are available and usually prove quite helpful. Patients with recurrent yeast infections may have an underlying condition that is causing the infections and should be evaluated by a skilled clinician.

Any patient with a vaginal discharge that is colored (e.g., yellow, green, gray, etc.); has a strong odor (i.e., "fishy"); or has moderate lower abdominal pain or pain during intercourse may have a sexually transmitted infection and should be evaluated as soon as possible to avoid further complications.

Any patient in acute pelvic or lower abdominal pain should be seen ASAP. Table 3-22 lists the tasks, questions, responses, and actions for vaginal screenings.

Table 3-22
VAGINAL SCREENINGS

Task or Question	Response	Action
1. List date and time of call or visit.		
2. Give a brief description of patient's complaint using the patient's own words.		
3. Does patient have a discharge?		
Is the discharge yellow, green, gray, or brown with an unpleasant odor?	Yes	(24–48)
Is the discharge white with a cottage-cheese texture accompanied with itching and vaginal redness?	Yes	PC (24–48)
Are the symptoms not responding to OTC treatment?	Yes	

4. List date of onset.		
5. Does patient have any urinary symptoms? (Turn to urinary symptoms for a complete list of urinary symptoms.)	**Yes**	**SDA**
6. Does patient have a fever?	**Yes**	**SDA**
7. Does patient have abdominal pain, nausea, or vomiting in conjunction with symptoms?	**Yes**	**SDA**
8. Is there a possibility of a sexually transmitted disease?	**Yes**	**(24–48)**
9. Does patient have any lesions or warts inside, surrounding, or outside the vaginal area?	**Yes**	**(24–48)**
10. Record all OTC and prescribed medications currently being taken by the patient.		
11. List any drug allergies.		
12. List instructions given to patient and state where they came from (e.g., screening manual, provider).		
13. Record closing signature.		

Provider's Call

Home Care Instructions

1. Avoid tight underwear, pantyhose, and jeans.
2. Avoid using feminine hygiene products, bath gels, and bubble baths.
3. Good hygiene following sexual intercourse will help to cut down on the number of microorganisms that invade the vaginal tract.
4. Avoid douching because it removes the body's natural secretions that help to fight infection.

OTC—Over-the-Counter Medication

If patient has a thick white discharge that is odorless or has the odor of bread baking, along with vaginal redness and itching, check with physician to see if an OTC vaginal yeast product may be used.

CHARTING EXAMPLE

11/04/XXXX	*Pt. c/o vaginal discharge (frothy & yellow) × 3 days.*
8:15 a.m.	*⊕ fishy odor, ⊖ fever, ⊖ urinary sx, ⊖ abd. pain,*
	⊖ lesions or warts, 1 new sexual partner in last 6 months.
	OTC: None. ℞: Depo-Provera injections every 3 months,
	NKDA. Set pt. up for a 2:00 appointment on 11/06/XXXX,
	per screening manual, pg 37. K. Darst, RMA

Section 3-23

WOUNDS, ABRASIONS, BRUISES, LACERATIONS, AND PUNCTURES

Skin injuries are very common, especially among children. Most of these injuries can be treated at home, unless the area is gaping, something is embedded into the skin (e.g., gravel, etc.), uncontrollable bleeding occurs, the area appears to be infected, or the patient does not have an updated tetanus shot.

It is helpful if the screener understands the terminology involved when dealing with these types of injuries. The following descriptions give the screener some assistance.

- **Abrasion:** An abrasion usually refers to a scraping of the skin or mucous membrane, usually very painful. Patient should be seen if any foreign material is embedded into the skin. Abrasions can become infected. Patient should be seen if there is any sign of infection.

- **Contusion or Bruise:** A bruise is bleeding under the skin that usually occurs as a result of trauma to the area. Area is reddened at first, but will change within hours to a black, blue, yellow color. Some bruises will result in a hematoma, which is a collection of blood that makes the skin protrude outward.

- **Lacerations:** A laceration is a cut to the skin, usually the result of blunt force or a sharp object. If the laceration is gaping, the patient will need to be seen within 3–4 hours to suture the wound. If there is debris embedded into the laceration (e.g., gravel, dirt, etc.), the patient will need to be seen. The patient should be seen if the area looks infected or patient is behind on tetanus shot. Any loss of sensation would be considered an emergency.

- **Punctures:** A puncture wound is usually caused from a penetrating sharp object, like a nail or pin. Puncture wounds usually are not seen unless there are signs of infection, something lodged or embedded into the skin, or the patient is not up to date on tetanus shot. The patient should wash the area with soap and water.

Signs of Infection

Infection does not usually set in for at least 24 hours after the injury. The patient may have a light-colored drainage within the first 24 hours following an abrasion or laceration, but that is considered normal. An odiferous purulent drainage coming from the area, redness to the area that keeps getting worse, excessive swelling, and a streak running from the site of the injury are all reasons to have the patient evaluated. Table 3-23 lists the tasks, questions, responses, and actions for wound screenings.

Table 3-23
WOUND SCREENINGS

Task or Question	Response	Action
1. Record today's date and time of visit or call.		
2. Give a brief description of the patient's complaint using the patient's own words.		
3. Record date or time of injury.		
4. Does patient have uncontrollable bleeding coming from the area?	Yes	EMS
5. Has patient lost consciousness?	Yes	EMS
6. If patient has abrasion, does the area have any gravel or dirt embedded in it?	Yes	ASAP
If injury occurred >24 hours ago, does the area look infected?	Yes	SDA
7. If patient has a laceration and it is <4 hours old, is the area gaping?	Yes	SDA
Does patient have a complete loss of sensation?	Yes	STAT
8. Bruising: Does patient have a hematoma?	Yes	
Is it responding to ice?	No	SDA
If hematoma is on the head or scalp, is it getting larger or does patient have a horrible headache?	Yes	EMS
9. Puncture: Is anything embedded in the skin or does the area appear infected?	Yes	ASAP
10. What has patient done for injury?		
11. List all OTC and prescribed medications currently being taken by the patient.		

(continues)

(continued)

Task or Question	Response	Action
12. List any drug allergies.		
13. List instructions given to patient and state where they came from (e.g., screening manual, provider).		
14. List closing signature.		

Provider's Call

Home Care Instructions

Abrasions and Lacerations and Punctures: Once bleeding is controlled, wash area thoroughly with soap and water. Patient may cover area with a dressing. Applying ice to the area will help to reduce swelling. Change dressing when dirty or wet and at least once a day.

OTC—Over-the-Counter Medications

The doctor may want the patient to apply a skin antiseptic. Check with provider before encouraging the use of any medication.

Bruising: Apply ice to any hematomas.

Patients are to call if symptoms do not improve or worsen.

CHARTING EXAMPLE

| 02/14/XXXX 10:30 a.m. | TC: Pt. c/o a "goose egg" to forehead × 2 hours. Pt. ran head into the sliding glass doors. ⊕ HA (6), ⊖ gaping wound, ⊖ loss of consciousness. Pt. applied ice to the area, but the swelling is getting worse. ⊖ OTC, ℞: Proventil inhaler (PRN), Drug Allergies: Codeine. Instructed pt. to come in for an 11:30 a.m. appointment per screening manual, pg 34. N. Bradley, CMA (AAMA)———————— |

Section Four

ROUTINE CLINICAL PROCEDURES PERFORMED IN THE MEDICAL OFFICE

This section includes procedures routinely performed in the medical office. Specialized procedures that can be found in other sections include:

- Pediatric Procedures—Section 5
- OB-GYN Procedures—Section 6
- Medication Administration—Section 7
- Laboratory Procedures—Section 8
- Emergency Procedures—Section 10

Section 4-1

ASEPTIC PROCEDURES, INSTRUMENT IDENTIFICATION, CARE OF INSTRUMENTS, AND BIOHAZARD SPILLS

Aseptic Procedures

Procedure 4-1

MEDICAL ASEPTIC HANDWASH

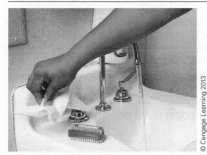

Figure 4-1: Prepare paper towels, use a towel to turn on the faucet, and adjust the water temperature.

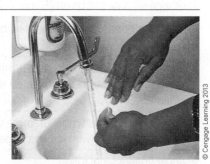

Figure 4-2: Use an orange stick to clean under the fingernails and around the cuticles for the first washing of the day.

(continues)

(continued)

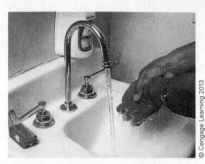

Figure 4-3: Rinse the hands with the fingers pointing downward.

Equipment and Supplies

Soap Antiseptic sink	Paper Towels	Orange Stick

1. Remove all jewelry.

2. Stand at the sink, but *do not* touch the rim of the sink with hands or clothing.

3. Turn on the faucet with a paper towel, adjust the water temperature, and discard the towel (Figure 4-1).

4. Wet the hands, wrists, and forearms and apply soap; using a circular motion and friction, scrub the backs and palms of hands, wrists, and forearms; interlace fingers and thumbs and rub back and forth to clean surfaces in-between; keep the hands pointing down during the entire washing process.

5. For the first handwashing of the day, clean the nails and cuticles with an orange stick or soft brush (Figure 4-2).

6. Rinse the hands and wrists well with the hands pointed downward (Figure 4-3).

7. Repeat the handwashing steps if this is the first handwashing of the day or when the hands are contaminated with blood or Other Potentially Infectious Material (OPIM).

8. Dry the hands, wrists, and forearms with a paper towel and discard the towel. Turn the faucet off with a clean paper towel.

9. Apply antibacterial lotion.

Procedure 4-2
REMOVING CONTAMINATED GLOVES

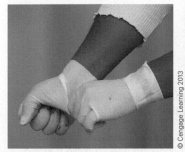

© Cengage Learning 2013

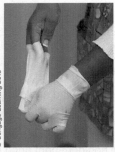

© Cengage Learning 2013

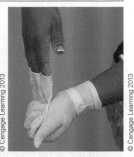

© Cengage Learning 2013

Figure 4-4: Grasp the palm of contaminated glove from the non-dominant hand with the glove from the dominant hand.

Figure 4-5: Start to remove the glove from the non-dominant hand turning it inside out.

Figure 4-6: Continue to remove the glove rolling it into a ball in the opposite glove.

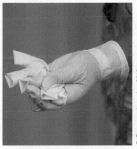

© Cengage Learning 2013

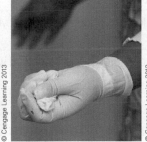

© Cengage Learning 2013

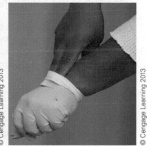

© Cengage Learning 2013

Figure 4-7: Glove is now completely removed and turned inside out in dominant gloved hand.

Figure 4-8: Crumple the contaminated glove and hold it in the dominant gloved hand.

Figure 4-9: Insert two fingers of ungloved hand between wrist and under cuff of contaminated glove.

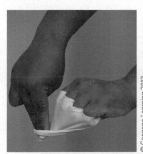

© Cengage Learning 2013

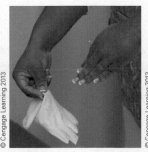

© Cengage Learning 2013

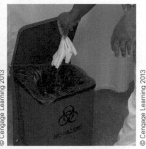

© Cengage Learning 2013

Figure 4-10: Turn the contaminated glove inside out over the other glove.

Figure 4-11: The contaminated surfaces of both gloves are now turned inside out.

Figure 4-12: Dispose of the gloves in biohazard container.

(continues)

(continued)

Equipment and Supplies

Biohazard waste container		

1. With the hands pointed downward and away from the body, grab the palm of the glove from your non-dominant hand with the dominant gloved hand (Figure 4-4).

2. Turn the glove from the non-dominant hand inside out and crumple it into a ball in the dominant hand (Figures 4-5, 4-6, 4-7, and 4-8).

3. While grasping the contaminated glove that has been removed in the gloved hand, insert two fingers of the ungloved hand between the wrist and under the cuff of the contaminated glove (Figure 4-9).

4. Turn the glove from the dominant hand inside out over the other glove (Figures 4-10 and 4-11).

5. Dispose of the contaminated gloves in a biohazard waste container (Figure 4-12).

Instrument Identification

The following are common instruments that are used.

INSTRUMENTS

Category: Description

Cutting and Dissecting

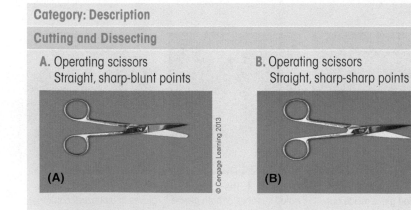

A. Operating scissors
   Straight, sharp-blunt points

(A)

© Cengage Learning 2013

B. Operating scissors
   Straight, sharp-sharp points

(B)

© Cengage Learning 2013

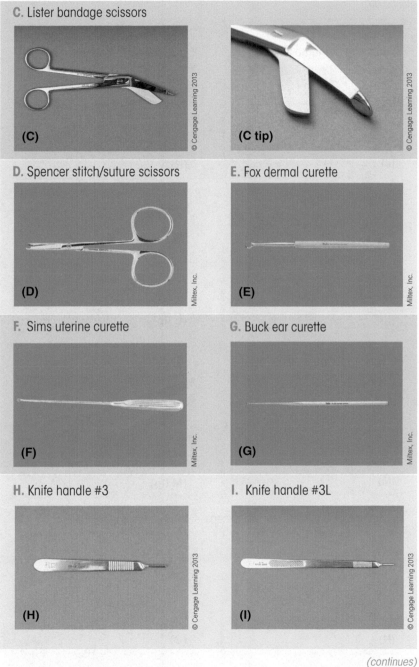

C. Lister bandage scissors

(C)

© Cengage Learning 2013

(C tip)

© Cengage Learning 2013

D. Spencer stitch/suture scissors

(D)

Miltex, Inc.

E. Fox dermal curette

(E)

Miltex, Inc.

F. Sims uterine curette

(F)

Miltex, Inc.

G. Buck ear curette

(G)

Miltex, Inc.

H. Knife handle #3

(H)

© Cengage Learning 2013

I. Knife handle #3L

(I)

© Cengage Learning 2013

(continues)

(continued)

Clamping and Grasping

J. Dressing or thumb forceps

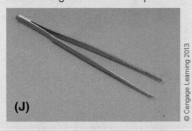

(J)

K. Adson tissue forceps

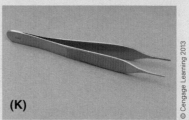

(K)

L. Allis tissue forceps

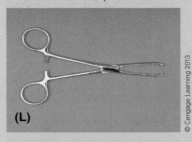

(L)

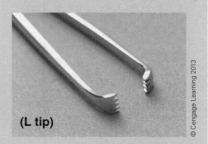

(L tip)

M. Forest sponge holding forceps

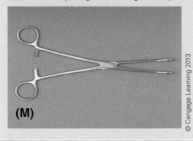

(M)

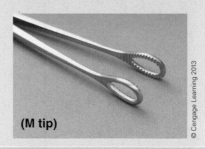

(M tip)

N. Hartman mosquito hemostatic forceps

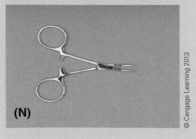

(N)

O. Kelly forceps

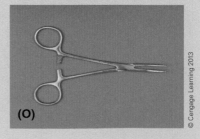

(O)

© Cengage Learning 2013

P. Olsen Hegar needle holder

Q. Backhaus towel forceps

Dilating, Probing, and Visualizing

R. Senn retractor

S. Ribbon retractor

T. US Army retractor

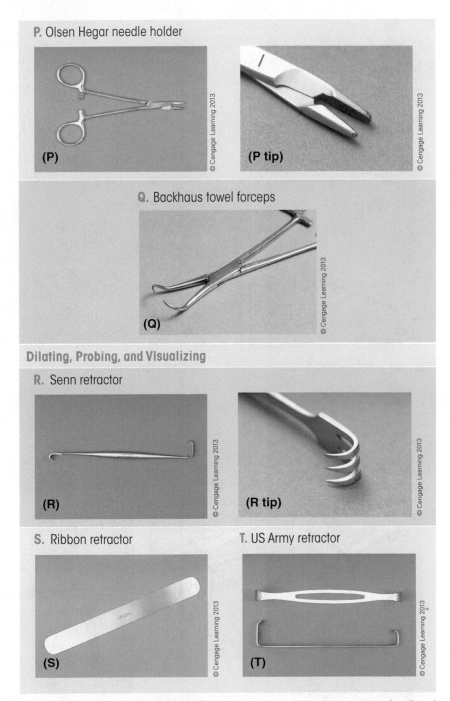

(P)

(P tip)

(Q)

(R)

(R tip)

(S)

(T)

© Cengage Learning 2013

(continues)

(continued)

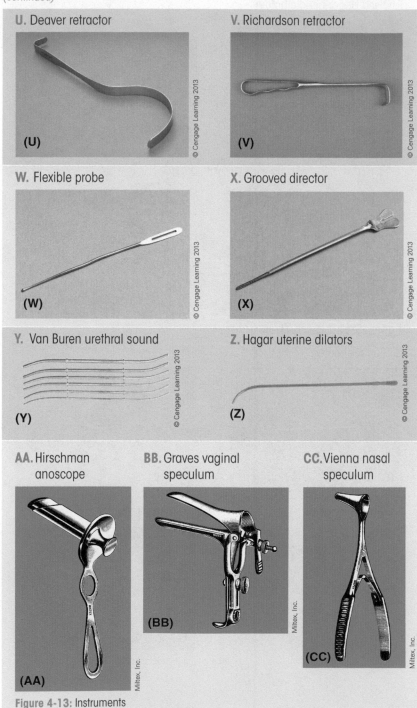

U. Deaver retractor

(U)

© Cengage Learning 2013

V. Richardson retractor

(V)

© Cengage Learning 2013

W. Flexible probe

(W)

© Cengage Learning 2013

X. Grooved director

(X)

© Cengage Learning 2013

Y. Van Buren urethral sound

(Y)

© Cengage Learning 2013

Z. Hagar uterine dilators

(Z)

© Cengage Learning 2013

AA. Hirschman anoscope

(AA)

Miltex, Inc.

BB. Graves vaginal speculum

(BB)

Miltex, Inc.

CC. Vienna nasal speculum

(CC)

Miltex, Inc.

Figure 4-13: Instruments

Instrument Cleaning and Care

Procedure 4-3

SANITIZATION AND LUBRICATION OF INSTRUMENTS

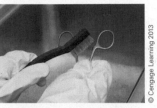

Figure 4-14: The medical assistant must scrub all parts of each instrument, especially in crevices, teeth, or serrations.

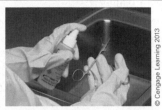

Figure 4-15: The medical assistant applies lubricating spray to the box lock of the instrument to keep it functioning correctly.

Equipment and Supplies

Sink Surgical soap or sanitizer Distilled or deionized water	Basins (one for soaking and one for washing) Scrub brush Waterproof drape	Lint-free cloth or equivalent Lubricating spray

1. Wash your hands and apply the appropriate personal protective equipment (PPE).

2. Soak items in a lined metal basin or plastic basin with deionized or distilled water.

3. Pour the water out of the first basin, protecting the instruments. Place the instruments into a new basin filled with warm water and an approved neutral cleanser made especially for surgical instruments.

4. Thoroughly scrub each part of the instruments. Pay close attention to parts of the instruments that contain crevices, teeth, and serrations (Figure 4-14).

5. Thoroughly rinse each instrument in distilled water or an approved rinsing solution.

6. Place each instrument on a waterproof drape until all instruments have been thoroughly sanitized and rinsed.

7. Dry each instrument with a muslin cloth or comparable material.

8. Inspect each instrument for any defects. Remove any instruments that are damaged.

(continues)

(continued)

9. Soak each instrument in lubricating solution or spray instrument lubricant directly onto any instruments with box locks to keep the instruments working properly (Figure 4-15).

10. Dry the lubricated instruments according to the instructions found on the lubricant label.

11. Prepare the instruments for disinfection or wrapping.

12. Clean the area using an approved disinfectant.

Procedure 4-4
CHEMICAL DISINFECTION

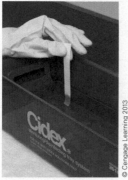

Figure 4-16: The disinfecting solution must be checked to be sure it meets minimum effective concentration level.

Equipment and Supplies

Chemical disinfectant	Chemical solution	Distilled water for rinsing
Disinfecting tray	indicator strip	Disinfecting log
Clean container (to	Lint-free cloth	
put items in after		
disinfection)		

1. Choose a room that is well ventilated and clean.

2. Wash your hands, gather the supplies, and apply the appropriate PPE. (Check the expiration dates on the indicator strips and disinfecting solution to make certain that neither is expired.)

3. Prepare and pour the solution into an acceptable disinfecting container following the manufacturer's instructions.

4. Record the date that the solution was opened on the bottle that houses the disinfectant and record the date that the solution was made on the disinfecting container. Place your initials on the disinfecting container.

5. Place a chemical indicator strip into the solution following the manufacturer's instructions (Figure 4-16). Remove and read the strip.

6. Place the instrument to be disinfected into the disinfecting tray and lower the tray so that the entire instrument is completely submerged in the disinfecting solution. Shut the lid on the solution so that it is secure.

7. Set the timer according to the manufacturer's instructions. Remove PPE and wash hands.

8. Record the date and time that the instrument was submerged into the instrument disinfecting log with your initials.

9. When the timer goes off, reapply PPE, lift the tray out of the disinfecting solution and rinse the item according to manufacturer's instructions.

10. Dry instrument with a lint-free cloth. (Handle items with clean gloves when moving to a storage container.)

11. Clean the area and return used supplies to storage. Remove PPE and wash your hands. Record the procedure in the instrument disinfection log.

INSTRUMENT DISINFECTING LOG

Date of Disinfection	Name of Instrument	Mec Control Result	Name and Strength of Solution	Start Time	End Time	Initials
01-12-XXXX	Nasal Speculum	Acceptable	Cidex Plus	9:30 a.m.	10:00 a.m.	MH, CMA

Table 4-1
GENERAL LENGTH OF TIME ITEMS SHOULD BE STERILIZED

Type of Item	Sterilization Time
Unwrapped items	20 minutes
Single wrapped items or items that are loosely wrapped	30 minutes
Double wrapped items or items that are tightly wrapped	40 minutes

Procedure 4-5
WRAPPING INSTRUMENTS AND RUNNING AUTOCLAVE

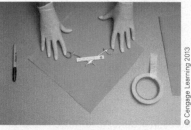

© Cengage Learning 2013

Figure 4-17: Place the instrument for sterilization in the center of the pack with a sterilization indicator.

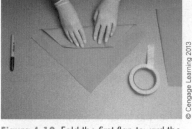

© Cengage Learning 2013

Figure 4-18: Fold the first flap toward the center leaving a small corner turned back on itself.

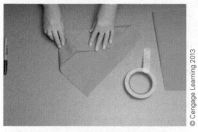

© Cengage Learning 2013

Figure 4-19: Fold one side flap toward the center, leaving a small corner turned back on itself.

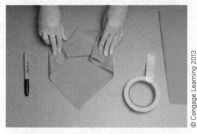

© Cengage Learning 2013

Figure 4-20: Fold the other side toward the center, leaving a small corner turned back on itself.

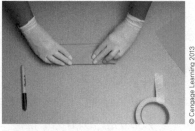

© Cengage Learning 2013

Figure 4-21: Fold the package up from the bottom and secure it.

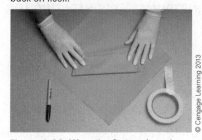

© Cengage Learning 2013

Figure 4-22: Wrap the first package in another wrap.

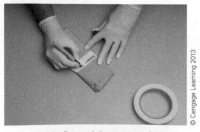

© Cengage Learning 2013

Figure 4-23: Record the name of the instrument, the expiration date, and your initials on the autoclave tape.

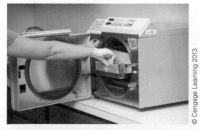

© Cengage Learning 2013

Figure 4-24: Place the packs so that they are in a vertical position at least 1 to 3 inches apart inside autoclave.

Equipment and Supplies

Sanitized instruments or items to be sterilized Wrapping materials (sterilization paper, muslin cloth, or plastic seal pouch)	Autoclave tape Sterilization indicator strip Permanent marker	Distilled water Potholder or thermal gloves

1. Wash your hands, gather supplies, and don a set of clean gloves.

2. Check the integrity of the wrapping materials for flaws and check the expiration date on the sterilization indicators.

3. Place the items on a clean, dry, flat surface.

Items to Be Wrapped in Paper or Muslin:

4. Place one or two sheets of paper or muslin cloth facing diagonally so that they resemble a diamond.

5. Place the sanitized instrument in the center of the paper. Completely open instruments with hinges and shield any sharp tips with a piece of gauze. Place a sterilization indicator beside the instrument (Figure 4-17).

6. Take the bottom edge of the paper that is facing you and fold it upward. Fold the top edge of the diagonal back toward you so that there is a flap (Figure 4-18).

7. Fold one side corner of the wrap toward the center line. Fold the tip back so that there is a flap (Figure 4-19).

8. Repeat step 7 for the other side (Figure 4-20).

9. Fold the pack upward from the bottom edge until the article is completely covered (Figure 4-21).

10. If double wrapping, place the wrapped item onto the center of a second piece of autoclave paper (Figure 4-22). Repeat steps for wrapping.

11. Secure the point that is left with autoclave tape. The following items should be recorded on the tape with permanent ink: the name of the instrument or pack, the date of sterilization, and your initials (Figure 4-23).

Items in Plastic Peel-Apart Wrap:

12. Write the name of the item on the envelope.

(continues)

(continued)

---

13. Place handled instruments in the envelope (handle first).

---

14. Pull the backing off of the adhesive strip and bend the adhesive flap downward so that it completely seals the envelope.

---

15. Finish wrapping all other items that are to be autoclaved and arrange the items on the autoclave trays so that the steam can penetrate all surfaces of each instrument. Packs should be placed in a vertical position and separated at least 1 to 3 inches (Figure 4-24). Jars should be placed on their sides with their lids ajar or removed altogether to facilitate complete sterilization of the contents within the jar.

---

16. Check the gauge of the autoclave reservoir and add distilled water to the fill-line (if applicable).

---

17. Place trays in the autoclave. Make any necessary adjustments to accommodate the proper positioning of the instruments on each tray. Close and latch the door according to manufacturer's instructions.

---

18. Select the appropriate sterilization cycle according to the load's contents and press the start button. The load will run through the entire cycle and will vent on its own.

---

19. Once the load has properly vented, open the door according to the manufacturer's instructions. If time permits, allow items to remain in the autoclave for an additional 20 to 30 minutes to facilitate drying.

---

20. Pull out the trays using caution. You may need to wear thermal gloves or use a towel to pull out the trays. (If the trays are allowed to cool before removing, just wear clean gloves to keep the outside of the packs as clean as possible.)

---

21. Remove the items and check to make certain that the stripes on the autoclave tape turned the appropriate color.

---

22. Store the items in a clean, covered environment.

INSTRUMENT AUTOCLAVE LOG

Date	Start Time	Finish Time	Items Autoclaved	Controls Used to Test Sterility	Results of Controls	Initials
01-12-XXXX	1:30 p.m.	2:15 p.m.	2 Laceration trays 2 Wrapped vaginal speculums	Autoclave tape Chemical indicator pellet	Both tape and indicator pellet positive for sterilization	DE, CMA

Biohazard Spills

Procedure 4-6
RESPONDING TO A BIOHAZARD SPILL

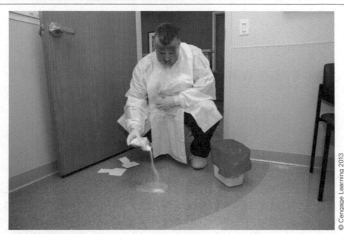

Figure 4-25: MA in full PPE with biohazard container next to him, opened spill kit and pouring coagulating powder on spill.

Equipment and Supplies

Hand sanitizer Commercailly prepared spill kit or germicidal cleaner	Paper towels	Biohazard waste container

1. Apply full PPE.

2. Pour coagulating powder from the spill kit over the spill (Figure 4-25). Carefully scoop contents of spill and coagulating powder with scooping device from spill kit.

3. Discard of the absorbent material and scooping device in a biohazard trash bag.

4. Spray the area with germicidal cleaner, and wipe with paper towels. Discard contaminated towels in a biohazard bag.

5. Remove PPE while gloves are still in place and discard contaminated items into biohazard waste container.

6. Discard gloves in biohazard trash and wash your hands.

Section 4-2

ASSESSMENT, WEIGHT AND HEIGHT, POSITIONING, AND VITAL SIGNS

Assessment

Procedure 4-7

CONDUCTING A PATIENT HISTORY

Equipment and Supplies

Patient history form	Writing instruments	

1. Wash hands and prepare the interview area. The interview area should be private, comfortable, and free of distractions. The furniture should be arranged to accommodate the patient and anyone who may be with the patient. The medical assistant's chair should be at least 4 to 12 feet away from the patient's chair.

2. Once the patient has been escorted to the examination room, identify yourself, list your title, and identify the patient using two different identifiers. Ask the patient if he has a certain preference for the way he wants to be addressed throughout the remainder of the interview and future visits.

3. Explain the purpose of the history and inform the patient that everything that is shared during the interview will remain confidential.

4. If the patient completed the form before the visit, review all information and check for possible omissions or incomplete responses. If the medical assistant is completing the entire form, address all questions on the form.

5. Properly develop all "Yes" responses in the past medical history section. List the exact name of the disease or condition, duration or onset of the disease, treatment, current status, and date of resolve, if applicable.

6. Properly expand on all "Yes" responses listed in the family and social history sections.

7. Make certain that either you or the patient lists all current prescribed medications and over-the-counter drugs that are being taken by the patient. List their strengths and how often the patient takes the medication.

8. Make certain that all drug and other types of allergies are listed under the appropriate section and that drug allergies are either highlighted or written in red ink.

9. Make certain that all hospitalizations and surgeries are listed on the medical history form.

10. List the patient's chief complaint.

11. Once the form is completed, summarize the information with the patient.

12. Ask the patient if he would like any additional information added to the history form.

13. Thank the patient for his assistance during the interview process.

14. Instruct the patient how to disrobe prior to the examination.

Weight and Height

Procedure 4-8
WEIGHT AND HEIGHT MEASUREMENT

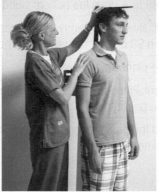

Figure 4-26: Adjust the height bar so it rests on the top of the patient's head.

Equipment and Supplies

Upright scale	Paper towel	Patient record

1. Place the scale weights at zero. Check that the scale is balanced and adjust, if necessary. Wash your hands.

2. Identify the patient using two identifiers, identify yourself, and explain the procedure.

(continues)

(continued)

3. Assess the stability of the patient.

4. Have the patient remove any unnecessary clothing, such as a jacket or sweater, as well as shoes.

5. Place a paper towel on the floor of the scale.

6. Assist the patient onto the scale, facing the weights.

7. Instruct the patient to stand on the center of the scale and to hold still. Slowly adjust the weights until the scale arrow is balanced.

8. Record the measurement, return the weights to zero, and then assist the patient off the scale.

9. Raise the calibrated height bar to a height that would be greater than the patient's height. Extend the bar used to measure to a horizontal position.

10. Assist the patient back onto the scale platform. Patient's back should be toward the measurement tool. Have the patient stand as erect as possible.

11. Lower the horizontal bar slowly and gently until it reaches the top of the patient's head, forming a 90-degree angle with the height bar (Figure 4-26).

12. Assist the patient off the platform.

13. Record the measurement. Place the measurement bar back to its original position and discard the paper towel.

14. Document the results in the patient record (if you didn't already). Convert weight into kilograms, if necessary.

Positioning and Draping

Procedure 4-9
POSITIONING AND DRAPING PATIENTS

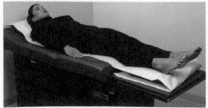

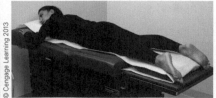

Figure 4-27: Supine or Horizontal Recumbent Position (Used for exams of the anterior body)

Figure 4-28: Prone (Used for exams of the posterior body)

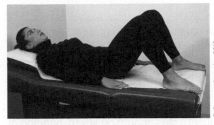

Figure 4-29: Dorsal recumbent (May be used for abdominal, pelvic or rectal exams)

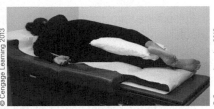

Figure 4-30: Sims' (Used for rectal exams, enemas and rectal procedures.)

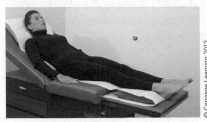

Figure 4-31: Semi-Fowler's (Used for patients with breathing problems or patients with back pain.)

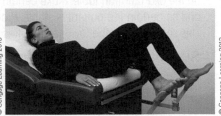

Figure 4-32: Lithotomy (Used for vaginal or rectal exams)

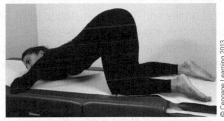

Figure 4-33: Knee-chest (Used for rectal exams)

Equipment and Supplies

Examination table Table paper	Patient gown	Paper or cloth drape

1. Wash your hands.

2. Prepare the examination room, positioning the table into a low, flat position, if applicable.

3. Identify the patient using two identifiers, identify yourself, and explain the procedure.

4. If a gown is to be used, provide this to the patient with instructions on opening in the front or rear. Allow the patient privacy to change into the gown. Provide assistance with gowning if requested.

(continues)

(continued)

5. Pull out the retractable step to allow the patient to step up and be seated safely on the examination table. Once the patient is seated on the examination table, push in the retractable step and assist the patient into one of the following positions:

Sitting position:

Explain to the patient how to sit. The patient's legs should be flexed, hanging at a 90-degree angle over the edge of the table. The thighs should be supported on the examination table. Make certain the patient is sitting in a stable manner and be certain the patient is stable. Provide a drape for privacy and comfort. This should cover the lower extremities and lap area.

Supine position: (Figure 4-27)

Ask the patient to sit at the end of the examination table. Have the patient lie back on the examination table and extend the table extension to rest the patient's legs on. Place a pillow under the patient's head and shoulders, for comfort. Place a drape over the torso and lower extremities for comfort and privacy.

Prone position: (Figure 4-28)

Ask the patient to sit on the end of the examination table. Have the patient lie back in the supine position and extend the table extension. Instruct the patient to roll toward you and lie on the stomach. Position the patient with the head turned to the side and the arms at the side or above the head. Place a drape on the torso and lower extremities for comfort and privacy.

Dorsal recumbent position: (Figure 4-29)

Ask the patient to sit on the end of the examination table. Have the patient lie back in the supine position and extend the table extension. Ask the patient to bend the knees and place the feet flat on the table. Push the table extension in. Drape the patient so that one corner of the drape points toward the head and covers the abdominal region and the opposite corner points toward the feet (known as the diamond drape).

Sims' position: (Figure 4-30)

Ask the patient to sit on the end of the examination table. Have the patient lie back in the supine position and extend the table extension. Ask the patient to roll toward you up onto the left side. Instruct the patient to place the left arm behind the body and the right arm in front of the body. Both legs are flexed slightly, with the top leg flexed at a more extreme angle. Drape the patient for comfort and privacy.

Semi-Fowler's position: (Figure 4-31)

Ask the patient to sit on the end of the examination table. Elevate the head of the table to the desired angle (Full Fowler's is a 90-degree angle and semi-Fowler's is a 45-degree angle). Drape the torso and lower extremities for comfort and privacy.

Lithotomy position: (Figure 4-32)
Ask the patient to lie on the examination table in the supine position, and pull out the table extension. Extend the stirrups at the end of the table and instruct the patient to scoot to the end of the table and place the feet in the stirrups; assist the patient, because this is sometimes difficult. Drape the patient with the diamond drape.

Knee-chest position: (Figure 4-33)
Ask the patient to lie on the examination table in the prone position. Instruct the patient to get on hands and knees and pull the knees as close to the chest as possible. Have the patient turn the head to the side and bend the arms and place them above the head. Drape the patient with the diamond drape.

6. Instruct the patient not to tuck the drape under or around body parts.

Vital Sign Measurements

Temperature

Table 4-2
NORMAL TEMPERATURE READINGS BY ROUTE

Oral	98.6° F	37.0° C
Aural	99.6° F	37.7° C
Rectal	99.6° F	37.7° C
Temporal	99.6° F	37.7° C
Axillary	97.6° F	36.3° C

Procedure 4-10
OBTAINING ORAL TEMPERATURE USING AN ELECTRONIC THERMOMETER

Equipment and Supplies

Patient chart	Electronic thermometer	Probe covers Alcohol wipes

1. Wash your hands. (Gloving is optional.)

2. Assemble the equipment. Ensure equipment is charged, clean, and in working order.

(continued)

---

3. Identify the patient using two identifiers, identify yourself, and explain the procedure.

---

4. Ask if the patient has ingested hot or cold food or beverages or smoked within the last half hour. (If the patient has ingested hot or cold items or smoked, use a different method for taking the patient's temperature or wait an appropriate amount of time prior to taking the patient's temperature.)

---

5. Select the blue oral probe and cover it with a disposable probe cover.

---

6. Place the thermometer in the patient's mouth under the tongue to the right or left side of the frenulum linguae.

---

7. Instruct the patient not to clench or bite down on the thermometer and to hold the mouth closed and breathe through the nostrils, not through the mouth.

---

8. Keep the thermometer in place until a tone or beep is heard.

---

9. Remove the thermometer and read the digital display.

---

10. Discard the used probe cover following institutional guidelines.

---

11. Place the electronic thermometer base back in the base holder for recharging.

---

12. Wash your hands and record the temperature reading in the patient record.

CHARTING EXAMPLE

04/27/XXXX	*T 99.9° F. Lilly Kelly, CMA (AAMA)* ————
9:30 a.m.	

Procedure 4-11
MEASURING TEMPERATURE USING A TYMPANIC THERMOMETER

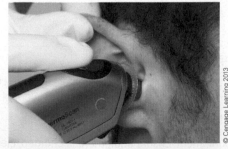

© Cengage Learning 2013

Figure 4-34: Gently insert the probe into the patient's ear canal. Pull the auricle up and back on an adult and down and back on an infant or young child.

Equipment and Supplies

Patient chart	Tympanic thermometer	Probe covers Alcohol wipes

1. Wash your hands. (Gloving is optional.)

2. Assemble the equipment. Ensure equipment is charged, clean, and in working order.

3. Identify the patient using two identifiers, identify yourself, and explain the procedure.

4. Place a clean probe cover over the tympanic probe and make certain the unit is turned on and in the "ready" mode.

5. Straighten the aural canal to best facilitate an accurate measurement. (Pull the auricle up and back on adults and children over the age of 3 years. Pull down and back on the auricle on anyone age 3 or younger.)

6. Place the covered probe into the patient's ear canal (Figure 4-34), forming a tight seal and pointing the probe toward the eardrum.

7. Activate the thermometer while having the patient quietly relax.

8. Leave the probe in place until the unit beeps. The temperature will be displayed digitally on the thermometer.

9. Discard the probe cover in the appropriate waste container. Return the thermometer to storage.

10. Wash your hands.

11. Document the results, including which ear was used for the measurement.

CHARTING EXAMPLE

11/04/XXXX 10:00 a.m.	T 99.2° F, TM, L. ear. Cassy Smith, RMA

Procedure 4-12

MEASURING TEMPERATURE USING A TEMPORAL ARTERY THERMOMETER

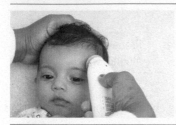

Figure 4-35: The medical assistant slides the probe across the forehead and ends with the probe over the temporal artery.

Equipment and Supplies

Patient chart	Temporal artery thermometer	Probe covers Alcohol wipes

1. Wash your hands. (Gloving is optional.)

2. Assemble the equipment. Ensure equipment is charged, clean, and in working order.

3. Identify the patient using two identifiers, identify yourself, and explain the procedure.

4. Remove hats or scarves on the side of the head that is to be measured and pull hair back, if applicable.

5. Check the forehead for perspiration. Wipe dry if perspiration is present.

6. Depress the scan button and begin by placing the probe at the midline of the forehead. Keep probe flush with the skin and slowly glide the thermometer across the forehead until the probe reaches the hairline on the side of the head over the temporal artery (Figure 4-35).

7. When the reading is complete, release the scan button, lift the probe from the patient's skin, and check the display for the reading. (Take a second reading behind the ear under the mastoid process, if necessary.)

8. Clean the probe and accurately document the reading and the method by which the reading was obtained in the patient record.

CHARTING EXAMPLE

10/10/XXXX 10:15 a.m.	T 98.6° F (TA). Kelly Leonard, CMA (AAMA)

Pulse

Table 4-3
PULSE RATES

Patient Population	Average Pulse Rate (Bpm)
Newborn	140
0–6 months	130
6–12 months	115
12–24 months	110
2–6 years	100
Early school age	95
Adolescence through adulthood	80
Geriatric	74
Athletes	60
Elite athletes	50

Procedure 4-13
MEASURING RADIAL PULSE

Equipment and Supplies

Patient chart	Watch with a second hand	

1. Wash your hands.

2. Assemble the equipment.

3. Identify the patient using two identifiers, identify yourself, and explain the procedure.

4. Place the patient in a calm, quiet environment. Allow the patient to relax in a sitting position with the arm in a comfortable location.

5. Locate the radial pulse with your index and middle fingers. The hand you use should be opposite from the hand on which you wear your watch. Never use your thumb when measuring the pulse.

6. Apply slight pressure onto the radial artery. Increase pressure until the pulse is felt.

(continues)

(continued)

7. Count the number of beats for a minimum of 30 seconds. Multiply this number by 2 for a full-minute rate.

8. Note if any irregular beats occur.

9. Maintain fingers on the pulse and begin counting respirations. (Refer to Procedure 4-16 for the respiration procedure.)

10. Wash your hands.

11. Document the results of the pulse in the patient record.

CHARTING EXAMPLE

10/04/XXXX 9:30 a.m.	P 84. M. Jones, CMA (AAMA)

Procedure 4-14
MEASURING APICAL PULSE

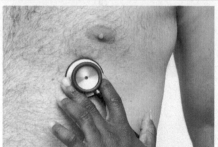

Figure 4-36: The apical pulse can be counted by placing the stethoscope over the apex of the heart.

Equipment and Supplies

Patient chart	Stethoscope	Watch with a second hand

1. Wash your hands. (Gloving is optional.)

2. Assemble the equipment. Ensure equipment is clean, and in working order.

3. Identify the patient using two identifiers, identify yourself, and explain the procedure.

4. Instruct the patient to expose the chest area by either unbuttoning the shirt or removing clothes from the waist up. Provide a gown for privacy.

5. Remove clothing, gown, or drape covering the left thoracic area.

6. Place the stethoscope in your ears correctly.

7. Locate the apical pulse.

8. After warming the diaphragm of the stethoscope, place it over the apex of the heart (Figure 4-36).

9. Count the beats for 1 full minute.

10. Note any irregularities, along with the quality of sound.

11. Remove the stethoscope.

12. Assist the patient in redressing or draping.

13. Wash your hands.

14. Record the results in the patient record.

CHARTING EXAMPLE

10/04/XXXX 9:30 a.m.	P 84 (apical). Nancy Smith, CMA AMA ——————

Procedure 4-15
ASSESSING THE PULSE USING A DOPPLER UNIT

Equipment and Supplies

Patient chart Hand sanitizer	Doppler unit	Coupling agent

1. Wash your hands. (Gloving is optional.)

2. Assemble the equipment. Ensure equipment is charged, clean, and in working order.

3. Turn on the doppler unit and apply coupling agent to the probe.

4. Identify the patient using two identifiers, identify yourself, and explain the procedure.

5. Position the probe so that it is at a 45-degree angle.

(continues)

(continued)

6. Position the probe over the artery where the sound is the most prominent.

7. Assess the patient's heart rate, rhythm, and volume.

8. Document the measurement in the patient's chart.

9. Cleanse the gel from the patient's skin and clean the probe as well following manufacturer's instructions.

CHARTING EXAMPLE

| 10/04/XXXX | P 16 (Doppler Method), rate and volume normal. Jan |
| 1:20 p.m. | Zachrich, CMA (AAMA)————— |

Respiration

Table 4-4
AVERAGE RESPIRATORY VALUES MEASURED IN BREATHS PER MINUTE

Age	Rate
Newborn	30–60/min
12–24 months	20–40/min
8–15 years	15–25/min
16 years–adult	16–20/min

Procedure 4-16
OBTAINING A RESPIRATION

Equipment and Supplies

Patient chart	Watch with a second hand	

1. Wash your hands. (Gloving is optional.)

2. Assemble the equipment.

3. Identify the patient using two identifiers, identify yourself, and explain the procedure.

4. Place the patient in a calm, quiet environment. Allow the patient to relax in a sitting position with the arm in a comfortable location.

5. Because the respiration is usually performed in conjunction with the pulse, your fingers should remain over the radial artery while observing respiration. (This way the patient will not know that you are watching his or her respiration.)

6. Note that when counting respirations, one respiration is equivalent to one inhalation and one expiration combined.

7. Count respirations for 30 seconds and multiply by 2. (If breathing pattern is irregular, count for a full minute.)

8. Document the rate of breathing and record any irregularities.

CHARTING EXAMPLE

| 10/04/XXXX | P 88 R 16, unlabored, and regular. W Howard, CMA |
| 1:20 p.m. | (AAMA) |

Blood Pressure

Table 4-5
CLASSIFICATIONS OF ADULT BLOOD PRESSURE

Classification	Systolic (mm Hg)	Diastolic (mm Hg)
Normal or ideal	<120	<80
Prehypertension	120–139	80–89
Stage 1 hypertension	140–159	90–99
Stage 2 hypertension	>159	>99

Source: Seventh Report of the Joint National Committee on Detection, Evaluation, and Treatment of High Blood Pressure (JNC 7).

Procedure 4-17

MEASURING A BLOOD PRESSURE (AUSCULTATORY METHOD)

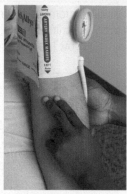

© Cengage Learning 2013

Figure 4-37: Palpate the brachial artery for a viable pulse.

Equipment and Supplies

Patient chart	Sphygmomanometer with appropriate cuff size	Stethoscope Alcohol wipes

1. Wash your hands. (Gloving is optional.)

2. Assemble the equipment. Ensure equipment is charged, clean, and in working order.

3. Identify the patient using two identifiers, identify yourself, and explain the procedure.

4. Position the patient's arm so that it is at heart level.

5. Remove clothing or pull sleeve of shirt up to expose the arm.

6. Center the cuff over the brachial artery.

7. Wrap the cuff around the patient's arm so that it is 1–2" above the bend of the elbow.

8. Palpate the brachial pulse with the index and middle finger of dominant hand (Figure 4-37).

9. Place the diaphragm of the stethoscope firmly against the brachial artery during the entire procedure.

10. Hold the air pump or bulb in your dominant hand and wrap your thumb and index finger around the valve.

11. Tighten the screw and rapidly inflate the cuff to 180 mm/hg on the dial or following institutional policy.

12. Open the valve to release air at a rate of 2 to 4 mm Hg per second.

13. Note the measurement at which you hear the first clear beat. This is the systolic reading!.

14. Continue to listen to the beat as you deflate the cuff.

15. Note the reading on the manometer when you hear the last beat. Open the valve and quickly deflate the cuff.

16. Remove the cuff and squeeze remaining air from the bladder of the cuff.

17. Return equipment to its proper place and wash your hands.

18. Document the reading and the position patient was in, if other than sitting.

CHARTING EXAMPLE

03/02/XXXX 4:30 p.m.	BP 142/82 L. arm. T CMA (AAMA)

Procedure 4-18
MEASURING A BLOOD PRESSURE USING THE PALPATORY METHOD

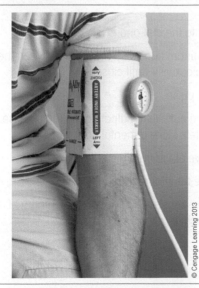

© Cengage Learning 2013

Figure 4-38: Blood pressure cuff should be placed so that the arrow lines up with the artery.

(continues)

(continued)

Equipment and Supplies

Patient chart	Sphygmomanometer with appropriate cuff size	Stethoscope

1. Wash your hands. (Gloving is optional.)

2. Assemble the equipment.

3. Identify the patient using two identifiers, identify yourself, and explain the procedure.

4. Test the equipment to make sure the bulb and gauge are in working order.

5. Assess the patient's upper arm diameter to determine if the size of the cuff selected is adequate.

6. Position the patient in a quiet, comfortable position.

7. Expose the arm by rolling up the patient's sleeve or removing any clothing or garments from the arm that will be used for obtaining the blood pressure.

8. Palpate the brachial artery for a viable pulse.

9. With the patient's palm facing upward, wrap the cuff around the upper arm 1 to 2 inches above the bend of the elbow (Figure 4-38). Position the arm so that it is at heart level.

10. Adjust the manometer so it is clipped to the cuff and is in clear view.

11. Hold the bulb in the palm of your dominant hand with the valve between the thumb and first finger. Turn the valve clockwise until closed.

12. With the other hand, locate the radial pulse.

13. Using the bulb, squeeze and inflate the cuff while palpating the radial pulse. Continue until the pulse is no longer felt. Make a mental note.

14. Open the valve completely and remove all air from the cuff.

15. After waiting 1 minute, prepare to take the blood pressure.

16. Place the stethoscope correctly in your ear canals. Place the diaphragm of the stethoscope securely over the brachial artery.

17. Tighten the valve and pump the cuff rapidly up to 30 mm Hg above the palpated pressure.

18. Begin to release the pressure in the cuff by slowly turning the valve counterclockwise, 2 to 4 mm Hg per second. Observe the manometer carefully. Note the measurement when the first beat is heard. This is the systolic pressure.

19. Continue to deflate the cuff. Observe the manometer carefully and note the measurement when the sound ceases. This is the diastolic pressure.

20. Open the valve completely to deflate the cuff quickly and remove all air from the cuff.

21. Remove the stethoscope from your ears and cuff from patient's arm. Squeeze out any excess air from the cuff.

22. Return equipment and wash your hands.

23. Record the results in the patient record, including the patient's position, if other than sitting.

CHARTING EXAMPLE

| 03/02/XXXX | BP 142/82 L. arm. Tim Hall, CMA (AAMA) —————— |
| 4:30 p.m. | |

Pulse Oxymetry

Procedure 4-19

MEASURING OXYGEN SATURATION RATE USING A PULSE OXIMETER

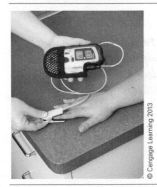

© Cengage Learning 2013

Figure 4-39: The medical assistant places the pulse oximeter probe on the patient's finger.

(continues)

(continued)

Equipment and Supplies

| Patient chart | Pulse oximeter unit/ finger probe | Nail polish remover (if indicated) |

1. Wash your hands. (Gloving is optional.)

2. Assemble the equipment. Ensure equipment is charged, clean, and in working order.

3. Identify the patient using two identifiers, identify yourself, and explain the procedure.

4. Have the patient remove nail polish, if necessary, and wash the hands. Hands should be rinsed well and dried to remove any dirt or lotions.

5. Apply the pulse oximeter probe (Figure 4-39) and observe the perfusion indicator. Observe both the heart rate and the SpO_2 levels.

6. Leave the oximeter probe attached to the patient and give the findings to the provider. If the saturation rate is below 90%, notify the provider as soon as possible.

7. Continue to monitor as long as the provider wants the patient monitored. (The patient may need to receive oxygen if oxygen is poor.)

8. Remove the probe once the provider orders the probe to be removed.

9. Record the results in the chart and assist the patient.

CHARTING EXAMPLE

| 02/14/XXXX 2:15 p.m. | Pulse oximetry per Dr. Simon. Patient washed hands prior to application. Hands completely dried. Applied unit to pt.'s right 3rd digit. Pulse rate: 98, SpO_2 96%. Informed provider of results. Ulisha Thompson, CMA (AAMA) |

Pain Assessment

Procedure 4-20

MEASURING PAIN USING PAIN ASSESSMENT SCALE

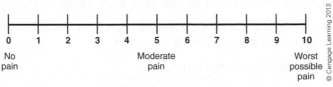

Figure 4-40: Numeric pain intensity scale to use with patients who can read and understand numbers.

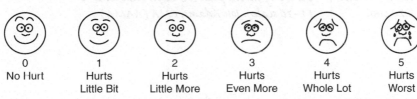

0	1	2	3	4	5
No Hurt	Hurts Little Bit	Hurts Little More	Hurts Even More	Hurts Whole Lot	Hurts Worst

Figure 4-41: Wong-Baker FACES Pain Rating Scale to use with children or patients with language barriers to rate their pain.

From Hockenberry MJ, Wilson D. Wong's essentials of pediatric nursing, ed. 8, St. Louis, 2009, Mosby. Used with permission. Copyright Mosby.

Equipment and Supplies

Patient record	Wong-Baker FACES or Pain Rating Scale	

1. Wash your hands.

2. Assemble supplies.

3. Identify the patient using two identifiers, identify yourself, and explain the procedure.

4. Ask patient for the exact location of the pain.

Measuring Pain Using a Number Scale

A1. Have the patient rate pain intensity on a scale of 1 to 10 (Figure 4-40), with one (1) being no pain, five (5) being moderate pain, and ten (10) the worst possible pain.

A2. Record the patient pain rating in chart.

(continues)

(continued)

Measuring Pain Using the Wong-Baker FACES (Used for children or patients with Limited English)

B1. Show the patient the six FACES pain rating scale (Figure 4-41).

B2. Explain what each face on the pain scale represents. Ask patient to point to the face that best describes his or her pain.

5. Record the patient pain rating in chart.

CHARTING EXAMPLE

| *03/19/XXXX* | *Pt. c/o of throat pain x 5 days. Pain level "6"* |
| *3:20 p.m.* | *(1–10 scale). Jon Adams, CMA (AAMA)* ———— |

Section 4-3

CARDIAC PROCEDURES

Procedure 4-21

PERFORM A STANDARD ELECTROCARDIOGRAM (ECG)

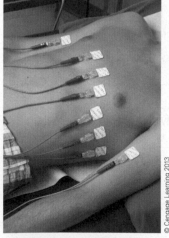

© Cengage Learning 2013

Figure 4-42: Chest electrode placement.

Lead	Description
V-1	(4th intercostal space, right margin of sternum)
V-2	(4th intercostal space, left margin of sternum)
V-3	Midway between Leads V2 and V4
V-4	(5th intercostal space, mid clavicle)
V-5	(Same horizontal level as V4, L. anterior axillary line)
V-6	(Same horizontal level as V4 and V5, midaxillary line)

Equipment and Supplies

Table with pillow and
    drape
Patient gown
Aniseptic wipes
	Tissues
	Razor
	ECG machine with
	    patient cable
		Disposable electrodes
		ECG tracing paper
		Mounting form
		    (if applicable)

1. Wash your hands.

2. Assemble the equipment.

3. Identify the patient using two identifiers, identify yourself, and explain the procedure.

4. Perform the ECG in a quiet, warm, and comfortable room away from other electrical equipment.

5. Explain to the patient why it is important not to move or talk during the tracing.

6. Instruct the patient to remove all clothing from the waist up and to expose the lower legs. Provide female patients with a gown that opens in the front. Provide all patients with a drape for warmth.

7. Prepare the patient's skin by scrubbing the areas where the electrodes are to be placed with skin antiseptic and allowing area to dry. (Dry shave areas on men that are particularly hairy.)

8. Place the electrodes on the fleshy part of the upper arm and the inner part of the calf midway between the knee and the ankle.

9. Place all six chest electrodes in the correct positions on the chest by counting down the intercostal spaces and locating the proper landmarks (Figure 4-42). *Do not trust your eyes alone.*

10. Securely connect all lead wires to the corresponding electrodes. Ensure that lead wires are pointed downward on the legs and upward on the arms and chest. The patient cable should rest on the table or the patient's abdomen.

11. Connect the patient cable to the machine and turn machine to the "ON" position. Enter the patient's data into the unit by using the keypad. Requested information may include the patient's name, age, gender, height, weight, and any cardiac medications currently being taken. (This step may be performed at beginning of procedure.)

12. Press the Auto Run button on the machine and allow the tracing to be recorded. Observe the standardization mark for accuracy.

(continues)

(continued)

---

13. Observe the tracing for problems or artifacts. Determine if any changes are needed with regard to the amplitude of the beats (gain or sensitivity control) or the heart's rhythm (paper speed). Normal sensitivity is 1 and normal paper speed is 25 mm/second.

---

14. Allow the provider to briefly scan the tracing before disconnecting the patient from the machine.

---

15. Disconnect the lead wires and remove the electrodes from the patient.

---

16. Clean the equipment following manufacturer's guidelines. Replace tracing paper as needed.

---

17. Wash your hands and document the procedure.

---

18. Place the tracing in the patient's chart.

CHARTING EXAMPLE

10/03/XXXX	12-lead EKG per Dr. Zeller. Pt. tol. well. Lillian Kelly,
10.30 a.m.	CMA (AAMA)

Procedure 4-22
APPLY A HOLTER MONITOR

Zymed EASI Lead Placement

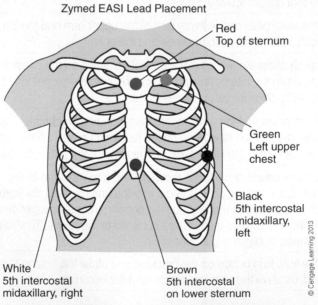

Red
Top of sternum

Green
Left upper
chest

Black
5th intercostal
midaxillary,
left

White
5th intercostal
midaxillary, right

Brown
5th intercostal
on lower sternum

© Cengage Learning 2013

Figure 4-43: Electrodes must be properly placed according to the manufacturer's directions to ensure an accurate tracing.

Equipment and Supplies

Antiseptic wipe	Electrodes	Carrying case
Razor (If applicable)	New battery	Patient activity diary
Holter monitor/cable	Recording Device or Tape	Gauze pads

1. Wash your hands.

2. Assemble the equipment and ensure it is in proper working order.

3. Identify the patient using two identifiers, identify yourself, and explain the procedure.

4. Place a recording device and a new battery in the monitor.

5. Accurately complete the information in the patient activity diary and instruct the patient to disrobe from the waist up. Provide gown and drape for patient.

6. Prepare the patient's skin: Dry shave hair, if necessary, and rub the area of skin where electrodes will be placed with an alcohol swab. Next, abrade the skin with dry gauze or pre-packaged pads.

7. Peel the backing from the electrode and check to make certain the electrolyte is moist. Correctly place disposable electrodes on the proper landmarks of the chest according to manufacturer's directions (Figure 4-43).

8. Be sure the electrodes adhere firmly to the skin by applying gentle pressure with your fingers, starting at the center of the electrode and working toward the outer edges.

9. Connect lead wires to the electrodes. Reinforce the electrodes to the skin with a piece of non-allergenic tape if necessary.

10. Instruct the patient to dress and plug the electrode cable into the monitor. Check the recorder by running a baseline test strip. Place the unit on the patient.

11. Note the start time. Explain the importance of the activity diary to the patient and how to accurately complete all information.

12. Specify the exact time the patient should return to the office for removal of the monitor.

13. Wash your hands and document the procedure in the patient's chart.

CHARTING EXAMPLE

| 09/03/XXXX 9:30 a.m. | *Holter monitor application per Dr. Beavers. Test strip satisfactory. Instructed patient on proper management of unit and items to enter in activity diary. Pt. instructed to return at 9:30 a.m. on 09/04/XXXX for monitor removal. Lillian Kelly, CMA (AAMA)* ———— |

Section 4-4

EYE AND EAR PROCEDURES

Eye Procedures

Procedure 4-23

SCREENING DISTANCE VISUAL ACUITY

Equipment and Supplies

| Patient chart | Snellen eye chart | Occluder Alcohol wipes |

1. Wash your hands.

2. Assemble the equipment.

3. Identify the patient using two identifiers, identify yourself, and explain the procedure.

4. Clean the occluder with an alcohol wipe and allow it to dry.

5. If the patient wears contact lenses, testing should be conducted with contacts. If the patient wears glasses, testing may be conducted both with and without glasses.

6. In a well-lit area, instruct the patient to stand at the mark placed 20 feet from the eye chart. Ask the patient to cover the left eye with the occluder but to keep the eye open. Ask the patient to read the chart aloud beginning with the 20/200 line or with one of the several lines above the 20/20 line.

7. Stand next to the chart and point to each line during testing.

8. Record the results as the last line the patient can read without errors. Acuity is recorded as a fraction: R. eye 20/10, L. eye 20/30, both eyes 20/20.

9. The patient should be observed during the screening for signs of difficulty such as squinting, watering of the eyes, or repositioning of the head.

10. After screening the right eye, repeat the procedure for the left eye and then with both eyes.

11. Point to the red line and ask the patient to repeat the color; do the same with the green line.

12. Clean the occluder with alcohol, wash your hands, and document results in the patient's chart.

CHARTING EXAMPLE

08/12/XXXX 1:10 p.m.	Snellen visual screening per Dr. Kelly. R. eye 20/10, L. eye 20/30, both eyes 20/20. Patient was observed squinting during testing of both eyes. Color vision normal. Lillian Kelly, CMA (AAMA)

Field Tip

It's always good to record the date of the patient's last eye examination and who it was with for patients who wear corrective lenses.

Procedure 4-24
SCREENING NEAR VISUAL ACUITY

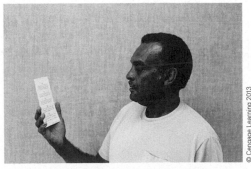

© Cengage Learning 2013

Figure 4-44: The patient's near visual acuity is assessed using the Jaeger chart.

(continues)

(continued)

Equipment and Supplies

Occluder	Alcohol wipes	Jaeger near visual acuity chart

1. Wash your hands.

2. Assemble the equipment.

3. Identify the patient using two identifiers, identify yourself, and explain the procedure.

4. Clean the occluder with an alcohol wipe.

5. With the patient in a sitting position, instruct the patient to hold the card approximately 14 inches from the eyes (Figure 4-44).

6. Instruct the patient to cover the left eye with the occluder and read the chart (out loud) with the right eye.

7. Record the results as the last line the patient can read without errors.

8. Repeat the procedure for the left eye and both eyes together. The patient should be tested with and without corrective lenses, if worn. (Do not have the patient remove contacts.)

9. Wipe the occluder with an alcohol wipe.

10. Wash your hands and document results in the patient's chart.

CHARTING EXAMPLE

11/08/XXXX 12:30 p.m.	Jaeger near visual acuity screening per Dr. Price. R. eye, No. 10 (2.25M), L. eye, No. 7 (1.5M), both eyes, No. 6 (1.25M) with corr. Lillian Kelly, CMA (AAMA) ———

Procedure 4-25

ISHIHARA TESTING FOR COLOR VISION

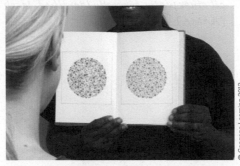

Figure 4-45: The patient's color vision acuity is tested using Ishihara plates.

Equipment and Supplies

Ishihara plates	2 Pairs of gloves for both the patient and you (optional)	

1. Wash your hands. (Gloves may be worn to keep the book from getting dirty.)

2. Assemble the equipment.

3. Identify the patient using two identifiers, identify yourself, and explain the procedure.

4. Conduct the test in a room illuminated by daylight or good overhead lighting.

5. Starting with the practice plate as an example, hold the plate 30 inches from the patient and at a right angle to the patient's field of vision. Instruct the patient to identify the number formed by the colored dots (Figure 4-45). Patient should only have 3 seconds to read each line.

6. Repeat the procedure with all plates. **Note:** Some lines will have a winding line that the patient will need to trace rather than a number to read. Record the results after each plate. (Patient should also wash their hands and apply gloves if he or she will be touching the pages of the book.)

7. Protect the plates from light when not in use.

8. Wash your hands and document results in the patient's chart.

01/11/XXXX 11:30 a.m.	*Ishihara color vision screening per Dr. Bell. Plate 4:X, all other plates correctly identified. Jacob Heller, CMA (AAMA)*

Procedure 4-26
EYE INSTILLATION

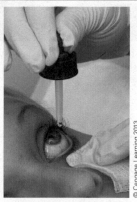

Figure 4-46: The patient looks up as the medical assistant instills eyedrops.

Equipment and Supplies

Disposable gloves	Gauze Tissues	Disposable eye dropper ophthalmic medication

1. Wash your hands.

2. Assemble the equipment.

3. Identify the patient using two identifiers, identify yourself, and explain the procedure.

4. Check medication against the provider's orders and look for the word *ophthalmic* on the label. Check the expiration date and check the label three times before administration.

5. If the medication has been refrigerated, it must come to room temperature before instilling.

6. Wash hands and apply gloves.

7. Place the patient in a sitting or lying position and prepare the medication. For eye drops, withdraw the medication into a sterile dropper (If applicable). For eye ointment, remove the cap from the tube.

8. Instruct the patient to look up at the ceiling. With your fingers over a gauze pad, gently pull down on skin to expose the lower conjunctival sac (Figure 4-46).

9. Instill the correct number of drops into the center of the eye or place a thin line of ointment along the lower surface of the conjunctiva. *Do not touch the tip of the medication applicator to the eye.*

10. Instruct the patient to close the eye and roll the eyeball around.

11. Dab excess solution from the eyelid with gauze or tissue.

12. *If applicable, do not return any unused medication to the bottle.* Discard the unused medication, and return the dropper to the bottle without touching the dropper to the outside of the bottle.

13. Discard used equipment and supplies.

14. Remove gloves and wash your hands.

15. Record the procedure in the patient's chart.

CHARTING EXAMPLE

12/14/XXXX 12:15 p.m.	*Visine, 2 gtt, R. eye per Dr. Gamble. Pt. tolerated procedure well. Pt. to RTO in 10 days. Anne Zeller, CMA (AAMA)*

Procedure 4-27
EYE IRRIGATION USING A WATER PICK

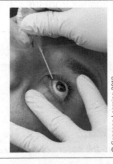

© Cengage Learning 2013

Figure 4-47: The medical assistant performs an eye irrigation using a water pick.

(continues)

(continued)

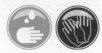

Equipment and Supplies

Disposable gloves	Water pick	Disposable towel
Sterile irrigation solution	Basin	Sterile gauze
		Towel

1. Wash your hands.

2. Assemble the equipment.

3. Identify the patient using two identifiers, identify yourself, and explain the procedure.

4. **Note:** If both eyes are to be irrigated, separate supplies will be needed for each eye.

5. Place the patient in a sitting or supine position with the head turned toward the affected eye.

6. Place a towel on the patient's shoulder and place a basin beside or below the affected eye. Wash your hands again and apply gloves.

7. Cleanse the eyelid from the inner to outer canthus with moistened gauze. Discard the gauze after each cleansing.

8. Prepare a water pick with irrigating solution and hold the eye open with the index finger and thumb.

9. Rest the bulb of the water pick on the bridge of the patient's nose. Be careful not to touch the eye or conjunctiva with the tip of the water pick.

10. Instruct the patient to stare at a fixed spot and open the water pick valve, allowing the solution to flow along the lower conjunctiva from the inner to outer canthus and into the basin (Figure 4-47).

11. After irrigation is complete, dry the eyelid and eyelashes from the inner to outer canthus with gauze.

12. Discard supplies in an appropriate container.

13. Remove gloves, wash your hands, and document the procedure in the patient's chart.

CHARTING EXAMPLE

5/22/XXXX 2:30 p.m.	Eye irrigation. 600 mL normal sterile saline, L. eye per Dr. Black. Return solution clear. Pt. tolerated procedure well. Jane Barnes, CMA (AAMA)

Ear Procedures

Procedure 4-28
EAR INSTILLATION

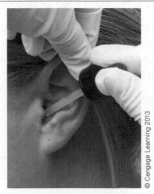

Figure 4-48: Eardrops are instilled into the ear canal.

Equipment and Supplies

Disposable gloves	Otic solution or medication	Sterile ear dropper (If applicable) Cotton balls

1. Wash your hands.

2. Assemble the equipment.

3. Identify the patient using two identifiers, identify yourself, and explain the procedure.

4. Check the medication against the provider's orders and check the medication three times. Check the expiration date of the medication and verify that the medication is for otic use.

5. Instruct the patient to lie on the unaffected side or sit with head slightly tilted toward the unaffected side. Place a towel on the patient's shoulder.

6. Apply gloves and withdraw the medication into a sterile dropper.

7. Grasp the top of the ear and pull up and back for adults, or grasp the earlobe and pull down and back for children under the age of 3 years (Figure 4-48).

(continues)

(continued)

8. Instill the prescribed amount of medication into the ear canal by depressing the rubber bulb of the dropper. *Do not touch the tip of the dropper to the ear.*

9. Instruct the patient to keep the head tilted for approximately 5 minutes.

10. Insert a slightly moistened cotton ball into the ear canal per the provider's orders and instruct the patient to leave it in place for 15 minutes. (This keeps the solution in the ear and prevents the cotton from soaking up the medication you just instilled.)

11. Dispose of used equipment and supplies.

12. Remove gloves and wash your hands.

13. Document the procedure in the patient's chart.

CHARTING EXAMPLE

12/20/XXXX 10:15 a.m.	Auralgan, 3 gtt, both ears per Dr. Leonard. Pt. given home instructions. Andy Price, RMA ——————————

Procedure 4-29
EAR IRRIGATION USING ELEPHANT EAR WASH

Equipment and Supplies

Disposable gloves
Elephant ear wash
	Ear or emesis basin
	Irrigating solution
	  warmed to body
	  temperature
		Waterproof drape
		Towels
		Cotton balls
		Otoscope

1. Wash your hands and apply gloves.

2. Assemble the equipment.

3. Identify the patient using two identifiers, identify yourself, and explain the procedure.

4. Check the expiration date of the irrigating solution and check the label three times.

5. If ordered to so by provider, check the patient's ear with an otoscope so that you can identify where the wax is located and the amount of wax present.

6. Inform the patient there may be minimal discomfort and some dizziness resulting from the flow of solution against the tympanic membrane.

7. Place the patient in a sitting position with the head tilted to the affected side.

8. Place a towel on the patient's shoulder and instruct the patient to hold an ear basin under the affected ear and against the neck.

9. Fill (Elephant Earwash) sprayer bottle with irrigating solution (approximately 30 to 50 mL) warmed to approximately 99° F to 100° F (37° C to 38° C).

10. Cleanse the outer ear with a cotton ball moistened with irrigating solution and discard.

11. Gently tug the tip of the auricle up and back.

12. Insert the tip of the sprayer tubing into the ear canal. Slowly, spray irrigating solution so it flows up toward the roof of the ear canal.

13. Continue the process following the doctor's order or until the desired effects are obtained.

14. Dry the outer ear and check the inner ear with an otoscope to determine removal of foreign matter or have the provider check if it is the policy of the office.

15. Remove the towel and ear basin and have the patient lie on the affected side on the examination table for approximately 5 minutes. (A chuck or waterproof drape should be placed under head and ear for proper drainage.)

16. Have the patient sit up and make certain he or she is steady. (Dismiss according to doctor's orders.)

17. Dispose of used equipment and supplies.

18. Remove gloves and wash your hands.

19. Document the procedure in the patient's chart.

CHARTING EXAMPLE

02/24/XXXX 11:00 a.m.	Irrigated both ears with normal saline. Solution warmed to 99° F per Dr. Peters. Pt. tol. proc. well. No dizziness or nausea following irrigation. Return basin for L. ear had 2 large pieces of cerumen and one small piece. Return basin for R. ear had 1 large piece of cerumen and 2 smaller pieces. Post exam of ears with otoscope appeared clear per Dr. Peters. Miriam Pentella, CMA (AAMA)

Section 4-5

MINOR SURGICAL PROCEDURES, TRAY SETUPS, AND WOUND CARE

Minor Surgical Procedures

Procedure 4-30
APPLY SKIN CLOSURES

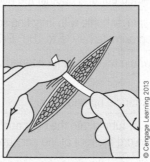

Figure 4-49: Apply the first skin closure strip in the center of the wound.

Equipment and Supplies

Hand sanitizer 2 Sterile 4×4s 1 Pack of skin antiseptic swabs 1 Pack of adhesive strips or closures (sized to match the patient's wound)	1 Bottle tincture of benzoin Sterile cotton-tipped applicators Sterile gloves	Bandage material (If necessary) Home care instructions Disinfectant Patient chart

1. Wash your hands and gather the supplies.

2. Identify the patient using two identifiers, identify yourself, and explain the procedure.

3. Make certain that the patient is not allergic to adhesive.

4. Inspect the wound and select the size of adhesive strips that best matches the patient's wound.

5. Position the patient so he is comfortable, and position the tray for easy access.

6. Clean the tray and set up the necessary items: Open all items in a sterile fashion so that they are completely open for easy access.

7. Wash your hands and apply sterile gloves.

8. Clean the patient's skin so that the cleansing extends at least 2 to 3 inches (5 to 7 cm) around the wound using sterile antiseptic swabs.

9. Allow the area to completely dry.

10. Apply a thin coat of tincture of benzoin to the periphery of the wound using a new sterile cotton-tipped applicator for each side. Do not allow the tincture of benzoin to touch the wound.

11. Follow the manufacturer's instructions for removing the strips.

12. If applying single strips, line the first strip up with the center of the wound (Figure 4-49). Firmly press one end of the strip on either side of the wound to secure it in place.

13. Gently stretch the strip while lining up both edges of the wound so that they come together. (You may need to use the other hand to help oppose the wound edges.)

14. Once the skin is lined up evenly on both sides, pull the tape to the opposite side while pressing down firmly on the skin.

15. Apply the next strip approximately ⅛ inch from the first strip on either side of the first strip.

16. Perform the same step on the opposite side of the wound.

17. Continue this process until the wound is completely closed.

18. If needed, apply one closure approximately ½ inch away from the strip's edges, running parallel to the wound on either side of the strips.

19. Make certain that there is good approximation of the wound.

20. Apply dressing, if necessary.

21. Remove gloves and wash your hands.

22. Give the patient home care instructions.

23. Document the procedure in the chart.

CHARTING EXAMPLE

10/12/XXXX 2:30 p.m.	*Steri-Strip application x 6 to pt's R. forearm per Dr. Kennedy. Cleaned surrounding area with iodine swabs. Applied tincture of benzoin and applied the strips. Good approximation of wound. Closed spiral dressing applied. Gave pt home care instructions to return in 5 days. Pt instructed to call if there are any concerns or complications. Chloe Brady CMA (AAMA)*

Procedure 4-31

SUTURE OR STAPLE REMOVAL

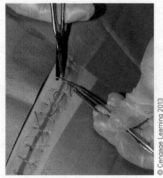

Figure 4-50: Pull up on one side of the knot and cut the suture as close to the skin as possible.

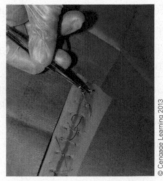

Figure 4-51: Remove the sutures by pulling toward the incision.

Equipment and Supplies

Hand sanitizer Suture removal kit or Staple removal kit Bandage scissors (if applicable) 4×4s	Skin antiseptic 2 Pairs of examination gloves Dressing supplies (if necessary)	Patient chart Disinfectant

1. Wash your hands and gather the supplies.

2. Identify the patient using two identifiers, identify yourself, and explain the procedure.

3. Ask if the patient took all of the antibiotic and whether all other home care instructions were followed, document your findings.

4. Examine the outside of the patient's bandage and make a mental note.

5. Wash hands again and apply clean examination gloves.

6. Remove the dressing and observe both the inside of the dressing and the wound area for any signs of infection. (If dressing is adhered to the wound, you may need to saturate the dressing with sterile saline to loosen it a bit before removal.)

7. Discard the dressing into the biohazard container, remove gloves, and wash your hands.

8. Have the provider observe the wound before starting the procedure.

9. Wash hands and apply gloves.

10. If the sutures are adhered to the skin by dried blood and other secretions, irrigate the wound according to the provider's instructions. Otherwise, cleanse area with a skin antiseptic.

11. If removing sutures, grasp one side of the first knot with the thumb forceps and gently tug upward on the end of the knot. Using the other hand, work the suture scissors under the knot as close to the skin as possible and cut the suture (Figure 4-50). Pull the knot toward the wound, making certain that no part of the suture that was on the outside goes through the inside of the wound (Figure 4-51). If removing staples, gently grasp the staple with the remover and squeeze the handle of the staple remover until the staple is pinched up and out.

12. Continue to remove the sutures or staples until all have been removed.

13. Make sure that the wound still has good approximation and that there is no gapping of the skin (notify the provider if there are any concerns).

14. Dress the wound according to the provider's instructions.

15. Remove gloves and wash your hands.

16. Give the patient any home care instructions and dismiss.

17. Clean the area with disinfectant and dispose of related items in the biohazard trash receptacle.

18. Document the procedure.

CHARTING EXAMPLE

12/12/XXXX 6:30 p.m.	Pt. here to have sutures removed from L. foot. Re- moved bandage and inspected wound. No exudates on bandage or coming from the wound, ⊖ erythema, ⊖ edema. Dr. Miller inspected wound and gave order to remove sutures. Removed all sutures (6 total). Good closure of wound following removal. Dressed site with adhesive bandage. Instructed pt. to remove bandage tomorrow and to call with any concerns. Scheduled pt. for a F/U appt. on 12/18/XXXX. Destiny Green, CMA (AAMA)

Procedure 4-32
PERFORM SURGICAL HANDWASH AND APPLY STERILE GLOVES

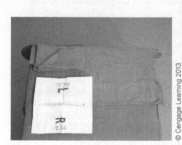 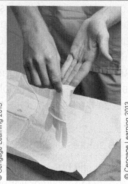 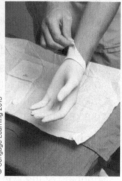

© Cengage Learning 2013

Figure 4-52: The sterile towel and gloves should be laid out prior to scrub itself.

Figure 4-53: Pick up first glove using your thumb, index finger, and middle finger by grasping the edge of the inside cuff with your nondominant hand.

Figure 4-54: Slide the glove onto your dominant hand by pulling the cuff in an upward motion.

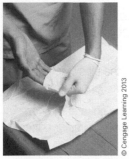

Figure 4-55: Pick up the second glove with your dominant hand by slipping the four fingers from the gloved hand underneath the cuff of the second glove.

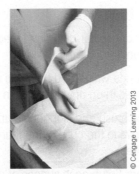

Figure 4-56: Lift up your hand to avoid dangling and with fingers still positioned on the inside of the cuff, roll back the cuff on the nondominant hand over the wrist. Do not allow the gloved thumb from the opposite hand to touch the inside of the cuff.

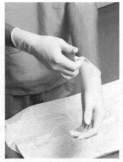

Figure 4-57: Repeat the same procedure for rolling back the cuff for the glove on the dominant hand.

Equipment and Supplies

Sterile brush impregnated with antiseptic soap/ fingernail cleaner	Sink/basin Sterile towel Sterile Drape	Package of sterile gloves

1. Peel apart the packet with the sterile towel without contaminating it and transfer towel to a sterile tray close to the area where the handwash is to take place.

2. Place gloves beside the sterile towel and remove them from the outer wrapper (Figure 4-52). Unfold the pack so that it lies flat. Carefully open each flap of the inner wrapper to expose the gloves without contaminating them or the sterile towel. The gloves should be positioned so that the cuffs are facing you, and the thumbs are pointing outward.

3. Open the sterile scrub pack containing the impregnated scrub brush and nail cleaner. Do not remove them yet. Place them in the sink area.

4. Remove all rings and watches and place them in your pockets. Turn on the water using the automatic sensor or foot or knee control and adjust the temperature (should be warm, not hot).

5. Rinse your hands under the water, keeping the hands and fingers pointed upward and the arms well above the waist.

(continues)

(continued)

---

6. Using just the nail stick and water, clean under each nail. Drop the nail stick in the sink and rinse hands.

---

7. Completely wet your hands, wrists, and forearms up to the elbow, keeping hands and fingers pointed in an upward position and well above the waist.

---

8. Obtain the impregnated brush and start the scrub on the palm of the non-dominant hand and move to the base of the thumb using a circular pattern. (Approximately 10 strokes)

---

9. Next, move to the fingers. Scrub each surface of each finger using several vertical strokes from the base of each finger to the tip (there are a total of four surfaces for each finger). Be certain to scrub the skin between the thumb and index finger as well. (Approximately 10 strokes per surface)

---

10. Once the fingers are completely scrubbed, turn the hand over and scrub the posterior portion of the hand extending to below the wrists using a circular pattern. (Approximately 10 strokes per surface)

---

11. Next, scrub the forearm using a circular pattern from the wrists to slightly above the elbow. Make certain to scrub all four surfaces. (Some professionals divide the forearm into thirds when scrubbing each surface.) (Approximately 10 strokes per surface)

---

12. Wash the dominant hand and arm using the same steps as the first arm. Drop the scrub brush in the sink and rinse thoroughly. The entire length of the scrub should be a minimum of 3 minutes.

---

13. Rinse each arm from the fingertips to above the elbows. (Keep fingers and hands facing upward and avoid touching or leaning into the sink.)

---

14. Turn off the water using the foot, knee, or sensor control when applicable.

---

15. Pick up the towel in your dominant hand by holding onto the corners. The towel should be several inches away from your body. Using just one side of the towel, start at the fingertips on your nondominant hand and pat dry all the way up to the elbow, making sure that you dry all four surfaces simultaneously. Remember to keep the arms and hands above the waist with fingers pointed upward.

---

16. Repeat the same procedure on your dominant hand using the opposite side of the sterile towel.

---

17. Once the hands are completely dried, walk to the sterile tray where the gloves are lying.

---

18. Pick up the first glove by the inside cuff using your non-dominant hand (Figure 4-53). Lift the glove up and away from the flat surface to avoid dangling the glove across a nonsterile surface. Slide the glove in an upward motion, over the hand (Figure 4-54).

---

19. Pick up the second glove with your dominant hand by slipping the four fingers from the gloved hand underneath the cuff of the second glove (Figure 4-55). Make certain that the thumb is facing outward. Slide the glove onto the hand without contaminating either glove.

20. Leaving your gloved fingers under the cuff, unfold the cuff so that it slides down over the wrist (Figure 4-56). Do not allow the gloved thumb from the opposite hand to touch the inside of the cuff. Repeat the same procedure for the first glove (Figure 4-57).

21. Examine both gloves for any tears or problems.

Procedure 4-33

PREPARE PATIENT'S SKIN FOR SURGERY USING ONE-STEP PROCEDURE

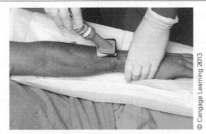

Figure 4-58: Apply the antiseptic scrub using either vertical strokes for narrow surfaces or concentric circles for wide surfaces.

Equipment and Supplies

Skin preparation kit Sterile gloves	Sterile drape	Fenestrated drape

1. Wash your hands and gather the supplies.

2. Identify the patient using two identifiers, identify yourself, and explain the procedure.

3. Verify that the patient followed the site-cleansing home instructions.

4. Expose the surgical site and drape the patient for modesty if necessary. Some facilities ask the patient to mark the area where the surgery is to take place with the patient's initials before preparing the skin.

(continues)

(continued)

5. Position the patient for comfort and place sterile drape under the area to be cleansed.

6. Adjust the light so that it illuminates the surgical site. Inspect the skin for any gross contamination. If any gross contamination is visible, the skin will have to be thoroughly cleansed before applying the antiseptic cleanser. (If the provider orders the area to be shaved, pull skin taut and shave in the direction that the hair grows. Shaving is usually not recommended unless absolutely necessary because of the danger of cuts.)

7. Open the skin preparation kit without contaminating the swab or the sponge applicator.

8. Wash your hands and apply sterile gloves.

9. Remove the swab or sponge, touching only the applicator or handle.

10. Apply the antiseptic scrub using vertical strokes (Figure 4-58) for narrow surfaces and concentric circles over wider areas.

11. Follow the manufacturer's instructions for length of scrub.

12. Apply fenestrated drapes and other surgical drapes according to the provider's preference.

13. Instruct the patient to keep hands below the drapes (when applicable).

Procedure 4-34

SET UP A COMPLETE STERILE TRAY

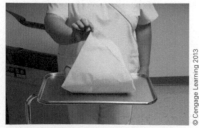

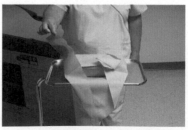

Figure 4-59: Using only your thumb and index finger to grasp the tip of the folded flap that was covered with tape and pull it away from you.

Figure 4-60: Using only right thumb and index finger, grasp the top of the folded-back flap on the right side and pull it all the way to the right.

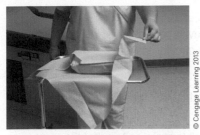

Figure 4-61: Using only the left thumb and index finger, grasp the tip of the folded-back flap on the left side and pull it all the way to the left.

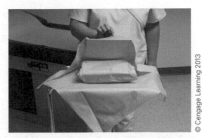

Figure 4-62: Using only the dominant thumb and index finger, grasp the tip of the last folded-back flap and pull it toward you without touching anything on the inside of the wrap.

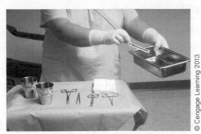

Figure 4-63: Once the field has been totally arranged, remove the sterilization indicator from the inside of the tray and make certain that it is the proper color.

Equipment and Supplies

Antibacterial hand sanitizer One wrapped tray of instruments with basins to pour the sterile solutions into	Mayo stand Small bottle of sterile saline Small bottle of sterile povidone-iodine 4×4s saturated with disinfecting solution	Package of sterile gloves or sterile transfer forceps

1. Perform an aseptic handwash.

2. Gather the supplies and place them on the side table.

3. Properly position the Mayo stand so that it is at your waist level.

(continues)

(continued)

---

4. Clean the Mayo stand with 4×4s that have been saturated with a disinfectant (but are not dripping), cleaning in a circular motion.

---

5. Allow the stand to dry.

---

6. Check the instrument pack and make certain that the integrity of the pack has not been compromised.

---

7. Check the tape on the outside of the pack to make certain that the stripes turned the correct color and that the pack has not reached its expiration date.

---

8. Pull the tape off of the pack and place it on the side table.

---

9. Place the sterile pack on the center of the Mayo stand so that the flap that was taped is facing you.

---

10. Using only your thumb and index finger, grasp the tip of the folded flap that was covered with tape and pull it away from you (Figure 4-59).

---

11. Using only your right thumb and index finger, grasp the tip of the folded-back flap on the right side and pull it all the way to the right (Figure 4-60).

---

12. Using only your left thumb and index finger, grasp the tip of the folded-back flap on the left side and pull it all the way to the left (Figure 4-61).

---

13. Using only your dominant thumb and index finger, grasp the tip of the last folded-back flap and pull it toward you without touching anything on the inside of the wrap (Figure 4-62).

---

14. Repeat steps 10 through 13 for the second layer of wrap. (The inner wrap will become your sterile drape.)

---

15. Move to the side table without turning your back on the field.

---

16. Open the pack of sterile gloves and remove them from the wrapper.

---

17. Open the inner wrapper without contaminating the gloves.

---

18. Wash your hands with alcohol-based hand sanitizer following the directions on the bottle.

---

19. Apply surgical gloves—remember to hold your hands above the waist.

---

20. Approach the field facing forward and stand a few inches away from the field. Remove the items from the inside of the tray and place them on the sterile field in a logical sequence. Place the basins for the sterile solution on the stand facing upward.

21. Once the field has been totally arranged, remove the sterilization indicator from the inside of the tray and make certain that it is the proper color (Figure 4-63).

22. Place the tray that held the instruments onto the side table. (Do not turn your body away from the sterile tray as you place the instrument tray on the side table.)

23. Remove gloves and wash your hands with hand sanitizer.

24. Pick up the brand new bottle of iodine and read the label. Make certain that you have the correct solution. Check the label to make certain that the solution has not passed its expiration date.

25. Now palm the label.

26. Remove the cap and place it to the side so that the lid is facing upward. Remove the protective seal and place it on the side table.

27. Move to the tray and approach the corner on which the basins are sitting.

28. Pour the iodine into the container labeled as iodine, pouring 2 to 6 inches above the field. Be careful not to allow the solution to splash. Fill to the desired level.

29. Repeat steps 24 through 28 with a new bottle of sterile saline, pouring into the container labeled as saline.

30. If the solutions are not used in their entirety, replace the caps and follow the institution's policy for storing the solutions. Keep in mind that these solutions should not be used for any future surgical procedures.

Procedure 4-35

SETTING UP A STERILE TRAY—APPLYING SINGLE INSTRUMENTS TO THE TRAY

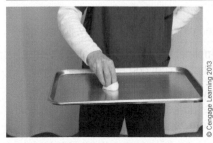

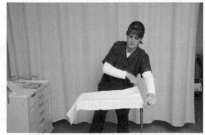

Figure 4-64: Sanitize and disinfect the Mayo tray.

Figure 4-65: Grasp the opposite corner of the unfolded drape and place the drape over the Mayo tray, without reaching over the drape.

(continues)

(continued)

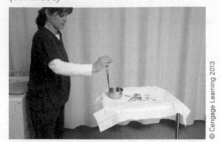

Figure 4-66: Transfer forceps (or sterile gloves) may be used to arrange the instruments on the tray in the proper order.

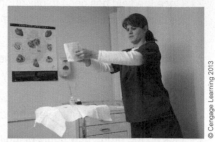

Figure 4-67: Turn the pack so that the instrument will fall easily onto the sterile field when released. Drop the instrument onto the sterile field.

Equipment and Supplies

Mayo stand
Antibacterial hand
  sanitizer
	4×4s saturated with
	  disinfecting solution
		Sterile drape
		Appropriate instruments
		  or supplies that are
		  wrapped in sterile
		  material

1. Wash your hands and gather the supplies.

2. Adjust the Mayo stand so that it is right about waist level.

3. Pick up the 4×4s saturated with disinfectant (but not dripping) by touching only the top side of the 4×4s. Clean the tray using the bottom side of the 4×4s using a circular motion until the whole tray is completely covered (Figure 4-64).

4. Allow the tray to air dry.

5. Select an appropriate sterile barrier and place it on a clean, dry, flat surface.

6. Peel back the top flap of the pack, completely exposing the drape. Make certain that the pack is positioned so that the cut corners are facing you.

7. Using your thumb and forefinger, gently pull up one of the top corner edges of the drape without touching any other part of the drape. Lift the drape well above the counter surface and away from you.

8. Grab the opposing corner so that both corners are now being held along the top edge of the drape. Keep the drape well above your waist and several inches away from your body.

9. Pull the drape over the Mayo stand so that the part of the drape that was facing you is lying against the surface of the tray and the part that was facing away from you is now facing upward on the tray (Figure 4-65).

Opening a Sterile Pack and Transferring Items to the Sterile Field
Using Sterile Transfer Forceps

10. Place a sterilized pack of transfer forceps on the side table.

11. Place the unopened sterilized instrument on the side table, examine the autoclave tape, and make certain that the stripes turned the appropriate color. Check the expiration date and the quality of the wrapper to make certain that the wrap has not been compromised.

12. Remove the tape from the packet and place it on the side table. Position the pack so that the flap that was taped is facing you.

13. Using only your thumb and index finger, grasp the tip of the folded flap that was covered with tape and pull it away from you.

14. Using only your right thumb and index finger, grasp the tip of the folded-back flap on the right side and pull it all the way to the right.

15. Using only your left thumb and index finger, grasp the tip of the folded-back flap on the left side and pull it all the way to the left.

16. Using only your dominant thumb and index finger, grasp the tip of the last folded-back flap and pull it toward you without touching anything on the inside of the wrap. The entire instrument should be exposed for easy retrieval later. Check the sterilization indicator in the pack to make certain it turned the appropriate color; if not, remove the pack and get a new one.

17. Move to the packet containing the sterile transfer forceps. Open the sterile transfer forceps the same way you opened the first pack.

18. Once the pack is opened, grasp only the handles of the sterile transfer forceps by placing your thumb in one ring and your index finger in the other ring. Do not touch any other part of the instrument. Lift the transfer forceps straight up, keeping the tips facing downward but well above the height of the side table.

19. Move the transfer forceps to the instrument that needs to be transferred to the sterile field. Once you are positioned in front of the sterile instrument, lower the transfer forceps to the sterile instrument and securely grasp the instrument. Lift the instrument well above the height of the side table and approach the sterile tray. Standing a few inches away from the field, gently lower the sterile instrument onto the tray (Figure 4-66). Do not allow your hand to drop below the level of the handle.

(continues)

(continued)

---

20. Once the instrument has been fully transferred to its appropriate place on the tray, pull the sterile transfer forceps up and away from the field and set them back down on the side table.

Opening a Peel-Apart Pack

---

21. Inspect the package and make certain that the integrity of the wrap has not been altered. Check the control strip to make certain that it turned the correct color. Check the expiration date to make certain that the pack is not expired.

---

22. Position yourself so that you are in front of the tray but several inches away from the field.

---

23. Grasp both the top edges of the peel-apart pack and carefully peel them apart by rolling the wrap downward on both sides.

---

24. Once the wrap has been peeled to the point that the item can be transferred to the field, turn your hands outward and push the pack forward so that the item is just slightly over the field (Figure 4-67). The hands should be well above the field. Gently drop the item onto the field.

Tray Setups

Table 4-6
ITEMS FOR A LACERATION REPAIR

Items Placed Directly on the Sterile Field	Items Placed on a Side Table
Sterile drapes	Sterile gloves
Needle holder	Bandage scissors
Appropriate suture material	Bandage material (gauze, tape, rolled gauze)
Surgical scissors	Antiseptic solution
Tissue forceps	Sterile water or saline
Sterile gauze pads	Appropriate anesthetic
Needle/syringe	Appropriate PPE
Two sterile cups or basins	Triple antibiotic cream/ointment
	Cotton-tipped applicators
	Biohazard and sharps container

Table 4-7

ITEMS FOR A SEBACEOUS CYST REMOVAL

Items Placed Directly on the Sterile Field	Items Placed on a Side Table
Sterile drapes	Appropriate PPE
Syringe and needle	Sterile gloves
Scalpel blade and handle	Anesthetic/alcohol wipe
Needle holder	Packing gauze (optional)
Appropriate suture material	Specimen container/lab form
Iris scissors	Sterile bandaging material
Hemostatic forceps	Antiseptic solution
Sterile gauze	Sterile water or saline
Hemostats (optional)	Biohazard and sharps containers
Suture material	
Two sterile cups or basins	

Table 4-8

ITEMS FOR A JOINT ASPIRATION TRAY

Items Placed Directly on the Sterile Field	Items Placed on a Side Table
Sterile drapes	Appropriate PPE
Syringe and needle	Sterile gloves
Aspiration needle	Anesthetic
Hemostat	Specimen container/culture transfer tube
Sterile gauze	Sterile bandaging material
Two sterile cups or basins	Antiseptic solution
	Sterile saline or water
	Biohazard and sharps containers

Table 4-9

ITEMS FOR AN INCISION AND DRAINAGE PROCEDURE

Items Placed Directly on the Sterile Field	Items Placed on a Side Table
Syringe and needle	Appropriate PPE
Scalpel blade and handle	Sterile gloves
Tissue forceps	Appropriate anesthetic
Sterile drapes	Packing gauze (iodoform or plain)
Dissecting scissors/hemostat	Sterile bandaging material
Sterile gauze	Penrose drain (up to the provider)
Two sterile cups or basins	Antiseptic solution
	Sterile saline or water
	Culture medium
	Biohazard and sharps containers

Table 4-10

ITEMS FOR SUTURE OR STAPLE REMOVAL TRAY

Items Placed Directly on the Sterile Field	Items Placed on a Side Table
Sterile suture removal scissors	PPE
Sterile dressing forceps	Sterile saline/skin antiseptic
Sterile bowl	Bandaging supplies
Sterile gauze pads	Triple antibiotic cream or ointment (if ordered)
	Biohazard container

Table 4-11
ITEMS FOR ELECTROSURGICAL TRAY

Items Placed Directly on the Sterile Field	Items Placed on a Side Table
Needle and syringe	PPE
Sterile gauze pads	Antiseptic solution/sterile saline
Cautery needles	Electrosurgical unit
Bovie pads	Disposable tips
Two sterile cups or basins	Specimen container
	Sterile gloves
	Triple antibiotic cream/ointment
	Gauze/tape
	Biohazard and sharps containers

Table 4-12
ITEMS FOR LASER SURGERY TRAY

Items Placed Directly on the Sterile Field	Items Placed on a Side Table
Sterile 4×4s	PPE
Sterile water (in sterile container)	Anesthetic
	Sterile syringe and needle
	Safety goggles for everyone involved in the procedure
	Laser instrument/tips
	Biohazard waste container

Wound Care

Procedure 4-36

REMOVE OLD DRESSING, IRRIGATE WOUND, AND APPLY NEW DRESSING

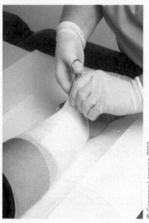

© Cengage Learning 2013

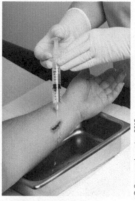

© Cengage Learning 2013

Figure 4-68: Cut the bandage with a pair of bandage scissors along the side of the wound. Carefully remove the bandage and dressing by pulling the corners of the bandage toward the wound.

Figure 4-69: Draw up irrigating fluid from the basin with the sterile syringe and irrigate the patient's wound, according to the physician's orders.

Equipment and Supplies

Waterproof pad	Sterile basins	Bandage scissors
Hand cleanser (alcohol-based)	Sterile 4×4s	Dressing and bandage material
Examination gloves	Sterile water or saline	Patient chart
Sterile gloves	20-mL syringe	Disinfecting solution

Removing an Old Dressing

1. Wash your hands and gather the supplies.

2. Identify the patient using two identifiers, identify yourself, and explain the procedure.

3. Check the patient's chart to determine the type and strength of irrigating solution and dressing to be used, and gather the supplies.

4. Ask the patient if he or she has had any problems since the surgery and make certain that the patient has been following all home care instructions.

5. Have the patient expose the area.

6. Place a waterproof pad under the wound area and position so that the work area is easily accessible.

7. Wash hands using aseptic technique and apply appropriate PPE (nonsterile examination gloves).

8. Inspect the outer covering of the bandage. Make a mental note of any concerns. Was the bandage torn, dirty, or wet?

9. Cut the bandage with a pair of bandage scissors along the side of the wound (Figure 4-68). Carefully remove the bandage and dressing by pulling the bandage toward the wound.

10. Inspect the inner portion of the bandage for any drainage or odor. Make a mental note of your findings. Discard the bandage material into a biohazard container.

11. Without touching the wound, look at the wound area and inspect it for any signs of infection, including edema, erythema, drainage, etc. Make a mental note of your findings.

12. Remove gloves and wash your hands. Follow office policy regarding having the provider check the wound before irrigating.

Irrigating the Wound

13. Properly position and clean the Mayo tray with the 4×4s containing disinfectant. Allow the stand to air dry.

14. Place one of the wrapped sterile basins on the center of the Mayo stand. Open using sterile technique.

15. Open the peel-apart package containing the sterile 4×4s and drop the contents from the packet onto the field.

16. Open sterile dressing and place it on the sterile field.

17. Open the sterile bandage material and place it on the sterile field.

18. Drop a sterile 20-mL syringe onto the sterile field.

19. Pour a small amount of sterile saline into the sterile basin.

(continues)

(continued)

---

20. Remove the other sterile basin from the side table and place it on the waterproof drape near the patient's wound. Open it in a sterile manner. Instruct the patient not to touch the basin or drape.

---

21. Thoroughly wash your hands using the alcohol-based sanitizer on the side table.

---

22. Don a pair of sterile gloves.

---

23. Arrange items on the tray for easy access.

---

24. Draw up irrigating fluid from the basin with the sterile syringe. Irrigate the patient's wound so that the water runs into the basin on the sterile field (Figure 4-69). Continue irrigating following provider's orders.

---

25. Dry the wound with sterile gauze.

Apply New Bandage

---

26. Pick up the sterile dressing and place it over the wound.

---

27. Choose a bandaging technique that best suits the patient's wound.

---

28. Throw away all trash into proper trash receptacles and give the patient home care instructions and any prescriptions.

---

29. Dismiss the patient and clean the room.

---

30. Document the procedure.

CHARTING EXAMPLE

04/15/XXXX *2:30 p.m.*	*Pt. here for a dressing change following last week's injury to L arm. Pt. states that she took all of her antibiotic and dressed wound according to home-care instructions. Dressing was clean and dry. A small amount of serosanguineous exudate present on the inside portion of the dressing. ⊖ Erythema or edema over the wound area. Irrigated wound with 40 mL of sterile saline. Dried area with sterile gauze. Applied a sterile collagen dressing to the area per Dr. Jones. Reinstructed pt. on proper wound care. Pt. to return next week. Jeanine Ruh, CMA (AAMA)*

Section 4-6

PHYSICAL AGENTS

Procedure 4-37
ADMINISTER HEAT THERAPY TREATMENTS

Equipment and Supplies (Refer to Each Individual Section)

1. Assemble the supplies and wash your hands.

2. Identify the patient using two identifiers, identify yourself, and explain the procedure.

3. Instruct the patient to remove clothing and put on a gown, if necessary, exposing the area to be treated.

4. Place the patient in the proper position for the treatment.

5. Administer heat therapy as ordered:

Heating Pad (Supplies: Heating Pad and Cover)

A1. Place the protective covering over the heating pad.

A2. Connect the cord to an electrical outlet and set the control to the setting indicated by the provider.

A3. Place the heating pad on the affected area (do not allow the patient to lie on the heating pad) and ask the patient how the temperature level feels.

Hot Water Bottle (Supplies: Hot Water Bottle and Cover)

B1. Fill the hot water bottle approximately half full with water [the water temperature should be between 105° F and 110° F (40.5° C and 43° C)].

B2. Compress the air out of the bottle and close the lid tightly.

B3. Cover the water bottle with a cloth or towel.

B4. Leave in place for the prescribed amount of time.

Hot Compress (Supplies: Basin, Thermometer, Cloth or Gauze, Plastic Covering)

C1. Fill a basin with hot water [between 105° F and 110° F (40.5° C and 43° C)].

C2. Soak cloth or gauze in hot water and wring out excess moisture.

C3. Cover the compress with a plastic covering. Place the compress over the affected area.

C4. Re-wet the compress to maintain the correct temperature.

(continues)

(continued)

C5. Replace the compress every few minutes for the amount of time prescribed by the provider.

Hot Pack (Supplies: Hot Pack and Pad)

D1. Hot packs are soaked in hot water, allowed to drain, and covered with a pad. They are used on larger areas of the body, such as the back or shoulder.

Hot Soak (Supplies: Soaking Container, Prescribed Solution, Towels)

E1. Fill an appropriate-sized container with hot water [approximately 105° to 110° F (40.5° to 43° C)] and add medication to the water if ordered by the provider.

E2. Place the body part in the water for the prescribed amount of time.

E3. After the prescribed amount of time, remove the body part from the soak and dry with a towel. Inspect the area for any redness or damage

Paraffin Bath (Supplies: Paraffin Tank, Mineral Oil, [Foil, Plastic Wrap, or Cloth] Sheet or Blanket, and Towels)

F1. A paraffin bath, composed of water and mineral oil, should be heated to approximately 127° F (53° C) but follow doctor's specific orders for temperature.

F2. Dip the affected body part in the paraffin until a thick coating of wax builds up.

F3. Wrap the body part in foil, plastic wrap, or a cloth for 30 minutes.

F4. Take the covering off and peel away the wax.

6. Check with the patient periodically during any heat treatment. The patient may feel chilled during the treatment, so cover the patient with a sheet or blanket.

7. Check the treatment area for signs of damage such as redness, blisters, or irritation.

8. Assist the patient with dressing, if needed.

9. Clean the area and wash hands.

10. Document treatment in the patient's chart.

CHARTING EXAMPLE

08/12/XXXX 1:30 p.m.	Hot compress applied to right forearm x 10 minutes per Dr. Cho's orders. No blistering or redness observed after treatment. Pt. tolerated procedure well. Ryan Leonard, CMA (AAMA)

Procedure 4-38
ADMINISTER COLD THERAPY TREATMENTS

Equipment and Supplies (Refer to Each Individual Section)

1. Assemble the supplies and wash your hands.

2. Identify the patient using two identifiers, identify yourself, and explain the procedure.

3. Instruct the patient to remove clothing and put on a gown, if necessary, exposing the area to be treated.

4. Place the patient in the proper position for the treatment.

5. Administer the cold therapy as ordered:

Ice Bag (Supplies: Ice Bag, Ice Cubes, and Towels)

A1. Check the ice bag for damage or leaks.

A2. Fill the bag approximately two-thirds full with small ice chips or cubes; refill as needed.

A3. Squeeze the bag to expel excess air and screw the top into place.

A4. Cover the pack with a towel for patient comfort and to help absorb any moisture.

A5. Keep the ice bag in place for the amount of time ordered by the provider (usually 15 to 30 minutes).

Commercial Ice Pack (Supplies: Ice Pack and Protective Covering)

B1. Place the gel pack in the freezer for the amount of time recommended by the manufacturer.

B2. If pack has a protective covering over it, place it on the affected area.

B3. If there is no covering on the pack, cover the pack with a cloth or towel before applying.

B4. Leave the pack in place for the prescribed amount of time.

B5. Place the bag in the freezer after use.

Chemical Ice Pack (Supplies: Chemical Ice Pack and Protective Covering)

C1. Inspect the bag for leaks.

C2. Squeeze the bag and shake.

(continues)

(continued)

C3. Cover the pack with a protective covering.

C4. Apply the pack to the affected area for the amount of time prescribed by the provider.

C5. Discard the pack after use.

Cold Compress (Supplies: Washcloth, Ice Cubes, Basin, and Ice Pack)

D1. Place a small volume of water in a basin, and add large ice cubes to the water.

D2. Soak a washcloth or gauze pad in the water and wring out any excess.

D3. Place an ice pack over the compress.

D4. Re-wet, as needed, to maintain the temperature of the compress.

D5. Repeat application every 2 to 3 minutes for the amount of time prescribed by the provider.

Ice Massage (Supplies: Ice Cup and Towels)

E1. Fill a paper cup three-fourths full of water and place in the freezer. Once frozen you may use for treatment.

E2. Expose the area to be treated and squeeze the paper cup so the ice cube is exposed.

E3. Move the ice cube in a circular motion over the affected area for the prescribed amount of time stop procedure if patient complains of numbness or burning in the area.

6. Check the treatment area following the procedure for paleness, redness, blueness, or any other signs of damage.

7. Assist the patient with dressing, if needed.

8. Clean the work area and wash hands.

9. Document the treatment in the patient's chart.

CHARTING EXAMPLE

08/16/XXXX 12:30 p.m.	Applied cold compress to left forearm, as per Dr. May's orders. Pt. tolerated procedure well. Notable decrease in swelling. Pt. noted a definite decrease in pain as well. Dawn Carter, RMA

Section 4-7

RESPIRATORY PROCEDURES

Procedure 4-39
INSTRUCT PATIENT HOW TO USE A PEAK FLOW METER

Equipment and Supplies

Peak flowmeter	Disposable mouthpiece	Documentation journal Patient chart

1. Wash your hands, and gather the equipment.

2. Greet and identify the patient using two identifiers, introduce yourself and explain the procedure.

3. Put on gloves.

4. Assemble the peak flow meter and disposable mouthpiece.

5. Pick up the meter and explain the proper way to set the gauge following each reading. Start pointer on flow meter on zero.

6. Hand meter to patient and ask patient put the peak flow meter mouthpiece in the mouth behind the teeth, with lips tightly sealed around the tube.

7. Instruct patient to take a deep breath and to blow out as hard as possible.

8. Instruct patient to read the result by noting where the sliding gauge stopped following expiration into the tube. Reset the gauge to zero.

9. Instruct patient to perform three consecutive tests, once in the morning and once in the evening and to record only the highest reading.

10. Give patient proper cleansing instructions for the meter. Explain how to clean the mouthpiece; instruct patient not to immerse flow meter in water.

11. Document the procedure.

CHARTING EXAMPLE

10/18/XXXX	Instructed pt. in the correct use of her new peak
2:00 p.m.	flow meter per Dr. Wong. Pt. was able to correctly
	demonstrate the procedure back to me. Gave pt.
	homecare instructions and instructed to call if she
	had any questions. F. Stout, CMA (AAMA) ————

Field Tips

Significance of a Peak Flow Reading

Because everyone has a different lung capacity, everyone has a different "personal best" peak flow reading. The provider will help the patient come up with what is considered a "personal best" reading, based on the patient's readings in the office and the patient's personal medical condition. Generally, patients that have a peak flow rating that is 80% or better of their personal best are well controlled and do not need immediate treatment. If the reading falls between 50% to 79% of the patient's personal best, it means that the patient needs to take a quick-relief medication. Anything below 50% means that the patient should immediately seek emergency care.

Procedure 4-40
PERFORM A PULMONARY FUNCTION TEST

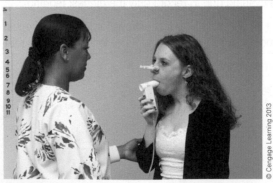

Figure 4-70: Instruct the patient to tightly seal the lips around the mouthpiece of the spirometer tube so that no air escapes.

Equipment and Supplies

Patient record	Disposable mouthpiece	Disposable tubing
Scales	Disposable nose clips	Spirometer calibration
Spirometer		syringe

1. Wash your hands and gather the equipment. (Calibrate the machine if applicable)

2. Greet and identify the patient using two identifiers, introduce yourself, and explain the procedure.

3. Put on gloves.

4. Measure the patient's height and weight if not already performed.

5. Have the patient remove constricting clothing, such as belts and sports bras.

6. Position the patient in a seated position.

7. Program the unit with the patient's information. Information may include the patient's name, sex, height, weight, and medication information.

8. Place the nose clip on the patient's nose.

9. Have the patient place the mouth piece in the mouth and to securely fasten lips around the tube. Seal lips securely around the mouthpiece (Press the start button according to manufacturer's instructions.)

10. Ask patient to take in a deep breath and to blow out as hard and long as possible (Figure 4-70).

11. Repeat the test two more times. Record the results from the spirometer and attach the printout to the chart.

12. If ordered, provide medication to the patient.

13. Repeat the spirometry procedure, if ordered.

14. Document procedure and make results available for provider.

15. Discard the disposable test supplies and clean the equipment.

CHARTING EXAMPLE

10/14/XXXX 2:30 p.m.	Wt. 125 lbs. Ht. 66″ T98.8, P 92, R20, BP 142/88: Spirometry testing per Dr. Wong. Dr. Wong ordered inhalation therapy after viewing results: Three puffs of Ventolin administered one minute apart. Spirometry testing repeated. Patient tolerated well. Dr. Wong given the results once again. Results normal. Jacob Green, CMA (AAMA)

Table 4-13

DEFINITIONS OF MEASUREMENTS FROM PULMONARY FUNCTION TESTS

Test	Definition
Forced expiratory volume after 1 second (FEV$_1$)	The total amount of air forcefully exhaled during the first second of testing. (Patients with healthy lungs should be able to force out 70 to 75% of the air in their lungs within that first second of testing, emphasizing the need for appropriate education and coaching. Any type of a blockage or restriction may cause the result to drop.)
Forced vital capacity (FVC)	The maximum amount of air forced out of the lungs, when the patient exhales as rapidly and forcefully as possible into the tube, after taking in a deep inhalation (usually expressed in liters).
Tidal volume (V$_t$)	The amount of air during inspiration and expiration when breathing normally.
Inspiratory reserve volume (IRV)	The additional amount of air a patient could potentially inhale.
Expiratory reserve volume (ERV)	The additional amount of air a patient could potentially exhale.

Residual volume (RV)	The air that is left in the lungs after the patient forcibly exhales all the air the patient can.
Total lung capacity (TLC)	The amount of air the lungs are able to hold.
Vital capacity (VC)	The maximum amount of air the patient is able to inhale and exhale.
Functional residual capacity (FRC)	The amount of air that is left in the lungs after the patient normally exhales.

Procedure 4-41
ADMINISTER A NEBULIZER TREATMENT

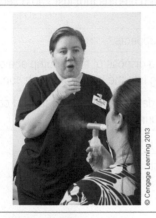

Figure 4-71: The patient is instructed to take in slow, deep breaths during the treatment.

Equipment and Supplies

Patient record Nebulizer	Disposable mouthpiece or face mask Disposable connecting tubing	Disposable medication dispenser Medication/diluent (if applicable)

1. Wash your hands and gather the equipment.

2. Greet and identify the patient using two identifiers, introduce yourself, and explain the procedure.

(continues)

(continued)

3. Put on gloves.

4. Check order (three times) and pour the correct amount of medication and diluent into the medication dispenser. Screw the lid on the dispenser and gently mix the medication.

5. Connect the medication dispenser to the mouthpiece or face mask.

6. Connect the disposable tubing to the medication dispenser and nebulizer.

7. Place the patient in a full-Fowler's position or upright position.

8. Turn the nebulizer on. When you turn the nebulizer on, you should see a mist.

9. If using a face mask, place it over the patient's face so that it fits comfortably. If using a mouthpiece, instruct patient to place it in the mouth between the teeth and to purse the lips over the mouthpiece making a seal.

10. Instruct the patient to take in slow, deep breaths that last 2 to 3 seconds (Figure 4-71).

11. Continue treatment until the mist disappears.

12. Turn off the nebulizer and remove and dispose of the mouthpiece or face mask, medicine dispenser, and tubing into the biohazard trash can.

13. Instruct the patient to take in several deep breaths and to try and cough up any secretions that were loosened during the treatment.

14. Wash your hands and document the procedure.

15. Give the patient home care instructions.

CHARTING EXAMPLE

| 12/12/XXXX 10:15 a.m. | Nebulizer treatment, Albuterol, 2.5 mg per Dr. Jones. Pt. tolerated procedure well. Following treatment patient brought up some mucus secretions that were white and tinged with a bit of green mucus. Pt. reported feeling much better following the treatment. Provider followed up with pt. Jay Craig, RMA |

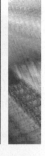

Section Five
PEDIATRIC SCREENINGS AND PROCEDURES

ASSISTING IN A PEDIATRIC OFFICE

INTRODUCTION

Pediatrics is a rewarding profession, but it is not a field for everyone. To work in pediatrics, you must enjoy children and have a great deal of patience. You must be caring and empathetic, but not highly emotional. You must possess a great deal of energy and have the ability to communicate with children from infancy through adolescence (Fig 5-1a and b).

(a)

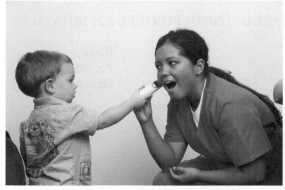

Figure 5-1: (a) The medical assistant communicates with the toddler by getting down to his level and allowing him to examine the equipment.

© Cengage Learning 2013

(b)

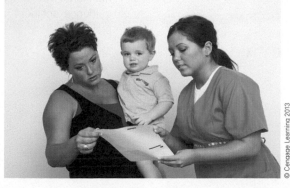

Figure 5-1: (b) The medical assistant adopts a more professional demeanor when communicating with the patient's mother.

© Cengage Learning 2013

209

Section 5-1

ROUTINE PROCEDURES FOR DIFFERENT PEDIATRIC INTERVALS

Well child check-ups provide the opportunity for providers and staff to provide anticipatory guidance and education as the child grows. For easy reference, Table 5-1 lists common abbreviations that are used within Table 5-2. Table 5-2 lists routine procedures that are performed at different age intervals.

Table 5-1

COMMON ABBREVIATIONS USED IN PEDIATRICS

Abbreviations	
HC—Head circumference	WT—Weight
HT—Height	PP—Plot percentiles

Table 5-2

ROUTINE PROCEDURES FOR DIFFERENT PEDIATRIC AGE INTERVALS

Age	HC	WT	HT	PP	Laboratory Tests	Routine Procedures/ Education
Newborn	X	X	X	X	Newborn screening	Apgar scores, anticipatory guidance, safety issues (circumcision for some males)
1 mo	X	X	X	X	Newborn screening	Anticipatory and nutrition guidance, accident prevention
2 mo	X	X	X	X		Anticipatory guidance
4 mo	X	X	X	X		Anticipatory guidance

6 mo	X	X	X	X	Optional hematocrit and hemoglobin for low-birth-weight babies	Anticipatory guidance
9 mo	X	X	X	X	Optional hematocrit and hemoglobin	Anticipatory guidance, safety information, poison control kit from pharmacy
12 mo	X	X	X	X		Anticipatory guidance
15 mo	X	X	X	X		Anticipatory guidance
18 mo	X	X	X	X		Anticipatory guidance
4–6 yr		X	X	X	Optional urinalysis, hematocrit, and hemoglobin	Vision and hearing screening, blood pressure, pulse, and respiration
11–12 yr		X	X	X	Optional urinalysis, hematocrit, and hemoglobin	Blood pressure, pulse, and respiration
14–16 yr		X	X	X	Optional urinalysis, hematocrit, and hemoglobin	Blood pressure, pulse, and respiration

Section 5-2

OBTAIN LENGTH, WEIGHT, AND HEAD CIRCUMFERENCE ON AN INFANT AND CHILD

Accurate measurement of length, weight and head circumference assists the provider to determine if there is normal growth of an infant (0 to 12 months of age) and child (12 months to puberty) (Figure 5-2).

Procedure 5-1

OBTAIN LENGTH, WEIGHT, AND HEAD CIRCUMFERENCE ON AN INFANT AND CHILD

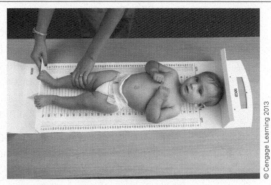

© Cengage Learning 2013

Figure 5-2: Recumbent length measurement using a caliper.

Equipment and Supplies

Measuring caliper	Measuring tape	Growth chart	Infant scale	Protective sheath

Steps

1. Wash hands and assemble equipment.

2. Identify the patient using two identifiers (name and date of birth).

3. Ask caregiver to remove infant's clothing down to the diaper.

4. Obtaining the Length

4a. Place infant on examination table or scale with a measuring caliper.

4b. Place the top of the infant's head flush with the top of the measuring bar of the caliper.

4c. Gently stretch the infant's leg to full length and place the sole of the foot flush with the bottom of measuring bar.

4d. Document length.

5. Obtaining Weight Using a Digital Scale

5a. Zero scale after placing protective sheath on the scale. (Have caregiver remove the infant's diaper just before measurement.)

5b. Keep infant in the center of scale and make certain infant is safe.

5c. Once the weight is obtained note the reading and have caregiver remove the infant from the scale.

5d. Document both the length and the weight in the patient's chart.

6. Procedure for HC

6a. Using a non-stretching measuring tape, wrap measuring tape around the widest circumference of the head. (Widest portion of the forehead and around the widest part of the back of the head.)

6b. Note measurement.

6c. Record measurement in the patient's chart.

7. Plotting Growth Percentiles

7a. Select the appropriate gender growth chart.

7b. Find the infant or child's age on the horizontal axis.

7c. Find the weight, length, or head circumference (HC) on the vertical axis. Use a straight edge to draw a horizontal line across until it intersects the vertical line. Place a dot where the two lines intersect. Some providers may have you record the date above the dot.

ITEMS TO BE DOCUMENTED

1. Today's date and time.

2. Record chief complaint or examination interval.

3. Record patient's length or height.

4. Record patient's weight.

5. Record patient's HC.

6. Sign off the note using an approved exit signature.

CHARTING EXAMPLE

02/13/XXXX 9:30 a.m.	Pt here for 6-month male well baby check. Length 26", Wt 18# and HC 17.5" M. Livingston CMA (AAMA)—

EMR Application

Documenting growth statistics in the electronic medical record is very easy. You just bring up the appropriate growth chart, enter in the requested information and it plots the percentiles for you.

Section 5-3

NORMAL PEDIATRIC VITAL SIGN RANGES AND TIPS FOR TAKING VITAL SIGNS ON PEDIATRIC PATIENTS

Pediatric vital sign ranges are different from normal ranges for adults. Table 5-3 lists pediatric ranges.

Table 5-3

**NORMAL PULSE, RESPIRATION AND BLOOD PRESSURE
RANGES FOR PEDIATRIC AGE INTERVALS**

Age (Yr)	Heart Rate (Beats/Min)	Respirations (Breaths/Min)	Blood Pressure (Average) Systolic/Diastolic
<1 year	100–160	30–60	Not usually measured in an office setting, 80–100/45–65
1–2 years	90–150	24–40	90/60
2–5 years	80–140	22–34	90/60
6–12 years	70–120	16–30	100/60
>12 years	60–100	12–16	100/60

Field Tip

Allowing the pediatric patient to play with the equipment before the measurements will promote trust and help the child to relax for the measurements.

Field Tip

To obtain an accurate pulse on a young child or infant, you should perform an apical pulse with your stethoscope.

Section 5-4

PEDIATRIC IMMUNIZATION (IMZ) SCHEDULES

Disease prevention is the key to public health. It is always better to prevent a disease than to treat it. Vaccines prevent disease in people and protect those who come into contact with unvaccinated individuals. Vaccines are responsible for the control of many infectious diseases that were once common in this country, including polio, measles, diphtheria, pertussis (whooping cough), rubella (German measles), mumps, tetanus, and *Haemophilus influenzae* type b (Hib).

This section lists the different age intervals when immunizations should be administered (Figures 5-3–5-5). (Please note that the IMZ schedule is subject to change. Refer to the CDC website (http://www.cdc.gov/va) for the most current guide. You should check the schedule annually.)

Figure 5-3: Recommended immunization schedule for persons aged 0 through 6 years.

National Immunization Program, Centers for Disease Control and Prevention; pulled from http://www.cdc.gov/vaccines/recs/schedules/child-schedule.htm

Vaccine ▼　　Age ▶	Birth	1 month	2 months	4 months	6 months	9 months	12 months	15 months	18 months	19–23 months	2–3 years	4–6 years
Hepatitis B[1]	Hep B	HepB			HepB							
Rotavirus[2]			RV	RV	RV							
Diphtheria, tetanus, pertussis[3]			DTaP	DTaP	DTaP		see footnote[3]	DTaP				DTaP
Haemophilus influenzae type b[4]			Hib	Hib	Hib		Hib					
Pneumococcal[5]			PCV	PCV	PCV		PCV				PPSV	
Inactivated poliovirus[6]			IPV	IPV		IPV						IPV
Influenza[7]						Influenza (Yearly)						
Measles, mumps, rubella[8]							MMR			see footnote[8]		MMR
Varicella[9]							Varicella			see footnote[9]		Varicella
Hepatitis A[10]							Dose 1[10]				HepA Series	
Meningococcal[11]							MCV4 — see footnote[11]					

Legend:
- Range of recommended ages for all children
- Range of recommended ages for certain high-risk groups
- Range of recommended ages for all children and certain high-risk groups

This schedule includes recommendations in effect as of December 23, 2011. Any dose not administered at the recommended age should be administered at a subsequent visit, when indicated and feasible. The use of a combination vaccine generally is preferred over separate injections of its equivalent component vaccines. Vaccination providers should consult the relevant Advisory Committee on Immunization Practices (ACIP) statement for detailed recommendations, available online at http://www.cdc.gov/vaccines/pubs/acip-list.htm. Clinically significant adverse events that follow vaccination should be reported to the Vaccine Adverse Event Reporting System (VAERS) online (http://www.vaers.hhs.gov) or by telephone (800-822-7967).

1. **Hepatitis B (HepB) vaccine.** (Minimum age: birth)

   At birth:
   - Administer monovalent HepB vaccine to all newborns before hospital discharge.
   - For infants born to hepatitis B surface antigen (HBsAg)–positive mothers, administer HepB vaccine and 0.5 mL of hepatitis B immune globulin (HBIG) within 12 hours of birth. These infants should be tested for HBsAg and antibody to HBsAg (anti-HBs) 1 to 2 months after completion of at least 3 doses of the HepB series, at age 9 through 18 months (generally at the next well-child visit).
   - If mother's HBsAg status is unknown, within 12 hours of birth administer HepB vaccine for infants weighing ≥2,000 grams, and HepB vaccine plus HBIG for infants weighing <2,000 grams. Determine mother's HBsAg status as soon as possible and, if she is HBsAg-positive, administer HBIG for infants weighing ≥2,000 grams (no later than age 1 week).

   Doses after the birth dose:
   - The second dose should be administered at age 1 to 2 months. Monovalent HepB vaccine should be used for doses administered before age 6 weeks.
   - Administration of a total of 4 doses of HepB vaccine is permissible when a combination vaccine containing HepB is administered after the birth dose.
   - Infants who did not receive a birth dose should receive 3 doses of a HepB-containing vaccine starting as soon as feasible (Figure 3).
   - The minimum interval between dose 1 and dose 2 is 4 weeks, and between dose 2 and 3 is 8 weeks. The final (third or fourth) dose in the HepB vaccine series should be administered no earlier than age 24 weeks and at least 16

7. **Influenza vaccines.** (Minimum age: 6 months for trivalent inactivated influenza vaccine [TIV]; 2 years for live, attenuated influenza vaccine [LAIV])
   - For most healthy children aged 2 years and older, either LAIV or TIV may be used. However, LAIV should not be administered to some children, including 1) children with asthma, 2) children 2 through 4 years who had wheezing in the past 12 months, or 3) children who have any other underlying medical conditions that predispose them to influenza complications. For all other contraindications to use of LAIV, see MMWR 2010;59(No. RR-8), available at http://www.cdc.gov/mmwr/pdf/rr/rr5908.pdf.
   - For children aged 6 months through 8 years:
     — For the 2011–12 season, administer 2 doses (separated by at least 4 weeks) to those who did not receive at least 1 dose of the 2010–11 vaccine. Those who received at least 1 dose of the 2010–11 vaccine require 1 dose for the 2011–12 season.
     — For the 2012–13 season, follow dosing guidelines in the 2012 ACIP influenza vaccine recommendations.

8. **Measles, mumps, and rubella (MMR) vaccine.** (Minimum age: 12 months)
   - The second dose may be administered before age 4 years, provided at least 4 weeks have elapsed since the first dose.
   - Administer MMR vaccine to infants aged 6 through 11 months who are traveling internationally. These children should be revaccinated with 2 doses of MMR vaccine, the first at ages 12 through 15 months and at least 4 weeks after the previous dose, and the second at ages 4 through 6 years.

(continues)

(continued)

weeks after the first dose.

2. **Rotavirus (RV) vaccines.** (Minimum age: 6 weeks for both RV-1 [Rotarix] and RV-5 [Rota Teq])
   - The maximum age for the first dose in the series is 14 weeks, 6 days; and 8 months, 0 days for the final dose in the series. Vaccination should not be initiated for infants aged 15 weeks, 0 days or older.
   - If RV-1 (Rotarix) is administered at ages 2 and 4 months, a dose at 6 months is not indicated.

3. **Diphtheria and tetanus toxoids and acellular pertussis (DTaP) vaccine.** (Minimum age: 6 weeks)
   - The fourth dose may be administered as early as age 12 months, provided at least 6 months have elapsed since the third dose.

4. **Haemophilus influenzae type b (Hib) conjugate vaccine.** (Minimum age: 6 weeks)
   - If PRP-OMP (PedvaxHIB or Comvax [HepB-Hib]) is administered at ages 2 and 4 months, a dose at age 6 months is not indicated.
   - Hiberix should only be used for the booster (final) dose in children aged 12 months through 4 years.

5. **Pneumococcal vaccines.** (Minimum age: 6 weeks for pneumococcal conjugate vaccine [PCV]; 2 years for pneumococcal polysaccharide vaccine [PPSV])
   - Administer 1 dose of PCV to all healthy children aged 24 through 59 months who are not completely vaccinated for their age.
   - For children who have received an age-appropriate series of 7-valent PCV (PCV7), a single supplemental dose of 13-valent PCV (PCV13) is recommended for:
     — All children aged 14 through 59 months
     — Children aged 60 through 71 months with underlying medical conditions.
   - Administer PPSV at least 8 weeks after last dose of PCV to children aged 2 years or older with certain underlying medical conditions, including a cochlear implant. See MMWR 2010:59(No. RR-11), available at http://www.cdc.gov/mmwr/pdf/rr/rr5911.pdf.

6. **Inactivated poliovirus vaccine (IPV).** (Minimum age: 6 weeks)
   - If 4 or more doses are administered before age 4 years, an additional dose should be administered at age 4 through 6 years.
   - The final dose in the series should be administered on or after the fourth birthday and at least 6 months after the previous dose.

9. **Varicella (VAR) vaccine.** (Minimum age: 12 months)
   - The second dose may be administered before age 4 years, provided at least 3 months have elapsed since the first dose.
   - For children aged 12 months through 12 years, the recommended minimum interval between doses is 3 months. However, if the second dose was administered at least 4 weeks after the first dose, it can be accepted as valid.

10. **Hepatitis A (HepA) vaccine.** (Minimum age: 12 months)
   - Administer the second (final) dose 6 to 18 months after the first.
   - Unvaccinated children 24 months and older at high risk should be vaccinated. See MMWR 2006;55(No. RR-7), available at http://www.cdc.gov/mmwr/pdf/rr/rr5507.pdf.
   - A 2-dose HepA vaccine series is recommended for anyone aged 24 months and older, previously unvaccinated, for whom immunity against hepatitis A virus infection is desired.

11. **Meningococcal conjugate vaccines, quadrivalent (MCV4).** (Minimum age: 9 months for Menactra [MCV4-D], 2 years for Menveo [MCV4-CRM])
   - For children aged 9 through 23 months 1) with persistent complement component deficiency; 2) who are residents of or travelers to countries with hyperendemic or epidemic disease; or 3) who are present during outbreaks caused by a vaccine serogroup, administer 2 primary doses of MCV4-D, ideally at ages 9 months and 12 months or at least 8 weeks apart.
   - For children aged 24 months and older with 1) persistent complement component deficiency who have not been previously vaccinated; or 2) anatomic/functional asplenia, administer 2 primary doses of either MCV4 at least 8 weeks apart.
   - For children with anatomic/functional asplenia, if MCV4-D (Menactra) is used, administer at a minimum age of 2 years and at least 4 weeks after completion of all PCV doses.
   - See MMWR 2011;60:72–6, available at http://www.cdc.gov/mmwr/pdf/wk/mm6003.pdf, and Vaccines for Children Program resolution No. 6/11-1, available at http://www.cdc.gov/vaccines/programs/vfc/downloads/resolutions/06-11mening-mcv.pdf, and MMWR 2011;60:1391–2, available at http://www.cdc.gov/mmwr/pdf/wk/mm6040. pdf, for further guidance, including revaccination guidelines.

This schedule is approved by the Advisory Committee on Immunization Practices (http://www.cdc.gov/vaccines/recs/acip), the American Academy of Pediatrics (http://www.aap.org), and the American Academy of Family Physicians (http://www.aafp.org).
Department of Health and Human Services • Centers for Disease Control and Prevention

Figure 5-4: Recommended immunization schedule for persons aged 7 through 18 years.

National Immunization Program, Centers for Disease Control and Prevention; pulled from http://www.cdc.gov/vaccines/recs/schedules/child-schedule.htm

Vaccine ▼ Age ►	7–10 years	11–12 years	13–18 years
Tetanus, diphtheria, pertussis[1]	1 dose (if indicated)	1 dose	1 dose (if indicated)
Human papillomavirus[2]	see footnote[2]	3 doses	Complete 3-dose series
Meningococcal[3]	See footnote[3]	Dose 1	Booster at 16 years old
Influenza[4]		Influenza (yearly)	
Pneumococcal[5]		See footnote[5]	
Hepatitis A[6]		Complete 2-dose series	
Hepatitis B[7]		Complete 3-dose series	
Inactivated poliovirus[8]		Complete 3-dose series	
Measles, mumps, rubella[9]		Complete 2-dose series	
Varicella[10]		Complete 2-dose series	

Legend:
- Range of recommended ages for all children
- Range of recommended ages for catch-up immunization
- Range of recommended ages for certain high-risk groups

This schedule includes recommendations in effect as of December 23, 2011. Any dose not administered at the recommended age should be administered at a subsequent visit, when indicated and feasible. The use of a combination vaccine generally is preferred over separate injections of its equivalent component vaccines. Vaccination providers should consult the relevant Advisory Committee on Immunization Practices (ACIP) statement for detailed recommendations, available online at http://www.cdc.gov/vaccines/pubs/acip-list.htm. Clinically significant adverse events that follow vaccination should be reported to the Vaccine Adverse Event Reporting System (VAERS) online (http://www.vaers.hhs.gov) or by telephone (800-822-7967).

1. **Tetanus and diphtheria toxoids and acellular pertussis (Tdap) vaccine.**
   (Minimum age: 10 years for Boostrix and 11 years for Adacel)
   - Persons aged 11 through 18 years who have not received Tdap vaccine should receive a dose followed by tetanus and diphtheria toxoids (Td) booster doses every 10 years thereafter.
   - Tdap vaccine should be substituted for a single dose of Td in the catch-up series for children aged 7 through 10 years. Refer to the catch-up schedule if additional doses of tetanus and diphtheria toxoid–containing vaccine are needed.
   - Tdap vaccine can be administered regardless of the interval since the last tetanus and diphtheria toxoid–containing vaccine.

2. **Human papillomavirus (HPV) vaccines (HPV4 [Gardasil] and HPV2 [Cervarix]).** (Minimum age: 9 years)
   - Either HPV4 or HPV2 is recommended in a 3-dose series for females aged 11 or 12 years. HPV4 is recommended in a 3-dose series for males aged 11 or 12 years.
   - The vaccine series can be started beginning at age 9 years.
   - Administer the second dose 1 to 2 months after the first dose and the third dose 6 months after the first dose (at least 24 weeks after the first dose).
   - See *MMWR* 2010;59:626–32, available at http://www.cdc.gov/mmwr/pdf/wk/mm5920.pdf.

- For children aged 6 months through 8 years:
  - For the 2011–12 season, administer 2 doses (separated by at least 4 weeks) to those who did not receive at least 1 dose of the 2010–11 vaccine. Those who received at least 1 dose of the 2010–11 vaccine require 1 dose for the 2011–12 season.
  - For the 2012–13 season, follow dosing guidelines in the 2012 ACIP influenza vaccine recommendations.

5. **Pneumococcal vaccines (pneumococcal conjugate vaccine [PCV] and pneumococcal polysaccharide vaccine [PPSV]).**
   - A single dose of PCV may be administered to children aged 6 through 18 years who have anatomic/functional asplenia, HIV infection or other immunocompromising condition, cochlear implant, or cerebral spinal fluid leak. See *MMWR* 2010:59(No. RR-11), available at http://www.cdc.gov/mmwr/pdf/rr/rr5911.pdf.
   - Administer PPSV at least 8 weeks after the last dose of PCV to children aged 2 years or older with certain underlying medical conditions, including a cochlear implant. A single revaccination should be administered after 5 years to children with anatomic/functional asplenia or an immunocompromising condition.

6. **Hepatitis A (HepA) vaccine.**
   - HepA vaccine is recommended for children older than 23 months who live in areas where vaccination programs target older children, who are at

(continues)

3. **Meningococcal conjugate vaccines, quadrivalent (MCV4).**
- Administer MCV4 at age 11 through 12 years with a booster dose at age 16 years.
- Administer MCV4 at age 13 through 18 years if patient is not previously vaccinated.
- If the first dose is administered at age 13 through 15 years, a booster dose should be administered at age 16 through 18 years with a minimum interval of at least 8 weeks after the preceding dose.
- If the first dose is administered at age 16 years or older, a booster dose is not needed.
- Administer 2 primary doses at least 8 weeks apart to previously unvaccinated persons with persistent complement component deficiency or anatomic/functional asplenia, and 1 dose every 5 years thereafter.
- Adolescents aged 11 through 18 years with human immunodeficiency virus (HIV) infection should receive a 2-dose primary series of MCV4, at least 8 weeks apart.
- See MMWR 2011;60:72–76, available at http://www.cdc.gov/mmwr/pdf/wk/mm6003.pdf, and Vaccines for Children Program resolution No. 6/11-1, available at http://www.cdc.gov/vaccines/programs/vfc/downloads/resolutions/06-11mening-mcv.pdf, for further guidelines.

4. **Influenza vaccines (trivalent inactivated influenza vaccine [TIV] and live, attenuated influenza vaccine [LAIV]).**
- For most healthy, nonpregnant persons, either LAIV or TIV may be used, except LAIV should not be used for some persons, including those with asthma or any other underlying medical conditions that predispose them to influenza complications. For all other contraindications to use of LAIV, see MMWR 2010;59(No.RR-8), available at http://www.cdc.gov/mmwr/pdf/rr/rr5908.pdf.
- Administer 1 dose to persons aged 9 years and older.

increased risk for infection, or for whom immunity against hepatitis A virus infection is desired. See MMWR 2006;55(No. RR-7), available at http://www.cdc.gov/mmwr/pdf/rr/rr5507.pdf.
- Administer 2 doses at least 6 months apart to unvaccinated persons.

7. **Hepatitis B (HepB) vaccine.**
- Administer the 3-dose series to those not previously vaccinated.
- For those with incomplete vaccination, follow the catch-up recommendations (Figure 3).
- A 2-dose series (doses separated by at least 4 months) of adult formulation Recombivax HB is licensed for use in children aged 11 through 15 years.

8. **Inactivated poliovirus vaccine (IPV).**
- The final dose in the series should be administered at least 6 months after the previous dose.
- If both OPV and IPV were administered as part of a series, a total of 4 doses should be administered, regardless of the child's current age.
- IPV is not routinely recommended for U.S. residents aged18 years or older.

9. **Measles, mumps, and rubella (MMR) vaccine.**
- The minimum interval between the 2 doses of MMR vaccine is 4 weeks.

10. **Varicella (VAR) vaccine.**
- For persons without evidence of immunity (see MMWR 2007;56[No. RR-4], available at http://www.cdc.gov/mmwr/pdf/rr/rr5604.pdf), administer 2 doses if not previously vaccinated or the second dose if only 1 dose has been administered.
- For persons aged 7 through 12 years, the recommended minimum interval between doses is 3 months. However, if the second dose was administered at least 4 weeks after the first dose, it can be accepted as valid.
- For persons aged 13 years and older, the minimum interval between doses is 4 weeks.

This schedule is approved by the Advisory Committee on Immunization Practices (http://www.cdc.gov/vaccines/recs/acip), the American Academy of Pediatrics (http://www.aap.org), and the American Academy of Family Physicians (http://www.aafp.org). Department of Health and Human Services • Centers for Disease Control and Prevention

Figure 5-5: Catch-up immunization schedule for persons aged 4 months through 18 years who start late or who are more than 1 month behind

National Immunization Program, Centers for Disease Control and Prevention, pulled from http://www.cdc.gov/vaccines/recs/schedules/child-schedule.htm

Vaccine	Minimum Age for Dose 1	Minimum Interval Between Doses			
		Dose 1 to dose 2	Dose 2 to dose 3	Dose 3 to dose 4	Dose 4 to dose 5
Persons aged 4 months through 6 years					
Hepatitis B[1]	Birth	4 weeks	8 weeks and at least 16 weeks after first dose; minimum age for the final dose is 24 weeks		
Rotavirus[1]	6 weeks	4 weeks	4 weeks[1]		
Diphtheria, tetanus, pertussis[2]	6 weeks	4 weeks	4 weeks	6 months	6 months[2]
Haemophilus influenzae type b[3]	6 weeks	4 weeks if first dose administered at younger than age 12 months / 8 weeks (as final dose) if first dose administered at age 12–14 months / No further doses needed if first dose administered at age 15 months or older	4 weeks[3] if current age is younger than 12 months / 8 weeks (as final dose)[3] if current age is 12 months or older and first dose administered at younger than age 12 months and second dose administered at younger than 15 months / No further doses needed if previous dose administered at age 15 months or older	8 weeks (as final dose) This dose only necessary for children aged 12 months through 59 months who received 3 doses before age 12 months	
Pneumococcal[4]	6 weeks	4 weeks if first dose administered at younger than age 12 months / 8 weeks (as final dose for healthy children) if first dose administered at age 12 months or older or current age 24 through 59 months / No further doses needed for healthy children if first dose administered at age 24 months or older	4 weeks if current age is younger than 12 months / 8 weeks (as final dose for healthy children) if current age is 12 months or older / No further doses needed for healthy children if previous dose administered at age 24 months or older	8 weeks (as final dose) This dose only necessary for children aged 12 months through 59 months who received 3 doses before age 12 months or for children at high risk who received 3 doses at any age	
Inactivated poliovirus[5]	6 weeks	4 weeks	4 weeks	6 months[5] minimum age 4 years for final dose	
Meningococcal[6]	9 months	8 weeks[6]	4 weeks		
Measles, mumps, rubella[7]	12 months	4 weeks			
Varicella[8]	12 months	3 months			
Hepatitis A	12 months	6 months			
Persons aged 7 through 18 years					
Tetanus, diphtheria/tetanus, diphtheria, pertussis[9]	7 years[9]	4 weeks	4 weeks if first dose administered at younger than age 12 months / 6 months if first dose administered at 12 months or older	6 months if first dose administered at younger than age 12 months	
Human papillomavirus[10]	9 years	Routine dosing intervals are recommended[10]			
Hepatitis A	12 months	6 months			
Hepatitis B	Birth	4 weeks	8 weeks (and at least 16 weeks after first dose)		
Inactivated poliovirus[5]	6 weeks	4 weeks	4 weeks[5]	6 months[5]	
Meningococcal[6]	9 months	8 weeks[6]			
Measles, mumps, rubella[7]	12 months	4 weeks			
Varicella[8]	12 months	3 months if person is younger than age 13 years / 4 weeks if person is aged 13 years or older			

(continues)

219

(continued)

1. **Rotavirus (RV) vaccines (RV-1 [Rotarix] and RV-5 [Rota Teq]).**
   - The maximum age for the first dose in the series is 14 weeks, 6 days; and 8 months, 0 days for the final dose in the series. Vaccination should not be initiated for infants aged 15 weeks, 0 days or older.
   - If RV-1 was administered for the first and second doses, a third dose is not indicated.

2. **Diphtheria and tetanus toxoids and acellular pertussis (DTaP) vaccine.**
   - The fifth dose is not necessary if the fourth dose was administered at age 4 years or older.

3. **Haemophilus influenzae type b (Hib) conjugate vaccine.**
   - Hib vaccine should be considered for unvaccinated persons aged 5 years or older who have sickle cell disease, leukemia, human immunodeficiency virus (HIV) infection, or anatomic/functional asplenia.
   - If the first 2 doses were PRP-OMP (PedvaxHIB or Comvax) and were administered at age 11 months or younger, the third (and final) dose should be administered at age 12 through 15 months and at least 8 weeks after the second dose.
   - If the first dose was administered at age 7 through 11 months, administer the second dose at least 4 weeks later and a final dose at age 12 through 15 months.

4. **Pneumococcal vaccines. (Minimum age: 6 weeks for pneumococcal conjugate vaccine [PCV]; 2 years for pneumococcal polysaccharide vaccine [PPSV])**
   - For children aged 24 through 71 months with underlying medical conditions, administer 1 dose of PCV if 3 doses of PCV were received previously, or administer 2 doses of PCV at least 8 weeks apart if fewer than 3 doses of PCV were received previously.
   - A single dose of PCV may be administered to certain children aged 6 through 18 years with underlying medical conditions. See age-specific schedules for details.
   - Administer PPSV to children aged 2 years or older with certain underlying medical conditions. See *MMWR* 2010;59(No. RR-11), available at http:// www.cdc.gov/mmwr/pdf/rr/rr5911.pdf.

5. **Inactivated poliovirus vaccine (IPV).**
   - A fourth dose is not necessary if the third dose was administered at age 4 years or older and at least 6 months after the previous dose.
   - In the first 6 months of life, minimum age and minimum intervals are only recommended if the person is at risk for imminent exposure to circulating poliovirus (i.e., travel to a polio-endemic region or during an outbreak).
   - IPV is not routinely recommended for U.S. residents aged 18 years or older.

6. **Meningococcal conjugate vaccines, quadrivalent (MCV4). (Minimum age: 9 months for Menactra [MCV4-D]; 2 years for Menveo [MCV4-CRM])**
   - See Figure 1 ("Recommended immunization schedule for persons aged 0 through 6 years") and Figure 2 ("Recommended immunization schedule for persons aged 7 through 18 years") for further guidance.

7. **Measles, mumps, and rubella (MMR) vaccine.**
   - Administer the second dose routinely at age 4 through 6 years.

8. **Varicella (VAR) vaccine.**
   - Administer the second dose routinely at age 4 through 6 years. If the second dose was administered at least 4 weeks after the first dose, it can be accepted as valid.

9. **Tetanus and diphtheria toxoids (Td) and tetanus and diphtheria toxoids and acellular pertussis (Tdap) vaccines.**
   - For children aged 7 through 10 years who are not fully immunized with the childhood DTaP vaccine series, Tdap vaccine should be substituted for a single dose of Td vaccine in the catch-up series; if additional doses are needed, use Td vaccine. For these children, an adolescent Tdap vaccine dose should not be given.
   - An inadvertent dose of DTaP vaccine administered to children aged 7 through 10 years can count as part of the catch-up series. This dose can count as the adolescent Tdap dose, or the child can later receive a Tdap booster dose at age 11–12 years.

10. **Human papillomavirus (HPV) vaccines (HPV4 [Gardasil] and HPV2 [Cervarix]).**
    - Administer the vaccine series to females (either HPV2 or HPV4) and males (HPV4) at age 13 through 18 years if patient is not previously vaccinated.
    - Use recommended routine dosing intervals for vaccine series catch-up; see Figure 2 ("Recommended immunization schedule for persons aged 7 through 18 years").

Clinically significant adverse events that follow vaccination should be reported to the Vaccine Adverse Event Reporting System (VAERS) online (http://www.vaers.hhs.gov) or by telephone (800-822-7967). Suspected cases of vaccine-preventable diseases should be reported to the state or local health department. Additional information, including precautions and contraindications for vaccination, is available from CDC online (http://www.cdc.gov/vaccines) or by telephone (800-CDC-INFO [800-232-4636]).

Section 5-5

PEDIATRIC INJECTIONS

Administering injections to newborns, infants, and children can be challenging. *Vaccines and medications will be given by various routes.* The majority of vaccines are given intramuscularly, but others are given the subcutaneous route. Table 5-4 lists specifics about each site used in pediatrics.

Table 5-4
ADMINISTRATION SITES

Patient Age	Injection Site	Needle Size
Newborn (0–28 days)	Anterolateral thigh muscle (vastis lateralis)	5/8 inch (22–25 gauge)
Infant (1–12 months)	Anterolateral thigh muscle (vastis lateralis)	5/8–1 inch (22–25 gauge)
Patient Age	Injection Site	Needle Size
Toddler (1–2 years)	Anterolateral thigh muscle (vastis lateralis)	5/8–1 inch (22–25 gauge)
Children (3–18 years)	Anterolateral thigh muscle (vastis lateralis) or deltoid if muscle mass is adequate	1–1¼ inch (22–25 gauge)

Field Tips

Tips for Administering Parenteral Medications on an Infant or Young Child

1. Prepare all syringes in the medicine room, out of the patient's view.
2. It is important to properly immobilize infants and young children during injections. Eliciting help from another staff member will aid in safe administration of medications.

(continues)

(continued)

3. When no assistance is available, you can secure an infant patient by placing your non-dominant hand over the knee to secure it and injecting with your dominant hand.

4. Distraction techniques sometimes work to alleviate anxiety; for example, having the child blow into a noisemaker during administration helps the child concentrate on something other than the needle.

Procedure 5-2

ADMINISTERING AN INTRAMUSCULAR INJECTION (IM) TO AN INFANT AND CHILD (ANTEROLATERAL THIGH OR DELTOID)

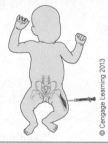

© Cengage Learning 2013

Figure 5-6: Vastus lateralis injectionsite in the pediatric patient.

Equipment and Supplies

Needle Syringe Vaccine information sheet (VIS)	Cotton ball/gauze Vaccine Authorization form	Adhesive bandage Gloves	Alcohol pad

Steps

1. Wash hands and assemble equipment.

2. Identify the patient with two identifiers (name and date of birth).

3. Provide the caregiver with a vaccine information statement (VIS) for each vaccine to be given and have the caregiver sign a consent form authorizing the patient to have the vaccines.

4. Lay the infant or child on a table to prevent movement while injecting the vaccine.

5. Wash hands and apply gloves.

6. If possible, have child relax the muscle before insertion. Insert needle at a 90-degree angle (in a rapid fashion) into the anterolateral thigh muscle or deltoid muscle above the level of the axilla and below the acromion process.
Check drug packaging insert regarding aspiration.

7. Withdraw needle and discard in the sharps container.

8. Apply bandage to injection site.

9. Remove gloves.

10. Wash hands.

11. Document the procedure.

ITEMS TO BE DOCUMENTED

1. Record date and time of administration.

2. Record name of medication and strength.

3. Record route of administration.

4. Record exact location of injection.

5. Record who ordered the medication.

6. If applicable, record the manufacturer's name, lot number on bottle, and expiration date.

7. If applicable, record VIS distribution information including the date on the VIS.

8. Record any complications or concerns.

9. Sign appropriate closing signature.

CHARTING EXAMPLE

| 12/14/XXXX 9:00 a.m. | Hepatitis B vaccine (#2) per Dr. Chase, 0.5 mL IM, R anterolateral thigh, VIS (May XXXX) given to mom prior to administration. Authorization form signed. No complications prior to or following the procedure. J. Dudy RN |

IMMUNIZATION LOG

Vaccine Name	Manufacturer Name	Lot No.	Expiration Date	Provider	Person who Administered
HBV	Merck	98786D	01/(XXXX)	Dr. Chase	J Dudy RN

EMR Application

Many EMR programs have a section that stores medication lot number information. Once the lot information has been entered, the assistant entering the information just pulls up the vaccine log and enters the lot number of the medication. The manufacturer's name, expiration date and route that the medication is given automatically populates, saving lots of time for the person recording the information.

Procedure 5-3

ADMINISTER SUBCUTANEOUS INJECTION TO AN INFANT OR CHILD

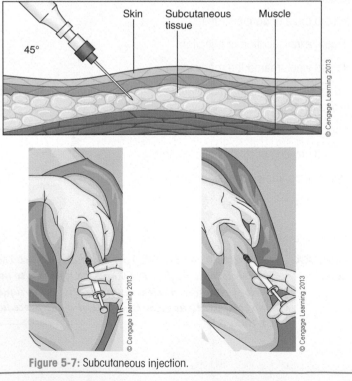

Figure 5-7: Subcutaneous injection.

Equipment and Supplies

Needle Syringe Vaccine Informa- tion Sheet	Cotton ball/gauze Vaccine/ medication Authorization forms	Adhesive bandage Gloves	Alcohol pad

Steps

1. Wash hands and assemble equipment (Medication is usually prepared in medication room).

2. Identify the patient with two identifiers (name and date of birth).

3. Provide the caregiver with a VIS for each vaccine given. Give caregiver instructions for signing consent form if applicable.

4. It is important that the infant or child is on a table to prevent movement while injecting the vaccine.

5. Rewash hands and Apply gloves.

6. Grasp the subcutaneous tissue and insert needle at a 45-degree angle to the skin (Figure 5-7a and b). (Check drug packaging insert regarding aspiration.)

7. Withdraw needle and discard in sharps container.

8. Apply bandage to injection site.

9. Remove gloves.

10. Wash hands.

Section 5-6

TELEPHONE SCREENING FOR THE PEDIATRIC PATIENT

Table 5-5 is designed to help the health care worker who will be screening phone calls in a pediatric setting. It is a quick-glance chart that categorizes the order in which patients with particular diseases and conditions should be seen. Check with providers in your particular practice for approval before implementing this chart.

Table 5-5

TELEPHONE SCREENING FOR THE PEDIATRIC PATIENT

Call EMS	Should Be Seen in Office ASAP	Should Be Seen the Same Day—24 Hours	Should Be Seen Within the Week
Any life-threatening injuries	Abdominal pain (acute), especially if right-sided, or if other sx are present	Abdominal pain (chronic), s̄ any other sx	Behavioral or emotional problems
Any life-threatening illnesses	Asthma (acute attack), but not severe	Cold sx with fever >100° F	Routine check-ups
Anaphylactic reactions (e.g., bee stings)	Burns on genitals, buttocks, hands, feet, or face	Diarrhea (chronic) s̄ any other sx	Routine general concerns
Asthma (severe attacks)	Cough that is productive or in association with fever or breathing problems	Fever <100.6° F under age of 2 mo (no other sx)	Usual follow-up examinations
Breathing difficulties	Croup, if in conjunction with other sx	Fever <103° F over the age of 6 mo.	
Burns that are severe	Diarrhea (acute) >4–6 stools in 12-hour period, or connected with acute pain or high fever	Fever connected to chronic illness	
Hemorrhaging	Possible Dehydration cases	Headache (chronic) s̄ other sx	
Poisonous substance ingestion	Ear pain	Prescription renewals	
Seizure (first time)	Eye infections or eye injuries	Rash (persistent diaper rash)	
Shock	Fever >100.6° F if under the age of 2 mo	Rash (asymptomatic)	

Unconscious patient	Fever >103° F if over the age of 6 mo	Seizure (follow-up if no current sx are present)
	Fever >101° F if in conjunction with acute illness	Stomach upset, any other sx
	Headache (migraine variant)	Stools (blood with no other sx)
	Headache, with high fever, stiff neck, visual disturbances, vomiting, or strange behavior	Strains (mild pain)
	Insect bites or stings that look suspicious or infected (any insect or animal bite)	Urinary sx (chronic back pain or fever)
	Lacerations that are gaping, other wounds that might be infected, dog bites that break the skin, or any red streaks that run upward from a wound	Vomiting (mild in nature), without severe pain, or high fever
	Poison follow-ups (if directed by Poison Control Center)	
	Rashes that are in conjunction with fever, earache, sore throat, or that might be related to a medication	

(continues)

(continued)

Call EMS	Should Be Seen in Office ASAP	Should Be Seen the Same Day—24 Hours	Should Be Seen Within the Week
	Sore throat with fever >100° F, pus patches, swollen glands, stiff neck, or acting very ill		
	Sprains or strains (possible), very painful		
	Unconscious (patient was unconscious and is now conscious)		
	Urinary symptoms, if in conjunction with fever, back pain, or vomiting, vaginal or penile discharge		
	Vomiting (severe) or blood present or persisting >24 hours		

Disclaimer: Provider Should Pre-approve Telephone Screening Chart Prior to Implementation.

Section 5-7

COMMON PEDIATRIC DISEASES AND DISORDERS

Table 5-6 lists common pediatric diseases and disorders. It defines each of the illnesses, lists the symptoms to look for, presents the usual treatments, and provides possible diagnostic testing that may be needed for each. Disclaimer: The following table is strictly a reference guide and is not intended to be used for diagnosing or prescribing. May be helpful in anticipating what the provider may order. (Do not perform any test or treatment without an order from the provider.)

Table 5-6

COMMON PEDIATRIC DISEASES AND DISORDERS

Disease	Definition	Symptoms	Usual Treatment
Asthma	A lung disease characterized by (1) airway(s) obstruction that is reversible, (2) airway(s) inflammation, and (3) increase in airway(s) responsiveness to a variety of stimuli	Will vary. Some airway obstruction of varying degree, hyperventilation, coughing and wheezing, inability to speak, fatigue, cyanosis, severe distress, confusion, and lethargy	Rescue medications: Bronchodilators—albuterol or Xopenex; drug therapy may include any of the following: long-acting beta-adrenergic agents and corticosteroids
Diagnostic Testing for Asthma Patients: May include any of the following: arterial blood gas (ABG) (hospital test), sputum analysis, chest x-ray, pulmonary function testing, and breath sounds			
Diaper dermatitis	A rash that can appear anywhere in the groin region or in the gluteal folds of the buttocks. It usually starts from a moist diaper that rubs against the skin. The rash may become infected with bacteria or yeast.	Skin will have patches of erythematous tissue that sometimes contain exudative patches varying in size and shape. Red base pustules may occur.	Air-drying the skin can help the rash, as can changing the diaper often and applying a protective barrier that contains zinc.
Eczema	Superficial skin inflammation that occurs in children who have a genetic tendency toward allergies	Inflamed skin characterized by vesicles, redness, edema, oozing, crusting, scaling. Itching may be a problem as well.	Removal of offending agent; oral and/or topical corticosteroids may also be used.
Diagnostic Testing for Eczema: May include patch testing			
Gastroenteritis	A syndrome of vomiting and diarrhea caused by pathogenic microorganisms that may lead to dehydration and an electrolyte imbalance	Will vary, but may include any of the following: diarrhea, vomiting, and dehydration; symptoms such as lethargy, anorexia, fever, oliguria, and weight loss	Oral rehydration therapy; antibiotic therapy in bacterial infections

(continues)

(continued)

Disease	Definition	Symptoms	Usual Treatment
Diagnostic Testing for Gastroenteritis: May include any of the following: hematocrit, serum electrolytes, urinalysis, stool cultures, and complete blood count (CBC)			
Impetigo	A bacterial vesicular skin infection that is usually caused from a break in the skin's surface or irritation of the nostril from a runny nose.	Lesions that may be located on the arms, legs, and face. Lesions may be from the size of a pea to very large. Exudate may be present and may crust over. Some itching may be present.	Systemic antibiotics and topical antibiotics
Otitis media	A bacterial or viral infection of the middle ear. Usually secondary to an upper respiratory infection (URI). Most common in ages 3 months to 3 years.	Severe earache, fever, nausea/vomiting, and diarrhea. May have a discharge when tympanic membrane is ruptured.	Antibiotic therapy
Pinworms (*Enterobius vermicularis*)	Small, white, thread-like worms that may enter the body through the oral route from food or from placing contaminated objects in the mouth. Eggs hatch in the intestines, where they quickly become adult worms and multiply rapidly. Female worms lay eggs near the anus at night, causing itching. The child scratches and picks up eggs on the fingers. The oral-fecal route is established; others are soon infected. Direct transfer of eggs is from the anus to the mouth; indirectly with eggs in clothing and sheets.	Severe anal itching, increased hunger, stomachache, restless sleep; observing worms around the anus during the night with a flashlight or before bowel movement (also irritability)	Oral medication for the entire family; topical medication for anal irritation; scrupulous hygiene; shorten fingernails; launder items in hottest water possible

Pityriasis rosea	A self-limited, mild, inflammatory skin disease characterized by scaly lesions, possibly due to an unidentified infectious agent	A "herald patch" or "mother patch" commonly found on the trunk. It is slightly erythematous and rose- or fawn-colored. It has a slightly raised border and resembles ringworm. Similar lesions may occur that can be anywhere from 0.5 to 2.0 cm in diameter. Patient may have some itching.	Usually none. Sunlight may help. Prednisone may be used in cases in which itching is a major factor.

Diagnostic Testing for Pityriasis Rosea: May include a serological test for syphilis because the lesions can resemble those that occur with secondary syphilis

Pneumonia	Acute infection of the lung parenchyma, including the alveolar spaces and interstitial tissue Usually secondary to an upper respiratory tract infection	Will vary, but may include fever, pain on breathing, dyspnea, chills, cough, sputum production, an increase in pulse and respiration, nausea, vomiting, malaise, and myalgias	Antibiotic therapy

Diagnostic Testing for Pneumonia: May include a chest x-ray and sputum analysis

Scabies	Caused by the itch mite *Sarcoptes scabiei.* The impregnated female mite tunnels her way into the epidermis and deposits her eggs along the burrow. Larvae hatch within a few days and congregate along the hair follicle.	Severe itching, which is intensified when the patient is in a supine position. Initial lesions are burrows that have fine, wavy, dark lines anywhere from a few millimeters to 1 cm long, with a minute papule at the open end. Lesions occur on the finger webs, wrists, elbows, axillary folds, trunk, and extremities.	5% permethrin cream; the whole family should be treated.

(continues)

(continued)

Disease	Definition	Symptoms	Usual Treatment
Streptococcal pharyngitis	Invasion of streptococcus in the throat region	Will vary. Sore throat, may have erythema, and/or pustules, high fever, possible rash	Antibiotic therapy, e.g., penicillin (G or V)
Diagnostic Testing for Streptococcal Pharyngitis: May include a throat culture and a rapid strep test			
Upper respiratory infection	Viral infection of the respiratory tract with inflammation in any or all of the airways	Nasal or throat discomfort followed by sneezing, rhinorrhea, and malaise	Rest, analgesics, nasal decongestants, and antihistamines
Diagnostic Testing for Upper Respiratory Infection: May include physical assessment and smear of any exudates			
Urinary tract infection	Invasion of bacteria in the urinary tract. May be asymptomatic or with the manifestation of cystitis or pyelonephritis	Will vary, but may include dysuria, urinary frequency, hematuria, urinary retention, suprapubic pain, urinary incontinence, or foul-smelling urine	Antibiotics with increased fluid intake
Diagnostic Testing for Urinary Tract Infections: May include urinalysis, culture, and sensitivity			

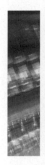

Section Six
ASSISTING IN AN OB-GYN PRACTICE

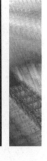

INTRODUCTION

This section is designed to assist those individuals who work in obstetrics and gynecology (OB-GYN) practices. Some of its content will also be useful for those working in internal medicine and family practice.

This section provides the medical assistant with screening questions to ask at the time of an annual examination, pelvic examination, and OB examination. Other features of this section include common diseases and disorders of the female reproductive system, common gynecological diagnostic testing, and common OB diagnostic testing.

Section 6-1
GYNECOLOGICAL SCREENINGS AND PROCEDURES

It is important to complete a thorough screening of GYN patients before examination. Responses gathered during the screening will affect the way the patient disrobes and the way the room is set up.

Assisting with a Pap Examination

A Papanicolaou (Pap) test is done to evaluate the cervical tissue for changes. The speculum is placed into the vagina and opened to expose the cervix. The provider will then take a few cells from inside and around the cervix. The cells are placed in a liquid medium or on a prepared slide. Table 6-1 provides information that should be documented before a Pap test.

Table 6-1

SCREENING INFORMATION THAT SHOULD BE DOCUMENTED BEFORE PAP PROCEDURES

1. Today's date and time

2. Last Pap test and results

3. Last mammogram and results

(continues)

(continued)

4. G P A
  • Gravida: Pregnancies
  • Para: Births
  • Abortions (Spontaneous/Elective)

5. Last menstrual period (LMP)

6. Form of birth control/hormone therapy

7. Any gynecological surgeries

8. Number of sexual partners (Provider may want to ask this!)

9. Any current problems including:
  • Vaginal discharge
  • Pain during intercourse
  • Vaginal redness, itching, or burning
  • Any urinary symptoms
  • Breast concerns (How often performing breast self-examinations?)

10. Closing signature.

CHARTING EXAMPLE

9-18-XXXX 10:30 a.m.	Pt. here for annual Pap & pelvic exam. Last Pap, 10-18-XXXX (normal), G: 3 P: 3 A: 0. LMP: 09-1-XXXX, BC: Ortho Evra, GYN Surg: None, Sex part (1), no breast concerns or changes, "Performs monthly BSE". Latania Carter, CMA (AAMA)

Figure 6-1 illustrates the items that should be on a Pap tray.

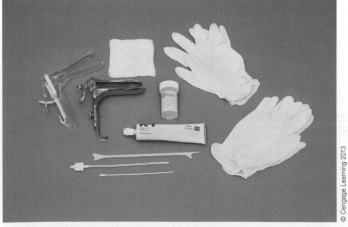

© Cengage Learning 2013

Figure 6-1: A tray setup for a pelvic examination and Pap test when using a liquid prep solution.

Procedure 6-1

ASSIST WITH A PAP EXAMINATION

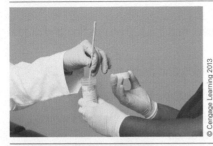

Figure 6-2: The medical assistant holds the vial for the provider as the provider places the broom into the ThinPrep solution.

© Cengage Learning 2013

Equipment and Supplies

	Conventional/direct method:	Liquid Medium method:
2 or 3 Pairs examination gloves Patient gown and drape Vaginal speculum/Light source Lubricant Culturing swabs (if applicable) Tissues Biohazard specimen bag Laboratory requisition	Glass slides Fixative Cervical spatula Endocervical brush Slide holder	Liquid Medium vial Cervical spatula Endocervical brush Endocervical broom (when using broom for collection)

1. Wash your hands and set up all needed equipment. Warm the speculum.

2. Label the specimens.

   Direct method: Label slides with the patient's name, the date, and source (V) = vaginal, (C) = cervical, or (E) = endocervical.

   ThinPrep method: Label the specimen container with the patient's name, date, and identification (ID) number (from laboratory request form).

3. Identify the patient using at least two identifiers, identify yourself, and instruct the patient to empty her bladder and collect the urine specimen in the event testing is necessary.

4. Obtain the patient's blood pressure and weight and update her medical and GYN history.

5. Explain the procedure to the patient and instruct her to undress completely and to put the gown on so that it opens correctly (check provider preference).

(continues)

(continued)

6. Instruct the patient to sit on the examination table until the provider enters the room.

7. After the provider enters, assist the patient into the supine position and drape for the breast examination.

8. Assist the patient into the lithotomy position and drape for privacy.

9. Hand the warmed vaginal speculum/light source to the provider.

10. Hand the spatula and brush to the provider when using the direct method, or the broom when using the ThinPrep method.

11. Apply clean gloves in order to receive the specimen(s).

   Direct method: Hold the slides so the provider can apply the collected cells to the slides. Immediately spray the slides with fixative from a distance of 6 inches. Allow the slides to dry for 10 minutes before placing in a holder.

   Liquid medium method: Hold the opened vial so the provider can place the broom in the vial (Figure 6-2). Agitate the broom in the solution until the entire specimen has been suspended in the liquid. Dispose of the broom in a biohazard container.

12. Squeeze lubricant on the provider's gloved fingers for the bimanual examination.

13. If applicable, supply the provider with culture swabs and put aside for processing.

14. After the provider completes the examination, assist the patient into a sitting position and give her tissues for lubricant removal.

15. Properly dispose of biohazardous wastes and other used supplies and soak the stainless steel speculum in a soapy solution. Sanitize and sterilize the speculum when convenient.

16. Instruct the patient to get dressed.

17. Prepare the specimen(s) and laboratory requisition for transport.

18. Remove gloves, wash your hands, and document the specimen preparation and the destination lab in the patient's chart.

Field Tip

Sometimes the provider will also perform a rectal examination toward the end of the pelvic examination. The medical assistant should be prepared to provide the provider with a new glove and lubricant following the vaginal examination. Also be prepared to hold an occult blood card out for the provider to smear a stool sample on at the conclusion of the rectal examination.

Breast Self-Examination

Breast self-examination (BSE) is an important part of a preventive health plan. Performing BSE on a monthly basis will increase your chances of detecting breast cancer in its early stages. According to the National Cancer Institute,

- One in eight women will be diagnosed with breast cancer in their lifetime.
- Over 200,000 women will be diagnosed with breast cancer this year.
- When breast cancer is detected early (localized stage), the 5-year survival rate is 98%.
- Over 30% of women are diagnosed after breast cancer has spread beyond the localized stage.

Patient Instruction 6-1
BREAST SELF-EXAMINATION

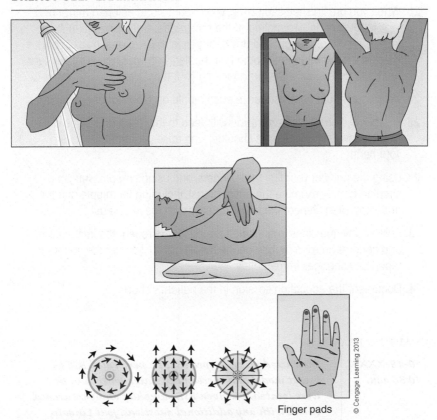

Finger pads

© Cengage Learning 2013

Figure 6-3: Three methods of BSE should be performed monthly in the shower, in front of mirror, and while lying down.

(continues)

(continued)

Equipment and Supplies

Pamphlet/shower hanger on BSE	Breast model

1. Greet the patient, identify yourself, and explain the purpose of BSE.

2. Give the patient a brochure and begin explaining the proper procedure for performing BSE. Explain to the patient that the breasts should be examined in the shower, in front of a mirror, and while lying down (Figure 6-3).

   Instruct the patient to do the following:

2a. Examine your breasts at the same time each month, preferably a few days to a week following your menstrual period. Start by covering the right breast with a soapy lather while you are in the shower and place your right arm over your head. Gently glide your fingers over the entire breast and axilla feeling for any lumps or thickening. Repeat the procedure with the left breast.

2b. When you are finished showering, you should stand before a mirror and look for puckering or dimpling of the skin, redness or a change in skin texture, nipple retraction, and any changes in the size or shape of your breasts. The examination should be repeated with your hands raised over her head and again with your hands on your hips.

2c. Next, you should gently squeeze each nipple and look for any discharge.

2d. For the next part of the exam, you will need to lay down and place a small pillow under your right shoulder and raise your right arm over your head.

2e. Using the pads of your first three fingers, and using firm pressure, in a circular motion, examine the entire breast, including the nipple and the underarm area. Repeat the entire process with the left breast.

3. Answer any questions and instruct the patient to repeat the instructions and perform an examination on the breast model. Instruct the patient to report any changes immediately.

4. Document the education session in the patient's chart.

CHARTING EXAMPLE

10-18-XXXX 10:30 a.m.	Instructed pt. on proper BSE. Pt. performed BSE on breast model and successfully stated where lumps were located. Pt. given BSE pamphlet and encouraged to call with any additional questions. Joni Lingale, RMA

Assisting with a Pelvic Examination

A pelvic examination is done to evaluate the size and position of the vagina, cervix, and uterus. It is important to explain the procedure to patients who have not had the procedure previously. A pelvic examination may be performed in conjunction with the Pap test or may be performed independently when the patient has urogential symptoms. Table 6-2 provides screening information to be documented before the pelvic examination.

Table 6-2

SCREENING INFORMATION TO BE DOCUMENTED BEFORE PELVIC EXAMINATIONS

1. Today's date and time

2. Form of birth control or other medications

3. Any drug allergies

4. LMP

5. Number of sexual partners

6. Current vaginal symptoms:
   - Vaginal discharge (Describe)
   - Vaginal itching or tenderness
   - Vaginal odor
   - Vaginal redness

7. Any abdominal pain? (Rate pain)

8. Any lower back pain? (Rate pain)

9. Any fever?

10. Any urinary symptoms?

11. Any rectal itching or pain?

12. What has patient done for symptoms? (Any relief?)

13. Closing signature.

CHARTING EXAMPLE

9-18-XXXX 10:30 a.m.	BC: None, Other meds: None, Drug allergies: Tetracycline. LMP: 09/05/XXXX, # of sexual partners: 1. Pt. c/o urogenital sx × 2 weeks. ⊕ vag discharge ("white and thick"), ⊕ vaginal itching, ⊕ redness, ⊖ odor. ⊖ abdominal or lower back pain. ⊖ fever, ⊖ urinary sx or rectal itching. Pt has not taken anything for sx. Azeller, CMA (AAMA)

Procedure 6-2

ASSIST WITH PELVIC EXAMINATIONS

Equipment and Supplies

2 or 3 Pairs examination gloves
Patient gown and drape
Vaginal speculum
Water-soluble lubricant
	Appropriate cultures
	Gauze squares/Tissues
	Cytology request/
	  Laboratory forms
		Biohazard container
		Transfer bag
		Urine container
		  (If applicable)

1. Wash your hands and set up all needed equipment. Warm the speculum.

2. Label the culture medium with the patient's name, date, and ID number.

3. Identify the patient using at least two identifiers, identify yourself, and instruct the patient to empty her bladder and collect urine specimen if urinary symptoms are present.

4. Obtain the patient's blood pressure and weight and update her medical and GYN history.

5. Explain the procedure to the patient and instruct her to undress from the waist down and to place a drape over her lap.

6. Instruct the patient to sit on the examination table until the provider enters the room.

7. After the provider enters, assist the patient into the lithotomy position and drape for privacy.

8. Hand the warmed vaginal speculum with light source to the provider.

9. Hand the provider any necessary culture swabs.

10. If provider chooses to perform a bimanual examination, squeeze lubricant on provider's gloved fingers for the examination.

11. After the provider completes the examination, assist the patient into a sitting position and give her tissues for cleansing the vaginal area.

12. Instruct the patient to get dressed and provide her with any parting instructions. Dismiss patient.

13. Properly dispose of biohazardous wastes and other used supplies and soak the stainless steel speculum in a soapy solution. Sanitize and sterilize the speculum when convenient.

14. Prepare the specimen and laboratory requisition for transport.

15. Remove gloves, wash your hands, and document the procedure in the patient's chart.

Assisting with a Colposcopy Procedure

A colposcopy is performed after an abnormal Pap test result. The procedure is usually done in the office with a setup similar to that for a Pap test or pelvic examination.

A colposcope is an electric microscope that is positioned approximately 30 cm from the vagina to view the cervix. A bright light on the end of the colposcope lets the provider clearly see the cervix.

Procedure 6-3

ASSIST WITH COLPOSCOPY AND CERVICAL BIOPSY

Equipment and Supplies

Instruments to Be Placed on the Sterile Field	Solutions and Supplies to Be Placed on the Field	Items to Be Placed to the Side of the Field
Sterile containers (3) Vaginal speculum Cervical punch biopsy forceps Uterine tenaculum Uterine dressing forceps	Acetic acid 3% or vinegar Normal saline solution Gram's iodine or Lugol's solution Sterile Sponges Cotton tipped applicators (sterile and long)	Colposcope Sterile gloves Labeled specimen container with preservative Silver nitrate sticks Tampons or pads Regular iodine product Lab requisition form

1. Wash hands and set up sterile tray and side table. Pour the acetic acid, saline and iodine into their respective containers. Cover tray with sterile drape if office policy.

2. Make certain light on colposcope is functional.

3. Explain procedure to patient and make certain consent form is signed.

4. Place patient into the dorsal lithotomy position and drape for privacy. If necessary, assist provider in positioning the colposcope.

5. If gloved and assisting provider, give provider sterile swabs immersed in appropriate solutions as requested.

(continues)

(continued)

6. If not already gloved, wash hands and glove to receive biopsy specimen.

7. If applicable, hand provider silver nitrate sticks to control bleeding.

8. Assist patient to a sitting position following the procedure and provide patient with home care instructions. Dismiss patient.

9. Label specimens, complete lab requisition forms and prepare specimens for transport.

10. Care for or dispose of equipment. Clean the room.

11. Dispose of biohazards and trash in proper receptacles and clean and disinfect colposcope and room.

12. Wash your hands and document the procedure in the patient's chart.

Field Tips

1. Procedure should be scheduled 1 week following the last day of patient's menstrual period.
2. Patient should be instructed not to douche or have intercourse 24 hours before procedure. (This could interfere with the testing process.)
3. Fill out requisition forms and label biopsy container before procedure.
4. Have patient sign consent form.
5. Check colposcope to make sure it is in working order at least 24 hours before the test and on the day of the test. If unit is not working properly, you may have time to repair it.
6. Be accessible to both the provider and patient during the procedure. Procedure may cause cramping; watch and listen for verbal and nonverbal messages.

CHARTING EXAMPLE

6-25-XXXX 10:30 a.m.	Follow-up on abnormal Pap exam. Pt. here to have colposcopy today. Explained procedure and homecare instructions. Consent form signed. Specimens sent to ABC lab. S. Mueller, CMA (AAMA)

Assisting with Cryosurgery or Cryotherapy

The purpose of this procedure is to freeze the cervix to stimulate new growth of tissue in patients who suffer from chronic cervicitis and erosion of the cervix. The cryotherapy unit may contain liquid nitrogen or carbon dioxide as the cooling agents.

Procedure 6-4

ASSIST WITH CRYOSURGERY OR CRYOTHERAPY

Equipment and Supplies

Items to Be Placed on the Sterile Field	Items to Be Placed at the Side of the Field
Sterile container/cup Vaginal speculum Cotton-tipped applicators (long and sterile) Sterile 4x4 with sterile lubricant	1. Cryosurgery unit and tips 2. Gloves (Both sterile and non-sterile) 3. Sanitary napkins 4. Acid-saline 5. Biohazard waste container 6. Silver nitrate sticks

1. Wash hands and set up sterile tray and side table. Pour acid-saline solution into sterile container.

2. Ascertain that cryosurgery unit is in good working order.

3. Explain the procedure to patient and have patient sign consent form.

4. Have patient disrobe completely from waist down. Provide patient with drape and exit room.

5. Upon re-entering the room, place the patient into the dorsal lithotomy position and drape for privacy.

6. Assist provider with cryotherapy unit as necessary.

7. Check on patient throughout the procedure. Patient may experience cramping.

8. When procedure is finished, assist patient to a sitting position. Provide home care instructions and dismiss patient.

9. Clean and disinfect any equipment used and the procedure room.

10. Wash hands and document any educational instructions or materials given to patient.

Section 6-2

GYNECOLOGICAL CONDITIONS

Gynecological infections are common among women of childbearing age. The risk for infection increases when a woman has a new sexual partner or more than one partner. GYN infections are usually manifested by odor

Field Tips

1. Inform patient of what to expect during the procedure. Patient may feel some cramping.
2. Be available to both the patient and the provider during the procedure.
3. Watch and listen for verbal and nonverbal messages from the patient.
4. Tell patient that she should refrain from intercourse for 1 month following the procedure.
5. Tell patient that she should expect a heavy watery discharge for the first 6 days that will subside but may continue for up to 4 weeks.
6. Tell patient that the first period may be heavier than normal and involve more cramping.

and discharge. Table 6-3 lists common vaginal infections. Table 6-4 lists common sexually transmitted infections.

Table 6-3

COMMON VAGINAL INFECTIONS

Possible Disorder/ Cause	Vaginal Symptoms	Diagnostic Testing
Trichomoniasis Cause: A parasite— Trichomonas vaginalis	Thin foamy vaginal discharge Color: Yellow-green Odor: Foul odor Pain: During intercourse lower belly pain may be present. (Considered a sexually transmitted infection STI.)	If sending out to a laboratory, place in sterile culture medium. If reading in office, set up a wet mount.
Candida moniliasis (yeast) Cause: A type of yeast— Candida albicans May be referred to as a candidal infection, or candidiasis.	Scanty discharge/ cottage cheese–like appearance. Color: White Odor: None Vaginal redness and itching.	If sending out to a laboratory, place proper medium. If reading in office, set up a KOH/and wet prep.

Bacterial Vaginosis	Watery vaginal	If sending out to a labo-
Cause: A change in the balance of bacteria that is present in the vagina	discharge *Color:* Milky *Odor:* Fishy *External genitalia:* Edema and itching (Not an STI)	ratory, place in proper culture medium. If reading in office, set up wet prep/mount, and whiff test.

Wet Prep Instructions: Place swabbed contents into 0.5 mL of saline. Hang swab over slide and let 1 drop fall onto slide. Place cover slip over drop and place under microscope.

KOH/Wet Prep: Follow instructions for wet prep but add 1 drop of KOH to the drop before placing cover slip over it.

Whiff Test: Place a couple of drops of KOH on speculum. Provider will check to see if there is a fishy odor present after KOH is applied.

Disclaimer: Never run any test without an order from the provider!

Table 6-4
COMMON SEXUALLY TRANSMITTED INFECTIONS

Infection	Symptoms	Diagnostic Testing
Gonorrhea	Initially: **Vaginal discharge:** Yellow and purulent **Urinary discomfort** and frequency may also be present. **Progressive symptoms:** Acute abdominal pain and fever (PID symptoms)	**Set up:** DNA probe or Thayer Martin Culture. (Agar plate should be stored in refrigerator, but brought to room temperature before it is plated.)
Chlamydia	Many patients are asymptomatic. If symptoms are present: Vaginal discharge which may be thick, and white or yellow in color. **Odor:** Usually negative **Progressive symptoms:** Acute abdominal pain and fever (pelvic inflammatory disease [PID] symptoms)	**Set up:** Viral transport medium **Blood work:** May order serum-antibody detection or direct-antigen detection

(continues)

(continued)

Infection	Symptoms	Diagnostic Testing
Herpes simplex, type II	**Initially:** Painful blisters on vulva. Outbreak may last 10 days to 2 weeks. Flu-like symptoms may follow. Virus will stay in body throughout the patient's life.	**Set up:** Herpes or viral culture. Provider may want to perform Tzanck smear; will look at the tissue taken from the sores.
Syphilis	**Initially:** Chancre sore on vulva, vagina, and cervix, anus, or lips or in the mouth. A rash may appear for a short time following the chancre. The spirochete can live in the body for years, destroying additional tissue.	**Blood work:** Rapid plasma reagin (RPR) test or Venereal Disease Research Laboratory (VDRL) test
Condyloma, genital warts, human papilloma virus (HPV)	**Tiny warts, bumps, or cauliflower growths:** Granules may be flat and barely visible. **Color:** Flesh-colored, pink, or darker than surrounding tissue. Virus stays in body forever and may cause abnormal Pap smear results.	**In office:** Pelvic examination or colposcopy for visual examination. May confirm through a Pap test **Treatment:** Provider may want assistant to set out a topical chemical such as podophyllin, or provider may decide to use heat, laser, or freezing as other methods to eliminate warts.
Acquired immunodeficiency syndrome (AIDS), the result of HIV infection	**Multiple symptoms:** Lymph node enlargement, fevers, persistent diarrhea, chronic fatigue, anorexia, arthralgia, and adenopathy **Progressive symptoms:** A host of opportunistic infections and diseases	**Blood work:** Initial: HIV test; if positive, enzyme-linked immunosorbent (ELISA) test; if that is positive, a Western blot test is performed to confirm diagnosis. *Confirmation of AIDS:* The presence of AIDS-related disorders and a T-cell count of 200 or less

| **Pelvic inflammatory disease (PID)** | Severe infections such as chlamydia or gonorrhea can lead to PID. The patient may experience severe lower abdominal pain or tenderness, cervical discharge, fever, and adjacent tenderness. PID is more common in young girls in their late teens and early 20s who are sexually active and have multiple sexual partners, but seen in other age-groups as well. | **Cultures:** Gonococcal (GC) and chlamydia culture or set out a DNA probe

Blood work: Complete blood count (CBC) and erythrocyte sedimentation rate (ESR)

Other diagnostic testing: Laparoscopy |

Disclaimer: Do not perform any testing without an order from a provider!

Section 6-3

GYNECOLOGICAL DIAGNOSTIC TESTS AND PROCEDURES

Diagnostic tests and procedures for gynecological issues are valuable to assist the provider in determining appropriate therapy. Some of the procedures listed in Table 6-5 are performed in the office setting and many others are performed in a procedure room or operating room.

Table 6-5

GYNECOLOGICAL DIAGNOSTIC TESTS AND PROCEDURES

Test Name	Description	Indicated Conditions
Colposcopy	Examination of the vaginal and cervical tissues using an instrument called a colposcope	Abnormal Pap smears: Used to select sites of abnormal cell growth, evaluate benign lesions, and define tumor extension
Loop electrosurgical excision procedure (LEEP)	LEEP quickly removes abnormal tissue from the cervix.	Dysplasia

(continues)

(continued)

Test Name	Description	Indicated Conditions
Hysteroscopy	A hysteroscope is inserted into the uterus to permit visual examination of the uterus and its surrounding tissue.	Uterine fibroids, bleeding, and other abnormalities. Abnormal tissue may be extracted for biopsy.
Pap smear	Cells are collected from the vagina and cervix and sent to a laboratory for analysis.	Prevention tool for vaginal, cervical, and uterine cancer
Endometrial biopsy	Removing tissue from the uterine endometrium for evaluative purposes	Abnormal uterine bleeding and infertility
Laparoscopy or pelviscopy	Abdominal exploration through a laparoscope. Allows provider to examine uterus, fallopian tubes, and ovaries through two tiny incisions	Adhesions, fibroids, cysts, endometriosis, and ectopic pregnancies Tubal sterilization and ovary removal are performed using this procedure.
Ultrasonography	Sound waves instead of x-rays to produce images of the uterus, ovaries, and fetus	Used to determine fetal age, size, and various fetal abnormalities Also used to detect abnormalities of the ovaries and uterus including tubal pregnancies, fibroids, and cysts
Dilation and curettage	Dilating the cervix and scraping a portion of endometrial lining	Heavy bleeding, miscarriages, and removal of small growths It also can provide biopsy samples for evaluation and diagnosis.
Dilation and evacuation	Evacuation of the products of conception from the uterine cavity	Missed abortion, elective termination of the pregnancy

| Endometrial ablation | The use of electric current or a laser to destroy the entire uterine endometrium | Used to control heavy bleeding
Pregnancy and child-birth are no longer possible after this procedure. |
| Hysterosalpingogram (HSG) | Radiographic study of the fallopian tubes into which a radiopaque dye is introduced to check tube patency | Performed on women who have a difficult time conceiving |

Section 6-4

ASSISTING WITH THE OBSTETRICAL EXAMINATION

This section will discuss preparing the pregnant women for a prenatal examination. Table 6-6 will assist you in obtaining a specific history based on the gestation age. The table also gives common advice provided to pregnant women who call the office with questions. The provider should review the table and approve the protocol listed before giving the patient instructions over the telephone.

Table 6-6

ASSISTING WITH OBSTETRICAL EXAMINATIONS AND TELEPHONE SCREENINGS

Documentation Information	Special Equipment, Supplies, or Procedures	Telephone Triage Information
Expected date of confinement (EDC) Ask for the LMP on the first visit.	Fetal Doppler ultrasound, ultrasonic gel, ultrasound unit, and tape measure	Follow office protocol for how soon the patient should be seen. First appointment is usually 4–6 weeks after first missed period. Patient may perform pregnancy test at home.

(continues)

(continued)

Documentation Information	Special Equipment, Supplies, or Procedures	Telephone Triage Information
Any swelling in hands, feet, or face? Is the edema pitting?	Assist patient to lie on her left side and keep feet elevated.	If patient has an increase in swelling or pitting edema, a same-day appointment should be set.
Any vaginal bleeding? List amount (describe amount by type and number of pads used.) Has patient passed any clots or other tissue? Any cramping?	Set up for pelvic examination or ultrasound.	If bleeding is a light flow and dark in color, have patient elevate feet and call office if it gets worse. All other bleeding should be evaluated either in the office or at the hospital. Follow office protocol.
Any chance of an amniotic leak? It may be light in color but cloudy. May contain some floating particles.	Set up the following: Pelvic tray pH paper Speculum Microscope slide	**After 36 weeks:** Send to hospital. **Before 36 weeks:** If patient is not experiencing any contractions, have patient come directly into office. If in combination with contractions, send directly to the hospital.
Any unusual vaginal discharge? List color and amount.	Set up for pelvic examination. pH paper Cultures	Set up an appointment within 24–48 hours.
Any headaches, dizziness, or vision problems?	Take patient's BP; if elevated, assist patient to lie on her left side.	If severe, set appointment for the same day. If mild, suggest comfort measures approved by the provider.
Any nausea or vomiting?	Give emesis basin and make patient as comfortable as possible.	Check office protocol. Provider may want patient to come in or call something in for the patient.

Diagnostic Tests and Procedures Routinely Performed During Pregnancy

Prenatal laboratory testing is essential for the care of both the mother and fetus. Initial laboratory studies help to identify prenatal issues that may be treated (Tables 6-7, 6-8, and 6-9).

Table 6-7

ROUTINE BLOOD WORK PERFORMED ON PRENATAL PATIENTS

Test Name	Description	When Performed
Human chorionic gonadotropin (hCG) or pregnancy testing	Hormone secreted during pregnancy hCG testing may be performed on urine or blood.	First visit
Complete blood count	Checks for anemia. Many patients become anemic during pregnancy.	First visit, at 28 weeks' gestation, and as needed.
Rh factor and ABO testing	Checks to see if there is the potential of a blood incompatibility problem between mother and baby	First visit
Rubella titer	Checks the level of antibody against rubella (German measles, which may cause birth defects if contracted during pregnancy)	First visit or prenatally when patient is considering pregnancy
VDRL or RPR	Screening test for syphilis, which can cause intrauterine death or severe birth defects if contracted during pregnancy	First visit
HIV	The virus that causes AIDS. It can be transferred to the fetus.	First visit (may not be performed without consent from the patient)

(continues)

(continued)

Test Name	Description	When Performed
Antibody screen	Evaluates antibody formation in the mother	First visit, and repeated at 28 weeks with Rh-negative patient
Glucose tolerance test (GTT)	Test to determine whether the patient has gestational diabetes. This test starts with a 1-hour test; if positive will be followed up with a 3-hour test.	GTT is usually done at week 28 of pregnancy. If there is a history of gestational diabetes, this test may be done sooner.
Alpha-fetoprotein analysis (AFP)	This test is done to detect neural tube damage.	Performed between weeks 15 and 18 of pregnancy. Must obtain patient's consent

Table 6-8
ROUTINE CULTURES PERFORMED ON PRENATAL PATIENTS

Test Name	Description	When Performed
Gonorrhea	Culture to detect gonorrhea. Could cause ophthalmia neonatorum in the newborn, which could result in blindness	First visit; repeated if first culture was positive or patient is at high risk
Chlamydia	An STI. The baby could contract pneumonia or neonatal conjunctivitis if mother has chlamydia when the baby is born.	First visit; repeated if first culture was positive or patient is at high risk
Pap smear	Determines cell abnormalities such as dysplasia	First visit, unless the patient has had a pap smear in the last 12 months.

Table 6-9

OTHER OBSTETRICAL DIAGNOSTIC TESTS

Test Name	Description	Indicated Conditions When Performed
Amniocentesis	The aspiration of amniotic fluid for diagnosis of certain chromosomal disorders. The test can determine the baby's sex by chromosomal analysis.	It may be offered to high-risk patients and patients who have a family history of genetic diseases. The test is usually performed between weeks 14 and 16 of pregnancy.
Biophysical profile	Ultrasound technique to evaluate fetal activities and amniotic fluid volume. With the nonstress test (NST) results, points are given based on baby's activities. Low points may mean poor fetal outcome.	High-risk OB patient with NST indications
Fetal heart rate monitoring or NST monitoring or NST	Performed later in pregnancy to detect placental function	Performed on patients with gestational diabetes, decreased fetal movement, or decreased amniotic fluid, and patients with hypertension
Fetal heart tones	Auscultation with Doppler or fetoscope. Normal fetal heart rate is between 120 and 160 beats/min. If rate falls below 120 beats, it could indicate fetal distress.	Performed routinely at OB visits after 8–10 weeks' gestation.
Fundal height measurement	The provider measures from the top of the pubic bone to the top of the fundus. Fundal height monitors the growth of the fetus.	Performed at every OB visit after 12 weeks

(continues)

(continued)

Test Name	Description	Indicated Conditions When Performed
Fetal kick counts	Counting fetal kick movements at a specific time each day, usually after a meal or snack	Evaluate fetal well-being
Obstetrical ultrasound testing	Use of sound wave frequency to produce an image of the baby	Detection of ectopic pregnancy, abnormal bleeding; evaluation of fetal growth and sex determination; indicates presence of multiple fetuses and placental positioning

Section Seven
PHARMACOLOGY PROCEDURES

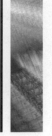

Section 7-1
DRUG CLASSIFICATIONS

This section is designed to assist those working in medical practices with spelling and classifying medications that are commonly prescribed, used over the counter, and injected into the patient. Prescription information is also found in this section.

Table 7-1
DRUG CLASSIFICATIONS AND THEIR ACTIONS

Note: Drugs that are capitalized indicate trade names. Drugs in parentheses indicate generic names.

Classification	Action	Examples
Analgesic	Relieves pain	***Non-opioid examples:*** Tylenol (acetaminophen) Bayer (aspirin) Motrin or Advil (ibuprofen) ***Narcotic examples:*** Hydrocodone w/APAP
Anesthetic	Produces a lack of feeling; may be local or general	***Local anesthetics:*** Novocain (procaine HCL) Xylocaine (lidocaine HCL) ***General anesthetic:*** Diprivan (propofol)
Angiotensin-converting enzyme (ACE) inhibitor (ACE-I)	Treats hypertension	Altace (ramipril) Prinivil (lisinopril) Vasotec (enalapril)
Antacid	Neutralizes stomach acid	Mylanta Maalox

(continues)

(continued)

Classification	Action	Examples
Antiacne	Treats acne	Accutane (isotretinoin) Differin Gel (adapalene gel)
Antianginal	Relieves the symptoms of angina	Imdur (isosorbide mononitrate) Isordil (isosorbide) Nitrostat (nitroglycerin)
Antianxiety	Relieves anxiety and muscle tension	Valium (diazepam) Xanax (alprazolam) Ativan (lorazepam)
Antiarrhythmic	Controls cardiac arrhythmias	Norpace (disopyramide) Procan SR (procainamide)
Antibiotic	Inhibits or destroys bacteria	Amoxil (amoxicillin) Bactrim (sulfamethoxazole/trimethoprim) Omnicef (cefdinir) Levaquin (levofloxacin)
Antibipolar agent	Treats bipolar disorders	Eskalith (lithium) Ability (aripiprazole)
Anticholinergic	Reduces muscle spasms in the bladder, lungs, intestines, and eye muscles (also known as an antispasmotic)	Ditropan (oxybutynin) Detrol (tolterodine)
Anticoagulant	Prevents or delays blood clotting at the platelet level	Coumadin (warfarin sodium) Dicumarol (heparin sodium) Lovenox (enoxaparin sodium)
Anticonvulsant	Prevents or relieves seizures	Keppra (levetiracetam) Neurontin (gabapentin) Tegretol (carbamazepine)
Antidepressant	Reduces or relieves symptoms of depression	Cymbalta (duloxetine) Celexa (citalopram) Effexor XR (venlafaxine) Wellbutrin-SR (bupropion)

Antidiabetic	Helps to lower blood glucose levels	***Oral hypoglycemics:*** Actos (pioglitazone) Glucophage (metformin) Micronase (glyburide) ***Forms of insulin:*** Lantus (long-acting insulin) Humulin R (short acting) Humulin N (long acting)
Antidiarrheal	Counteracts diarrhea	Kaopectate (kaolin/pectin) Pepto-Bismol (bismuth subsalicylate)
Antiemetic	Counteracts nausea and vomiting	Phenergan (promethazine) Compazine (prochlorperazine) Dramamine (dimenhydrinate)
Antiflatulant	Relieves gas and bloating in the GI tract	Gas-X (simethicone) Mylicon—infant drops
Antifungal	Reduces the growth of fungus	Diflucan (fluconazole) Monistat (miconazole) Nizoral (ketoconazole)
Antigout agent	Prevents or lessens the occurrence of gout attacks	Uloric (febuxostat) Benemid (probenecid) Zyloprim (allopurinol)
Antihistamine	Counteracts the effects of histamine in the body; helps to relieve symptoms of allergic reactions	Benadryl (diphenhydramine) Claritin (loratadine) Zyrtec (cetirizine)
Antihyperlipidemic or cholesterol-lowering agent	Helps to decrease cholesterol or lipid levels	Crestor (rosuvastatin) Lipitor (atorvastatin calcium) Zocor (simvastatin)
Antihypertensive	Reduces high blood pressure	Accupril (quinapril) Altace (ramipril) Vasotec (enalapril)
Anti-inflammatory	Reduces or relieves inflammation	Advil (ibuprofen) Motrin (ibuprofen) Bextra (naproxen) Celebrex (celecoxib)

(continues)

(continued)

Classification	Action	Examples
Antimigraine	Relieves migraines	Imitrex (sumatriptan)
Antineoplastic	Destroys or inhibits the growth of malignant cells	Avastin (bevacizumab) Cytoxan (cyclophosphamide)– Nolvadex (tamoxifen)
Antiparkinson's agent	Treats symptoms associated with Parkinson's disease	Sinemet (carbidopa/levodopa)
Antiprotozoal	Treats protozoan infections	Flagyl (metronidazole)
Antipsychotic	Treats schizophrenia and other associated brain disorders	Haldol (haloperidol) Seroquel (quetiapine) Zyprexa (olanzapine)
Antireflux agent	Reduces gastric acid secretion	Zantac (ranitidine) Prilosec (omeprazole) Protonix (pantoprazole)
Antiretroviral	Treats HIV infections	Retrovir (zidovudine)
Antispasmotic	Relieves cramps or spasms of the stomach, intestines, and bladder	Benlyl (dicyclomine)
Antitussive	Cough suppressant	Tussionex (hydrocodone polistirex and chlorpheniramine polistirex) Tessalon (benzonatate)
Antiviral	Reduces symptoms of a viral infection	Tamiflu (oseltamivir phosphate) Zovirax (acyclovir)
Bone resorption inhibitor	Treatment of osteoporosis	Evista (raloxifene) Fosamax (alendronate)
Bronchodilator	Improves breathing by dilating bronchial smooth muscle	Atrovent (ipratropium) Combivent (ipratropium and albuterol) Proventil (albuterol)
Cardiac glycoside	Strengthens the heart muscle; treats congestive heart failure	Digitek (digoxin) Lanoxin (digoxin)

Central nervous stimulant	Improves mental acuity in disorders such as attention deficit/ hyperactivity disorder (ADHD) and attention deficit disorder (ADD)	Adderall (amphetamine-dextroamphetamine) Strattera (atomoxetine HCl)
Contraceptive	Reduces conception	*Injectable:* Depo-Provera (medroxyprogesterone) *Oral:* Yaz (drospirenone and ethinyl estradiol)
Corticosteroid	Treats inflammation	Cortone (cortisone) Flovent (fluticasone), inhaled
Cough expectorant	Liquifies mucus and promotes its removal	Robitussin (guaifenesin)
Decongestant	Reduces nasal congestion and swelling	Mucinex (guaifenesin) Afrin (oxymetazoline) Sudafed (pseudoephedrine)
Diuretic	Increases urine output	Lasix (furosemide)
Hemostatic	Assists in blood coagulation or clotting	Vitamin K thrombin
Histamine (H_2) receptor antagonist	Blocks gastric acid secretion	Axid (nizatidine) Pepcid AC (famotidine)
Hormone replacement	Replaces hormones that are diminished (menopausal symptoms, thyroid disorder, etc.)	Premarin (conjugated estrogen) Prempro (conjugated estrogen/ progesterone)
Hypnotic	Produces sleep	Ambien (zolpidem)
Immunosuppressant	Suppresses the immune system (rheumatoid arthritis and transplant patients)	Neoral (cyclosporine) Sandimmune (cyclosporine)

(continues)

(continued)

Classification	Action	Examples
Laxative	Loosens stools and promotes normal bowel evacuation	Dulcolax (bisacodyl) Colace (docusate) MiraLAX (polyethylene glycol 3350)
Miotic	Contracts pupils of the eyes	Pilacar (pilocarpine) ophthalmic solutions
Mydriatic	Dilates pupils of the eyes	Neo-Synephrine (phenylephrine)
Muscle relaxant	Aids in relaxation of skeletal muscles	Flexeril (cyclobenzaprine) Robaxin (methocarbamol) Soma (carisoprodol)
Nonsteroidal anti-inflammatory drug (NSAID)	Relieves mild to moderate fever, pain, and inflammation	Aleve (naproxen) Celebrex (celecoxib) Relafen (nabumetone)
Sedative, hypnotic, tranquilizer	Produces a calming effect; used to treat insomnia	Ambien (zolpidem) Lunesta (eszopiclone)
Thrombolytic agents	Aids in dissolving blood clots	Activase (alteplase) Streptase (streptokinase)
Vasodilator	Produces relaxation of blood vessels; lowers blood pressure	Natrecor (nesiritide) Nitrostat (nitroglycerin) Apresoline (hydralazine)
Vasopressor	Produces constriction of blood vessels; elevates blood pressure and cardiac output	Intropin (dopamine)

Section 7-2

TOP 200 DRUGS

The following table represents the top 200 drugs with their generics and indications.

Table 7-2
TOP 200 DRUGS

Brand Name	Generic Name	Indication/(Drug Classification)
Ability	aripiprazole	Treatment of bipolar depression/(antipsychotic)
AcipHex	rabeprazole sodium	Antigastric acid/(proton pump inhibitor)
Actonel	risedronate sodium and calcium carbonate	Treatment of osteoporosis/(bisphosphonate)
Actonel 150	risedronate sodium and calcium carbonate	Treatment of osteoporosis/(bisphosphonate)
Actoplus MET	metformin and pioglitazone	Treatment of type 2 diabetes/(antidiabetic, combination medication)
Actos	pioglitazone	Treatment of type 2 diabetes/(antidiabetic)
Adderall XR	amphetamine and dextroamphetamine	Treatment of ADD and ADHD/(central nervous system stimulant) Drug Enforcement Agency [DEA] Schedule 2
AdvairDiskus	fluticasone + salmeterol	Treatment of asthma/(bronchodilator + corticosteroid)
Advair HFA	fluticasone + salmeterol	Treatment of asthma/(bronchodilator + corticosteroid)
Aggrenox	aspirin and dipyridamole	Reduces inflammation and blood clotting/(platelet aggregation inhibitor)
Ambien CR	zolpidem	Sleep aid/(miscellaneous anxiolytic, sedative, and hypnotics) (DEA Schedule 4)
Amitiza	lubiprostone	Treatment of chronic constipation/(chloride channel activator)
Androgen	methyltestosterone	Male testosterone replacement/(androgen hormone replacement agent)
Aricept	donepezil hydrochloride	Treatment of dementia—Alzheimer's type/(cholinesterase inhibitor)

(continues)

(continued)

Brand Name	Generic Name	Indication/(Drug Classification)
Arimidex	anastrozole	Treatment of postmenopausal women with hormone receptor–positive early breast cancer/(aromatase inhibitor, hormone/antineoplastic)
Arixtra	fondaparinux	Prevents the formation of blood clots/(anticoagulant)
Asacol	mesalamine	Treats ulcerative colitis/(anti-inflammatory agent)
Asmanex	mometasone	Treatment of asthma/(inhaled corticosteroid)
Atripla	efavirenz, emtricitabine, and tenofovir	Treatment of HIV/(antiviral combination)
Avalide	hydrochlorothiazide and irbesartan	Treatment of hypertension/(antihypertensive combination)
Avandia	rosiglitazone	Antidiabetic/(thiazolidinedione for type 2 diabetes)
Avapro	irbesartan	Antihypertensive/(angiotensin II receptor antagonist)
Avelox	moxifloxacin	Antibiotic/(fluoroquinolone)
Avodart	dutasteride	Treatment of prostate/(5-alpha-reductase inhibitor)
Avonex	interferon beta-1a	Treatment of patients with relapsing forms of multiple sclerosis/(interferon)
Azor	amlodipine and olmesartan	Antihypertensive/(calcium channel blocker)
Benicar	hydrochlorothiazide	Antihypertensive/(thiazide diuretic)
Benicar HCT	hydrochlorothiazide and olmesartan	Antihypertensive/(diuretic and angiotensin II receptor antagonist)
Betaseron	interferon	Antiviral/(interferon)

Boniva	ibandronate	Treatment of osteoporosis /(bisphosphonate)
Bystolic	nebivolol	Reduces heart rate/(beta blocker)
Caduet	amlodipine and atorvastatin	Treatment of elevated lipid levels and blood pressure/(antihyperlipidemic combination and antihypertensive combination)
Celebrex	celecoxib	Anti-inflammatory/(NSAID)
CellCept	mycophenolate mofetil	Antirejection/(selective immunosuppressants)
Chantix	varenicline	Treatment of smoking addiction/(smoking cessation agent)
Cialis	tadalafil	Treatment of erectile dysfunction/(impotence agent)
Ciprodex Otic	ciprofloxacin and dexamethasone otic	Treatment of otitis externa/(otic corticosteroid with anti-infective)
Clobex	clobetasol propionate	Treatment of skin inflammation/(topical corticosteroid)
Combivent	albuterol and ipratropium	Treatment of asthma/(bronchodilator combination)
Combivir	lamivudine and zidovudine	Treatment of HIV infections/(antiviral combination)
Concerta	methylphenidate	Treatment of ADD, ADHD/(central nervous system [CNS] stimulant)
Copaxone	glatiramer	Treatment of multiple sclerosis/(immunostimulant)
Coreg CR	carvedilol	Treatment of hypertension and congestive heart failure/(noncardioselective beta blocker)
Cozaar	losartan	Antihypertensive agent/(angiotensin II receptor antagonist)

(continues)

(continued)

Brand Name	Generic Name	Indication/(Drug Classification)
Creon	pancrelipase	Treatment of cystic fibrous/(digestive enzyme)
Cymbalta	duloxetine	Antidepressant/(selective serotonin reuptake inhibitor [SSRI])
Detrol LA	tolterodine	Treatment of bladder overactivity/(anticholinergic)
Dexilant	dexlansoprazole	Treatment of gastric acid reflux/(proton pump inhibitor)
Differin	adapalene	Antiacne/(topical acne agent)
Diovan	valsartan	Antihypertensive agents/(angiotensin II receptor antagonist)
Doryx	doxycycline	Antibiotic/(tetracycline)
Duragesic	fentanyl transdermal	Narcotic/(opioid)
Effexor XR	venlafaxine	Antidepressant/(SSRI)
Elmiron	pentosan polysulfate sodium	Treatment of bladder pain and discomfort caused by cystitis/ (anticoagulant)
Enablex	darifenacin	Treatment of bladder overactivity/(anticholinergic)
Enbrel	etanercept	Reduces immune response in rheumatoid arthritis/(antirheumatic, tumor necrosis factor [TNF]-alfa inhibitor)
Entocort EC	budesonide	Treatment of Crohn's disease/(corticosteroid)
Epipen	epinephrine	Treatment of anaphylactic reaction/(adrenergic bronchodilator)
Epzicom	abacavir and lamivudine	Treatment of HIV/(antiviral)

Evista	raloxifene	Treats or prevents osteoporosis in postmenopausal women and reduces risk for invasive breast cancer in postmenopausal women who have osteoporosis or who are at risk for invasive breast cancer/(hormone/antineoplastic, selective estrogen receptor modulator)
Exelon Patch	rivastigmine	Treatment of mild to moderate dementia of the Alzheimer's type/(cholinesterase inhibitor)
Exforge	amlodipine and valsartan	Treatment of hypertension/(antihypertensive, calcium channel blocker, angiotensin II receptor antagonist)
Femara	letrozole	Treatment of breast cancer/(hormone/antineoplastic)
Fentora	fentora	Treatment of severe pain due to cancer/(opioid analgesics)
Flector	diclofenac	Topical agent/(NSAID)
Flomax	tamsulosin	Treatment of BPH/(adrenergic agent, peripherally acting)
Flovent HFA	fluticasone inhalation	Fluticasone inhalation is used to prevent asthma attacks/inhaled corticosteroid
Forteo	teriparatide	Treatment of osteoporosis/(parathyroid hormone and analog)
Geodon	ziprasidone	Treatment of schizophrenia and the manic symptoms of bipolar disorder/(antipsychotic)
Humalog Mix 75/25	insulin lispro	Treats type 1 (insulin-dependent) diabetes in adults. Insulin lispro is a fast-acting form of insulin combined with long-acting insulin/(insulin)

(continues)

(continued)

Brand Name	Generic Name	Indication/(Drug Classification)
Humira	adalimumab	Antirheumatic, rheumatoid arthritis/(TNF-alfa inhibitor)
Humira Pen	adalimumab	Antirheumatic, rheumatoid arthritis/(TNF-alfa inhibitor), prefilled pen containing 40 mg
Humulin	insulin isophane and insulin regular	Antidiabetic/(long-acting form of insulin)
Hyzaar	hydrochlorothiazide and losartan	Reduces the risk for stroke in people with hypertension/(antihypertensive)
Intuniv	guanfacine	Treatment of attention deficit hyperactivity disorder/(antiadrenergic agent, centrally acting)
Invega	paliperidone	Treatment of schizophrenia/(atypical antipsychotic)
Isentress	raltegravir	Treatment of HIV/(integrase strand transfer inhibitor)
Janumet	metformin and sitagliptin	Treatment of type 2 diabetes/(antidiabetic combination)
Januvia	sitagliptin	Treatment of type 2 diabetes/(dipeptidyl peptidase 4 inhibitor)
Kadian	morphine extended-release	Treatment of moderate to severe pain/(opioid analgesics)
Kaletra	lopinavir and ritonavir	Treatment of HIV/(protease inhibitor)
Keppra	levetiracetam	Treatment of partial onset seizures/(pyrrolidine anticonvulsant)
Lamictal	lamotrigine	Treatment of seizures/(triazine anticonvulsant)
Lantus	insulin glargine	Treatment of types 1 and 2 diabetes/(insulin)
Levaquin	levofloxacin	Treatment of infections/(antibiotic, fluoroquinolone)

Levemir	insulin detemir	Treatment of types 1 and 2 diabetes/(insulin)
Lexapro	escitalopram oxalate	Treatment of depression/(SSRI)
Lialda	mesalamine	Treatment of ulcerative colitis/(5-aminosalicylate)
Lidoderm	lidocaine topical	Local anesthesia/(topical anesthetic)
Loestrin 24 Fe	ethinyl estradiol and norethindrone	Contraceptive/(sex hormone combination)
Lotrel	amlodipine and benazepril	Antihypertensive combination/(calcium channel blocker, ACE inhibitor)
Lovaza	omega-3 polyunsaturated fatty acids	Reduces the level of triglycerides/(nutraceutical product)
Lovenox	enoxaparin	Treatment of deep vein thrombus/(heparin)
Lumigan	bimatoprost ophthalmic	Treatment of glaucoma/(ophthalmic glaucoma agent)
Lunesta	eszopiclone	Treatment of insomnia/(miscellaneous anxiolytic, sedative, and hypnotic)
Lyrica	pregabalin	Treatment to control seizures and to treat fibromyalgia/(gamma-aminobutyric acid analog)
Maxalt	rizatriptan	Treatment of migraines/(antimigraine agents)
Maxalt MLT	rizatriptan	Oral disintegrating, treatment of migraines/(antimigraine agent)
Micardis	telmisartan	Treatment of hypertension/(antihypertensive)
Micardis HCT	telmisartan and hydrochlorothiazide	Treatment of hypertensive and fluid accumulation/(antihypertensive combination)

(continues)

(continued)

Brand Name	Generic Name	Indication/(Drug Classification)
Namenda	memantine	Treatment of moderate to severe dementia of the Alzheimer's type/ (miscellaneous central nervous system agent)
Nasonex	mometasone furoate	Treatment of seasonal or yearly allergies/(nasal corticosteroid)
Nexium	esomeprazole	Treatment of gastroesophageal reflux disease (GERD)/(proton pump inhibitor)
Niaspan	niacin	Improves cholesterol levels, reduces risk for a second heart attack/ (antihyperlipidemic agent)
Norvir	ritonavir	Antiviral, treatment of HIV/(protease inhibitor)
NovoLog	insulin aspart	Treats type 1, insulin-dependent diabetes in adults/(insulin)
NovoLog Mix 70/30	insulin aspart and insulin aspart protamine	Treats type 1 diabetes/(insulin)
NuvaRing	etonogestrel and ethinyl estradiol	Pregnancy prevention/(contraceptive)
Nuvigil	armodafinil	Treatment of excessive sleepiness caused by sleep apnea and narco- lepsy/(CNS stimulant)
Opana ER	oxymorphone	Treatment of severe pain/(opioid analgesic)
Oracea	doxycycline	Treatment of acne/(antibiotic, tetracycline)
Ortho Tri-Cyclen Lo	ethinyl estradiol and norgestimate	Pregnancy prevention/(contraceptive)
OxyContin	oxycodone	Treatment moderate to severe pain/(opioid analgesic)

Pataday	olopatadine	Once per day treatment of eye allergies/(ophthalmic antihistamine, decongestant)
Patanol	olopatadine	Twice per day treatment of eye allergies/(ophthalmic antihistamine, decongestant)
Plavix	clopidogrel	Prevention of blood clots/(platelet aggregation inhibitor)
Prandin	repaglinide	Treatment of type 2 diabetes/(meglitinide)
Premarin tabs	conjugated estrogen	Treatment symptoms of menopause/(estrogen)
Premarin vaginal	conjugated estrogen	Treatment of vaginal dryness/(estrogen)
Prempro	conjugated estrogen and medroxyprogesterone	Treatment of menopause symptoms/(sex hormone combination)
Prevacid	lansoprazole	Treatment of acid reflux disease/(protein pump inhibitor)
Prevacid SoluTab	lansoprazole	Quick-dissolving tablets for treatment of acid reflux disease/(protein pump inhibitor)
Prezista	darunavir	Treatment of HIV/(protease inhibitor)
Pristiq	desvenlafaxine	Antidepressant/(SNRI, selective serotonin and norepinephrine reuptake inhibitor)
ProAir HFA	albuterol	Rescue treatment of asthma/(bronchodilator)
Procrit	epoetin alfa	Treatment of anemia due to cancer/(recombinant human erythropoietin)

(continues)

(continued)

Brand Name	Generic Name	Indication/(Drug Classification)
Prograf	tacrolimus	Immunosuppressive agent/(calcineurin inhibitor)
Propecia	finasteride	Treatment of male pattern baldness/(5-alpha-reductase inhibitor)
Protonix	pantoprazole	Treatment of acid reflux disease/(proton pump inhibitor)
Proventil HFA	albuterol	Rescue treatment of asthma/(bronchodilator)
Provigil	modafinil	Treatment of excessive sleepiness/(CNS stimulant)
Pulmicort Respules	budesonide inhalation	Prevention of asthma attacks/ (inhaled corticosteroid)
Qvar	peclomethasone dipropionate	Prevention of asthma attacks/(inhaled corticosteroid)
Relpax	eletriptan	Treatment of migraines/(antimigraine agent)
RenaGel	sevelamer	Prevent hypocalcemia for chronic kidney disease/(chelating agent)
Renvela	sevelamer	Prevent hypocalcemia for chronic kidney disease/(chelating agent)
Restasis	cyclosporine	Treatment of chronic dry eye inflammation/(ophthalmic anti-inflammatory agent)
Reyataz	atazanavir	Treatment of HIV/(protease inhibitor)
Risperdal	risperidone	Treatment of mood disorders/(atypical antipsychotic)
Sensipar	cinacalcet hydrochloride	Reduces calcium levels in hyperparathyroidism disease/(miscellaneous uncategorized agent)

270

Seroquel	quetiapine	Treatment of schizophrenia and major depressive disorder/(atypical antipsychotic)
Seroquel XR	quetiapine, extended release	Treatment of schizophrenia and major depressive disorder/(typical antipsychotic)
Skelaxin	metaxalone	Treatment of muscle pain and inflammation/(skeletal muscle relaxant)
Singulair	montelukast sodium	Control of asthma and allergies/(leukotriene modifier)
Solodyn	minocycline	Treatment of moderate to severe acne/(antibiotic, tetracycline)
Spiriva	tiotropium bromide monohydrate	Treatment of asthma/(anticholinergic bronchodilator)
Strattera	atomoxetine	Treatment of ADD, ADHD/(CNS stimulant)
Suboxone	buprenorphine and naloxone	Treatment of narcotic addiction/(opioid analgesic combination)
Symbicort	budesonide and formoterol	Treatment of asthma/(bronchodilator combination)
Synthroid	levothyroxine	Treatment of hypothyroidism/(thyroid drug)
Tarceva	erlotinib	Chemotherapy/(epidermal growth factor receptor [EGFR] inhibitor)
Temodar	temozolomide	Treatment in conjunction with radiation therapy for brain tumors/ (alkylating agent)
Testim	testosterone	Treatment of low testosterone/(testosterone)
Topamax	topiramate	Treatment of seizure disorders/ (carbonic anhydrase inhibitor, anticonvulsant)

(continues)

(continued)

Brand Name	Generic Name	Incication/(Drug Classification)
Travatan Z	travoprost	Reduction of elevated intraocular pressure with open-angle glaucoma/ (ophthalmic glaucoma agent)
Tricor	fenofibrate	Treatment of high cholesterol and triglycerides/(fibric acid derivatives)
Trilipix	fenofibric acid	Treatment of high cholesterol and triglycerides/(fibric acid derivative)
Truvada	emtricitabine and tenofovir	Treatment of HIV/(antiviral combination)
Tussionex	chlorpheniramine and hydrocodone	Reduces cough/(upper respiratory combination)
Uroxatral	alfuzosin	Treatment of prostate symptoms/(alpha-adrenergic blocker)
Valcyte	valganciclovir hydrochloride	Treatment of cytomegalovirus (CMV) infection of the eye in adults with AIDS/(purine nucleoside)
Valtrex	valacyclovir hydrochloride	Treatment of viral symptoms/(purine nucleoside)
Vancocin HCl	vancomycin hydrochloride	Treatment of serious infections/(antibiotic, glycopeptide)
Ventolin HFA	albuterol	Rescue medication for asthma/(bronchodilator)
Veramyst	fluticasone	Treatment of allergies/(nasal corticosteroid)
Vesicare	solifenacin succinate	Treatment of bladder overactivity/(anticholinergic)
Viagra	sildenafil	Treatment of erectile dysfunction/(impotence agent)
Victoza	liraglutide	Treatment of type 2 diabetes/(incretin mimetic)
Vigamox	moxifloxacin hydrochloride	Treatment of bacterial conjunctivitis/(ophthalmic anti-infective)
Viread	tenofovir	Treatment of HIV/(nucleoside reverse transcriptase inhibitor [NRTI])

Vivelle	estradiol	Treatment of low estrogen levels/(estrogen)
Vytorin	ezetimibe and simvastatin	Transdermal medication for treatment of elevated cholesterol/(antihyperlipidemic combination)
Vyvanse	lisdexamfetamine dimesylate	Treatment of ADD, ADHD/(CNS stimulant)
Welchol	colesevelam hydrochloride	Treatment of elevated cholesterol/(bile acid sequestrant)
Wellbutrin XL	bupropion hydrochloride	Treatment of depression/(antidepressant)
Xalatan	latanoprost	Treatment of glaucoma/(ophthalmic glaucoma agent)
Xeloda	capecitabine	Treatment of breast and colon cancer/(antimetabolite)
Xopenex	levalbuterol	Rescue treatment of asthma/(bronchodilator)
Xyzal	levocetirizine	Treatment of allergies in adults and children 6 months old and older/(antihistamine)
Yaz	drospirenone and ethinyl estradiol	Prevention of pregnancy/(contraceptive)
Zetia	ezetimibe	Treatment of high cholesterol/(cholesterol absorption inhibitor)
Zovirax	acyclovir	Treatment of herpes viruses/(purine nucleoside)
Zyprexa	olanzapine	Treatment of schizophrenia and bipolar disorder/(atypical antipsychotic)
Zydis	olanzapine	Treatment of schizophrenia and bipolar disorder/(atypical antipsychotic)
Zyvox	linezolid	Treatment of resistant bacterial infections/(miscellaneous antibiotic)

Prescription Drug Information, Interactions & Side Effects. Available at http://drugs.com. Accessed September 22, 2011.

Section 7-3

TOP OVER-THE-COUNTER MEDICATIONS

The over-the-counter (OTC) chart in Table 7-3 will help health care professionals correctly spell common OTC medications. Non-licensed individuals need to be very careful about suggesting OTC medications to patients who ask for advice. Suggesting OTC medications without a license can put you in a compromising situation similar to prescribing medicine without a license. Some states allow nurses and other licensed individuals latitude in this area. Medical assistants should not suggest that a patient take any OTC medications unless they are following a specific protocol that has been developed or approved by the provider or other clinicians in the practice.

Check with your provider-employer before suggesting any OTC information.

Table 7-3

MOST COMMON OTC MEDICATIONS

Drugs in lowercase are generics.

Product Classification	Product Name
Acne preparations	benzoyl peroxide, Clean & Clear, Clearasil, Oxy 5/10
Adult cold: Capsule/tablet	Actifed, Advil Cold & Sinus, Comtrex, Dimetapp, Drixoral, Sudafed, Tavist
Adult cold: Liquid	DayQuil, Dimetapp, Naldecon DX, NyQuil, Robitussin CF, Triaminic, Vicks, Vicks 44
Adult cold: Nighttime	Benadryl, NyQuil, Tavist
Adult cough products	Benylin, DayQuil, Delsym, Dimetapp, Robitussin, Vicks 44
Allergy and hay fever remedies	Actifed, Benadryl, Chlor-Trimenton, Claritin, Dimetapp, NasalCrom, Sudafed
Antacids for heartburn	Axid AR, Gaviscon, Maalox, Mylanta, Pepcid AC, Pepcid Complete, Pepto-Bismol, Tums, Zantac
Antidiarrheals	Donnagel, Kaopectate, Immodium A-D, Pepto-Bismol

Antiflatulence	Alka-Selzer Gas Relief, Beano, Gas-X, Maalox-Antigas, Mylanta Gas, Phazyme
Arthritic, back, muscle pain: Topical products	Arthricare, Bengay, Flexall, Icy Hot (patch or cream), Thermacare Patch, Zostrix
Athlete's foot medicine	Desenex, Miactin, Lamisil AT, Lotrimin AF, Lotrimin Ultra, Tinactin
Burn preparations	Neosporin, Polysporin, Solarcaine
Calcium supplements	Caltrate, Citracal, Healthy Woman, Os-Cal, OsteoCal, Tums, Viactiv
Canker sore products	Anbesol, Campo-phenique, Gly-Oxide, Herpecin L, Kanka, Orabase, Tanac, Zilactin
Diabetic cough products	Diabetic Tussin, Naldecon, Robitussin Sugar Free, Safe Tussin, Scot-Tussin, Tussin DM
Diaper rash preparations	A & D Ointment, Balmex, Desitin
Fever sore and cold sore products	Abreva, Anbesol, Campho-phenique, Carmex, Herpecin, Orajel, Tanac, Zilactin
Headache products	Advil, Aleve, Bayer, Excedrin, Excedrin Migraine, Motrin, Motrin Sinus, Tylenol
Heart attack and stroke prevention	aspirin, Bayer, Ecotrin, Halfprin, St. Joseph
Hemorrhoidal preparations	Anusol, Nupercainal, Preparation H
Herbal supplements	Centrum, Nature Made, Nature's Resource, Nature's Solution, One-A-Day, Ricola, Your Life, Windmill Health Products
H-2 antagonists	Axid AR, Pepcid AC, Pepcid Complete, Tagamet HB, Zantac 75
Laxatives	Colace, Correctol, Doxidan, Exlax, Phillips Liqui-Gel, Surfak
Nasal decongestants (oral)	Dristan, Motrin-Sinus, Robitussin Cold, Sudafed, Tavist D, Triaminic, Tylenol Sinus

(continues)

(continued)

Product Classification	Product Name
Nasal decongestants (sprays)	4 Way, Afrin, Dristan, NasalCrom, Neo-Synephrine, Vicks Sinex, Zicam
Nasal strips	Breathe Right, Clear Passage
Poison ivy and oak topical remedies	Aveeno, Caladryl, Cortaid, Gold Bond Anti Itch, Ivarest, Ivy-block, Ivy-Dry, Tecnu
Scar treatment	Mederma, Rejuveness, Scar-Eeze, vitamin E
Sinus products	Advil Cold & Sinus, Benadryl, Drixoral, Motrin Sinus, Sinutab, Sudafed Sinus, Tavist Sinus, Tylenol Sinus
Smoking cessation products	NicoDerm CQ Patch, Nicorette Gum, Nicotrol Patch
Sleep aids	Alluna Sleep, Nytol, Sominex, Unisom
Sore throat liquids	Cepacol, Cepastat, Chloraseptic
Sore throat lozenges	Cepacol, Cepastat, Chloraseptic, Halls, NICE, Ricola, Spec T, Sucrets
Support hosiery	Bauer & Black, Futuro, Jobst, T.E.D.
Upset stomach remedies	Alka-Seltzer, Emetrol, Gaviscon, Maalox, Mylanta, Pepcid Complete, Pepto-Bismol, Tums
Vaginal antifungals	Femstat, Gyne-Lotrimin, Monistat, Mycelex, Vagistat
Vaginal moisturizers	Astroglide, K-Y Jelly, Lubrin, Replens, Summer's Eve, Vagisil

Section 7-4

TOP MEDICATION INJECTABLES

Table 7-4 lists the most common injectables used in ambulatory care settings.

Table 7-4

TOP MEDICATION INJECTABLES

Route Abbreviations: IM—intramuscular; Subcut—subcutaneous, IV—intravenous
Drug names that are capitalized are trade names. Drugs in italics and lowercase are generics.

Drug Name	Generic Name	Classification	Route
Avastin	bevacizumab	Chemotherapy	IV
Bicillin CR	penicillin G benzathine and procaine	Antibiotic	IM
Bicillin LA	penicillin G benzathine	Antibiotic	IM
Depo-Medrol	methylprednisolone	SAID (corticosteroidal anti-inflammatory drug)	IM
Depo-Provera	medroxyprogesterone	Contraceptive	IM
Depo-Testosterone	testosterone	HRT (hormone relacement therapy)	IM
Enbrel	etanercept	Antirheumatics	Subcut
EpiPen	epinephrine	Antianaphylaxis	Subcut, IM
Epogen	epoetin alfa	Treatment of severe anemia	IM
Herceptin	trastuzumab	Chemotherapy, HER2 inhibitors	IV
Humira	adalimumab	Antirheumatics	IV
Imitrex	sumatriptan	Antimigraine	Subcut
Kenalog	triamcinolone	SAID	IM
Xylocaine	lidocaine	Local anesthetic	Local
Xylocaine w/ epinephrine	lidocaine w/ epinephrine	Local anesthetic w/ vasoconstrictor	Local
NovoLog	Insulin	Treatment of type 1 and 2 diabetes	Subcut

(continues)

(continued)

Drug Name	Generic Name	Classification	Route
Phenergan	promethazine	Antihistamine w/ sedative, antispasmodic, and antiemetic effects	IM
Remicade	infliximab	Treatment of rheumatoid arthritis, psoriatic arthritis, ulcerative colitis, and Crohn's disease	IV
Rocephin	ceftriaxone	Antibiotic	IM
Solu-Medrol	methylprednisolone	SAID	IM
Toradol	ketorolac	NSAID	IM
Versed	midazolam	Anesthetic, sedative	IM
vitamin B_{12}	cyanocobalamine	Anemia Tx	IM
Zofran	ondansetron	Antiemetic	IM
Zosyn	piperacillin and tazobactam	Antiobiotic	IV

Section 7-5

COMMON MEASUREMENTS AND DOSAGE CALCULATIONS

Administering medications is a common task performed in ambulatory care. Before administering medications, you must be familiar with common measurement conversions and dosages calculation formulas (Tables 7-5, 7-6, and 7-7). This section provides reference information that will assist you in this endeavor.

Table 7-5
COMMON HOUSEHOLD MEASUREMENTS

60 drops = 1 teaspoon (tsp)
1 dash = less than 1/8 tsp
3 teaspoons = 1 tablespoon (tbsp)
2 tbsp = 1 ounce (oz)
4 oz = 1 juice glass
6 oz = 1 teacup
8 oz = 1 glass or cup
16 tbsp or 8 oz = 1 measuring cup
2 cups = 1 pint
2 pints = 1 quart
4 quarts = 1 gallon

Table 7-6
COMMON CONVERSIONS BETWEEN HOUSEHOLD MEASUREMENTS AND METRIC MEASUREMENTS

Household Measurement	Metric Measurement
1 teaspoon (tsp) and 1 dram	5 cc or 5 mL
1 tablespoon (tbsp)	15 cc or 15 mL
1 ounce (oz)	30 cc or 30 mL
1 cup (c)	180 cc or 180 mL
1 glass or 8 ounces (oz)	240 cc or 240 mL
2.2 pounds (lb)	1 kilogram (kg)
1 inch (in)	2.5 centimeter (cm)

Table 7-7
METRIC CONVERTER

Whole Numbers				Fractions or Decimals					
Increasing Value				←	→			Decreasing Value	
1000	100	10	1	1/ 10	1/ 100	1/ 1000	—	—	1/ 1,000,000
				0.1	0.01	0.001			0.000001
Kilo	Hecto	Deka	Standard unit (gram, liter and meter)	Deci	Centi	Milli	PH*	PH*	Micro
							—	—	
↑	↑	↑	↑	↑	↑	↑	↑	↑	↑

PLACE HOLDER COUNTING SECTION

This table is a metric converter for instances in which you need to convert within the metric system. Just place your finger on the arrow that describes the known value and count over the spaces it takes to get to the unknown value. You will move your decimal point the number of spaces it takes to get to the unknown value—in the same direction of the unknown value (i.e., 1 gram = __ mg). You place your finger on the arrow under "gram" and count over the spaces to "milli." You will move your decimal point three places to the right. The letters PH stand for "place holder." The majority of metric units are separated by one unit of 10; however, the separation between milli and micro jumps from 10 to 1000. So that you don't get confused, the placeholders between milli and micro serve as a reminder to move the decimal place three places between the two units.

Section 7-6

DOSAGE CALCULATIONS

This section lists formulas for calculating dosages when administering medications.

Adult Formula Method

The formula method of calculating adult dosages requires the use of the following mathematical formula:

$$\frac{\text{Amount Desired}}{\text{Amount Available}} \times \begin{array}{c} \text{Quantity (how it comes stocked, for example:} \\ \text{1 mL, 1 cap)} \end{array}$$

The physician orders 50 mg of Demerol. It comes stocked as 25 mg/mL, which means that there are 25 mg of Demerol in 1 mL of medication.

1. Determine if the dose desired is in the same units as the dose available or on hand. If not, convert so that they are in the same units (refer to Table 7-7.)

In this case, the desired amount is already in the same units as the available amount, so no conversion is necessary.

2. Next, use the formula listed below to calculate the dosage.

$$\frac{50 \; \cancel{mg} \; (\text{Desired})}{25 \; \cancel{mg} \; (\text{Available})} \times 1\,\text{mL} =$$

$$\frac{50}{25} \times 1\,\text{mL} =$$

$$2 \times 1\,\text{mL} = 2\,\text{mL}$$

(The unit mg cancels out.)

3. Round the calculation

The answer is the patient should receive 2 mL of Demerol. (There is no need to round this answer.)

Dosage Calculations: Pediatric Dosage by Kilogram of Body Weight

One way to calculate pediatric medication dosages is based on kilograms of body weight. Refer to the steps below:

Order: The provider orders ceftriaxone sodium (Rocephin) 50 mg/kg. The medication should be divided into equal doses every 12 hours (not to exceed 4 g) for Sandy Porter, who weighs 66 pounds. How many milligrams will Sandy receive?

1. Convert pounds into kilograms by dividing the number of pounds by 2.2. (Round the answer to the nearest hundredth.)

$$\frac{66 \; \text{lb}}{2.2} = 30 \; \text{kg}$$

(In this case, no rounding is necessary.)

2. Multiply the dose ordered by kilogram of body weight. (Cancel out like units.)

$$\frac{50 \text{ mg}}{\text{kg}} \times 30 \text{ kg} = 1500 \text{ mg} = 1.5 \text{ g}$$

3. If applicable, divide the child's dose by the number of equal doses to be given in a 24-hour period.

4. 1500 mg by 2 = 750 mg (Once you obtain the dosage, you will then use the adult formula to figure how many milliliters [mL] to give.)

Section 7-7

ADMINISTRATION OF MEDICATIONS

The administration of medications is a very important task. Table 7-8 lists the Seven Rights of Drug Administration that should be adhered to every time you give a medication, regardless of the route.

Table 7-8
THE SEVEN RIGHTS OF DRUG ADMINISTRATION

1. Right Patient
2. Right Medication
3. Right Dose
4. Right Time
5. Right Route
6. Right Technique
7. Right Documentation

Administering Oral Medications

Procedure 7-1
ADMINISTER AN ORAL MEDICATION

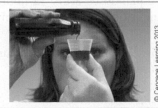

© Cengage Learning 2013

Figure 7-1: Pour the liquid medication so that it is at eye level.

Equipment and Supplies

Written medication order	Plastic medication cup	Water
Proper medication	Medication transport tray	Gloves (optional)

1. Verify the provider's order and institute the Seven Rights of Drug Administration.

2. Wash your hands and apply gloves (gloves are optional). Assemble the medication and supplies. Check the label on the medication bottle as you retrieve it from the cabinet (Medication check #1).

3. Compare the written drug order with the drug label before preparing the drug. Make certain that you have the right drug and the right dose (Medication check #2). Perform dosage calculation if necessary.

4. Check the expiration date of the drug.

5. Loosen the lid and remove it from the bottle. Place the lid on the counter so that the inside of the lid is pointing upward. Pour the correct amount of pills into the cap of the medication vial without contaminating the inside of the cap, and then into the medicine cup (Figure 7-1). *(When measuring a liquid form of medication, palm the label before pouring and hold the medication cup at eye level, as in Figure 7-1. Read the volume at the lowest point of the curve in the liquid, or at the meniscus.)*

6. Replace the medication in its proper storage area. Read the label once again before returning it to verify that it is the correct drug and dosage (Medication check #3).

7. Properly transport the medication to the patient. Be careful not to touch the medication or the inside of the container.

8. Identify the patient using a minimum of two identifiers.

9. Identify yourself and explain the procedure to the patient.

10. Give the patient the medication and water to swallow and observe the patient to make sure there is no difficulty in taking the medication. (Do not give water with medications that are liquids.)

11. Properly dispose of the medication cup and other disposable equipment into the garbage and remove gloves and wash hands.

12. Provide the patient with any relevant educational materials.

(continues)

(continued)

13. Document the procedure in the patient's chart.

07-12-XXXX 10:15 a.m.	Tylenol, 500 mg po per Dr. Legg. Observed pt swallow med. Gave pt. both verbal and written home care instructions for taking medication at home. Jane Barnes, CMA (AAMA)

Procedure 7-2
PREPARING A TOPICAL MEDICATION

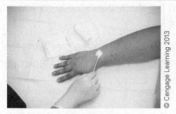
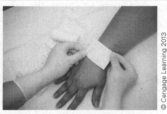

Figure 7-2: When applying a topical medication to an open area, use a sterile cotton-tipped applicator.

Figure 7-3: Apply a sterile dressing over the area.

Equipment and Supplies

Written medication order Proper medication	Sterile cotton-tipped applicator/sterile tongue depressor Disposable underpad (if applicable)	Gloves (optional) Drape (if applicable)

1. Verify the provider's order and institute the Seven Rights of Drug Administration.

2. Wash your hands and retrieve the medication and other necessary supplies. Check the label to determine that you have the correct medication before removing it from the shelf (Medication check #1).

3. Compare the written drug order with the drug label before preparing the drug (Medication check #2).

4. Check the expiration date of the drug.

5. Read the medication label again before placing it on the medication tray (Medication check #3).

6. Place all other supplies on tray, such as 4×4s, cotton-tipped applicators, tongue blades, etc.

7. Properly transport the medication to the patient.

8. Identify the patient correctly, using at least two identifiers.

9. Identify yourself and explain the procedure to the patient.

10. Ask the patient to expose the area where the medication is to be applied.

11. Wash your hands and apply gloves.

12. Place a pad under the area on which you are applying the medication.

13. Loosen the lid and remove the cap, placing it so that the inner part is facing upward before placing it on the table.

14. Remove the appropriate amount of medication from the container using a clean or sterile tongue depressor or cotton-tipped applicator.

15. Carefully apply the medication directly over the affected area, working from the inside out (Figure 7-2).

16. Ask if the patient is experiencing any pain or difficulty in tolerating the application of the medication.

17. Cover the area with a clean/sterile dressing (Figure 7-3) if necessary.

18. Properly dispose of the used disposable supplies.

19. Remove gloves and wash your hands.

20. Provide the patient with home care instructions and ask the patient to repeat the instructions.

21. Return the medication to the appropriate cabinet. (Make certain that the outside of the container is clean before replacing it back in storage.)

22. Document the procedure in the patient's chart.

| 09-18-XXXX 8:10 a.m. | *Silvadene ointment applied over burn on pt's R. forearm with a sterile cotton-tipped applicator per Dr. Jones. Sterile nonstick dressing applied to site. Pt given home care instructions and instructed to call with any concerns or questions. Pt appeared to understand the instructions. Kim Rippa, CMA (AAMA)* |

Procedure 7-3
ADMINISTER A TRANSDERMAL MEDICATION

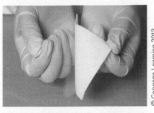

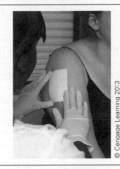

Figure 7-5: Apply the patch to the skin and press firmly on all corners of the patch to make certain it is completely adhered to the skin.

Figure 7-4: Peel the plastic backing off of the transdermal patch.

Equipment and Supplies

Written medication order	Transdermal patch	Gloves

1. Verify the provider's order and institute the Seven Rights of Drug Administration.

2. Wash your hands and retrieve the medication, checking the label before removing it from the shelf to make certain you have the correct medication and the correct dose (Medication check #1).

3. Assemble the equipment.

4. Remove an unopened transdermal patch from the box.

5. Compare the written drug order with the drug label (Medication check #2).

6. Check the expiration date of the drug.

7. Read the directions for proper application of the patch before returning the box to storage if you are unfamiliar with the procedure. Return other patches in the box to their proper storage area. When returning, read the label again to verify that you have the correct drug and dose (Medication check #3).

8. Place the unopened patch on a tray and transport the medication to the patient's room.

9. Correctly identify the patient by using a minimum of two identifiers.

10. Introduce yourself and explain the procedure to the patient.

11. Wash your hands and apply gloves.

12. Ask the patient to expose the area on which the medication is to be applied. Select an area that is free from hair growth, lesions, wounds, moles, or rashes. Never place a patch directly over the same site from which a patch was just removed. (Clean the skin with alcohol and allow to dry if the site is dirty or oily.)

13. Open the pack and peel off the protective plastic backing of the dermal patch (Figure 7-4).

14. Gently place the sticky side of the patch on the correct area. Apply gentle pressure to the patch to ensure the patch has adhered to the patient's skin properly (Figure 7-5).

15. Observe the patient for the appropriate time period for any signs of an allergic reaction.

16. Properly dispose of the medication package and other disposable supplies.

17. Remove gloves and wash your hands.

18. Provide the patient with verbal instructions and educational brochures and ask the patient to repeat back instructions if the patient is to apply the patch at home.

19. Dismiss the patient and chart the procedure.

| 03-21-XXXX 2:15 p.m. | Nitroglycerine transdermal patch, 0.4 mg—applied to upper right chest per Dr. Woo. Observed pt following administration for any problems. Neg reactions. Gave pt home care instructions and instructed pt to call with any questions. Pt appeared to comprehend instructions. Marcie Littlejohn, CMA (AAMA) |

Procedure 7-4
PREPARING MEDICATIONS (AMPULE OR VIAL)

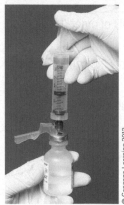

Figure 7-6: Inject air into the diluent vial.

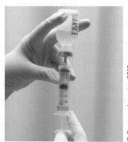

Figure 7-7: Hold the vial at eye level during withdrawal of the medication.

(continues)

(continued)

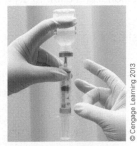

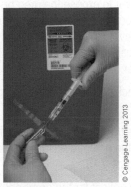

Figure 7-8: Flick the syringe to remove any air bubbles.

Figure 7-9: Completely draw up all medications into the syringe.

Equipment and Supplies

Vial of medication or with filter needle Ampule Antiseptic wipe	Needle and syringe appropriate for both procedures Gauze 2×2 sponge	Sharps container Medication tray

1. Wash your hands and apply gloves.

2. Assemble the equipment and institute the Seven Rights of Drug Administration (refer to Table 7-8).

3. Select the correct medication from the storage area and check the drug label (Medication Check #1).

4. Check the expiration date.

5. Compare the medication with the provider's possibility of order (Medication Check #2).

6. Calculate the correct dose to be given, if needed. Verify the correct calculations with the provider if necessary.

7. Open the syringe and attach the needle to the syringe. (If withdrawing from an ampule, attach a filter needle to syringe.)

Withdrawing Medication from a Vial
8. A1. Open the antiseptic wipe and clean the vial stopper.

A2. Holding the syringe at eye level, pull back on the plunger of syringe to draw an amount of air into the syringe equal to the amount of medication to be withdrawn from the vial.

A3. Check to make sure the needle is firmly attached to the syringe and remove the cap from the needle.

A4. Insert the needle through the rubber stopper until it reaches the empty space between the stopper and the fluid level.

A5. Push forward on the plunger to inject air into the vial (Figure 7-6). Keep the needle above the fluid level.

A6. Invert the vial while holding onto the syringe and plunger.

A7. Hold the syringe at eye level and withdraw the proper amount of medication (Figure 7-7).

A8. Keep the tip of needle below the fluid level.

A9. Remove any air bubbles in the syringe by tapping or flicking the side of the syringe where the bubbles are located (Figure 7-8).

A10. Remove any air remaining in the tip of the syringe.

A11. Replace the needle cap on the syringe or replace with a new needle and cap setup.

A12. Read the medication label and replace the medication vial in the correct storage cabinet (Medication Check #3).

A13. Place the syringe onto a clean tray with other items necessary for the injection, including an alcohol wipe, a cotton ball, and an adhesive bandage.

Withdrawing from an Ampule

B1. Tap the stem of the ampule lightly, or snap the wrist of the arm holding the ampule, to remove any medication in the neck of the ampule.

B2. Open the antiseptic wipe and clean the ampule container. Allow the ampule to dry completely.

B3. Place a piece of gauze around the neck of the ampule. Hold the ampule firmly between the fingers and the thumbs of both hands.

B4. Break off the stem by snapping it quickly and firmly away from the body. Discard the top in a sharps container and carefully set the ampule down on a flat, firm surface.

B5. Check to make sure the filter needle is firmly attached to the syringe and remove the cap from the needle.

(continues)

(continued)

B6. Insert the needle into the ampule below the fluid level. Hold the ampule at a slight angle while advancing the needle within the glass body. Completely draw up all the medication into the syringe (Figure 7-9).

B7. Remove the needle from the ampule without allowing the needle to touch the edges of the ampule.

B8. Dispose of the ampule into the sharps container. Check the medication label before discarding the ampule (Medication Check #3).

B9. Remove any bubbles in the syringe.

B10. Pull back slightly on the plunger to draw the medication from the needle into the syringe, engage the safety device, and remove the filter needle.

B11. Open a new needle for administering medication to the patient and attach it correctly to the syringe.

B12. Remove the cap from the needle and push slightly forward on the plunger to remove air that is within the tip of the syringe and shaft of the needle.

B13. Replace the needle cap on the syringe following institutional policy.

B14. Prepare the medication tray. Place a bandage, a gauze pad or cotton ball, an antiseptic wipe, and the syringe on a medication tray for transporting to the examination room to administer the injection to the patient.

Procedure 7-5
LOAD A CARTRIDGE OR INJECTOR DEVICE

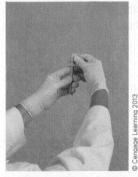

Figure 7-10: Turn the ribbed collar to the open position.

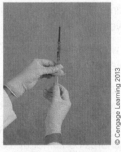

Figure 7-11: Thread the rod of the plunger into the cartridge unit until a slight resistance is felt.

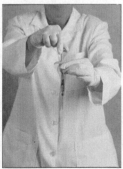

Figure 7-12: After the injection is given, disengage the plunger from the cartridge unit into the sharps container.

Equipment and Supplies

Prefilled cartridge of medication Cartridge holder	Antiseptic wipe Gauze 2×2 sponge	Sharps container Medication tray

1. Wash your hands and apply gloves.

2. Assemble the equipment and institute the Seven Rights of Drug Administration (refer to Table 7-8)

3. Select the correct medication from the storage area/refrigerator and check the drug label (Medication Check #1).

4. Check the expiration date.

5. Compare the medication with the provider's possibility of order. (Medication Check #2).

6. Calculate the correct dose to be given, if needed.

7. Pick up the cartridge unit holder (the injector).

8. Turn the ribbed collar toward the open position until it stops (Figure 7-10).

9. Hold the injector with the open end up and fully insert the sterile cartridge-needle unit.

10. Firmly tighten the ribbed collar of the unit at the syringe base by turning the ribbed collar toward the "close" arrow. (Hold the cartridge to prevent it from swiveling inside the holder while tightening.)

11. Thread the rod of the plunger into the cartridge unit until a slight resistance is felt (Figure 7-11).

12. Prepare the medication for injection into the patient at this time. Place a bandage, a gauze pad or cotton ball, an antiseptic wipe, and the syringe on a medication tray for transporting to the examination room. Check the medication label one last time (Medication Check #3).

13. After use, do not recap the needle.

14. Disengage the plunger rod from the cartridge unit holder while holding the needle down and away from the fingers or hands over a sharps unit (Figure 7-12).

15. Unscrew the ribbed collar of the cartridge unit holder.

16. Allow the needle cartridge unit to drop into the sharps container.

17. Cleanse the cartridge holder with an antiseptic cleanser and allow to dry.

18. Cleanse the work area and remove gloves and wash your hands.

Table 7-9

INTRADERMAL INJECTION SUMMARY CHART

Needle size	26–27 G, $^3/_8$″–$^5/_8$″
Syringe size	1 mL
Angle of insertion	10°–15°
Aspirate	No
Common medications or extracts given by this route	Allergy extract, Tuberculosis (TB) extract
Maximum amount of milliliters per location	0.1 mL
Massage	No

Procedure 7-6

PERFORMING AN INTRADERMAL INJECTION

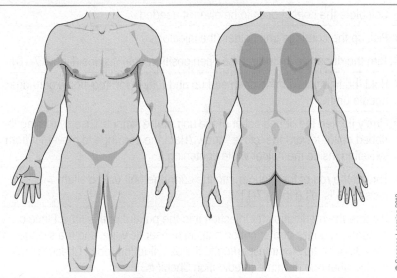

© Cengage Learning 2013

Figure 7-13: Sites for an intradermal injection include the inner forearm and the upper portion of the back.

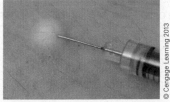

© Cengage Learning 2013

Figure 7-14: A wheal will form if the procedure was performed correctly.

Equipment and Supplies

Appropriate size needle and syringe unit with correct medication Antiseptic wipe	2×2 sponges Disposable gloves	Sharps container Medication tray

1. Complete steps 1 through 8 from Procedure 7-1.

2. Identify the patient using two identifiers, identify yourself, and explain the procedure to the patient.

3. Ask patient about drug allergies or latex allergies.

4. Select the proper injection site (anterior forearm or middle of back) (Figure 7-13).

5. Cleanse the site with antiseptic and allow to air dry completely. (Cleanse in a circular motion working outward to an area of 2 to 3 inches.)

6. Prepare the equipment and apply gloves.

7. Remove the needle cap. Pull the cap straight off, never twist.

8. Stretch the skin taut at the site of administration.

9. Insert the needle at a 10- to 15-degree angle with the bevel upward just under the skin.

10. Inject the medication slowly and steadily. A wheal should form (Figure 7-14).

11. Remove the needle quickly at the same angle of insertion.

12. Do not press on or massage the injection site. Do not apply a bandage to the site.

13. Properly engage the safety device on the needle and dispose of the needle-syringe unit in the sharps container.

14. Remove gloves and wash your hands.

15. Give proper patient education for caring for the site and inform the patient to wait 20 to 30 minutes.

16. Perform postinjection observation and document the procedure in the patient's chart and the appropriate logs.

05-22-XXXX 3:15 p.m.	Tubersol, 0.1 mL, ID , right lower forearm, per Dr. Jones. MFG: Kline Beecham, Lot number: K449. Neg. complications during postinjection observation. Sherri Jones CMA (AAMA)

Table 7-10
SUBCUTANEOUS INJECTION SUMMARY CHART

Needle size	23–25 G, $\frac{1}{2}$"–$\frac{5}{8}$"
Syringe size	1–3 mL (use an insulin syringe when giving insulin)
Angle of insertion	45 to 90 degrees
Aspirate	The majority of drugs given through this route should be aspirated, but aspiration is contraindicated in a select few drugs. Check the manufacturer's packaging information for specifics.
Common medications or extracts given by this route	Allergy injections; insulin injections; heparin; enoxaparin (Lovenox); mumps, measles, rubella (MMR) vaccine; smallpox vaccine; inactivated polio vaccine (IPV), varicella (VAR) vaccine
Maximum amount of milliliters per location	2 mL
Massage	Yes, except in a select few medications (read instructions)

Procedure 7-7
PERFORMING A SUBCUTANEOUS INJECTION

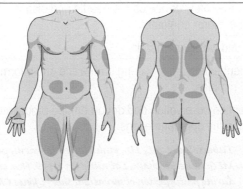

© Cengage Learning 2013

Figure 7-15: Common sites for a subcutaneous injection.

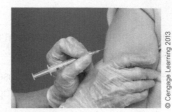

Figure 7-16: The proper angle of insertion for a subcutaneous injection.

Equipment and Supplies

Appropriate sized needle and syringe unit with correct medication Antiseptic wipe	Gauze 2×2 sponge Disposable gloves	Sharps container Medication tray

1. Complete steps 1 to 8 from Procedure 7-1.

2. Identify the patient using two identifiers, identify yourself, and explain the procedure to the patient.

3. Ask patient about drug allergies or latex allergies.

4. Select the proper injection site (fatty tissue of the arms, thighs, or stomach) (Figure 7-15).

5. Cleanse the site with antiseptic and allow to air dry completely. (Cleanse in a circular motion working outward to an area of 2 to 3 inches.)

6. Prepare the equipment and apply gloves.

7. Remove the needle cap. Pull the cap straight off, never twist.

8. Grasp or pinch the tissue lightly with one hand.

9. Insert the needle at a 45-degree angle with the other hand, using a quick and smooth motion (Figure 7-16).

10. Stabilize the needle within the tissue.

11. If indicated, aspirate to ensure the needle is not in a blood vessel.

12. Inject the medication slowly and steadily.

13. Remove the needle quickly at the same angle of insertion.

(continues)

(continued)

14. Place a cotton ball or gauze sponge over the injection site and gently massage the area, if applicable.

15. Properly engage the needle's safety device and dispose of the needle and syringe into the sharps container. Apply a bandage if applicable.

16. Remove gloves and wash your hands.

17. Give proper patient educational materials and waiting instructions.

18. Perform post-check of the patient and site 20 to 30 minutes after the procedure.

19. Chart the procedure correctly on the progress note and appropriate logs.

05-22-XXXX 3:15 p.m.	Varivax #1, 0.5 mL, subcut, right arm per Dr. Sullivan. MFG: Smith & CO Lot number: K449, exp. date – 12/XX. Pt. tolerated well, instructions given to pt. for site care and VIS (May XXXX) provided, consent form signed and filed in chart. Post injection follow-up, neg complications. Sherri Jones, CMA (AAMA)

Table 7-11

INTRAMUSCULAR INJECTION SUMMARY CHART

Needle size	20–23 G, 1–3
Syringe size	1–3 mL
Angle of insertion	90 degrees
Aspirate	Yes
Common medications or extracts given by this route	Most vaccines, analgesics, antibiotics, steroids, hormones
Maximum amount of milliliters per location	Deltoid: 1–2 mL; large muscles such as the dorsogluteal and vastus lateralis: 3 mL
Massage	Generally: yes; Z-track: no

Procedure 7-8
PERFORMING AN INTRAMUSCULAR INJECTION

(a)

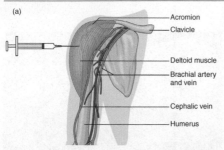

- Acromion
- Clavicle
- Deltoid muscle
- Brachial artery and vein
- Cephalic vein
- Humerus

(b)

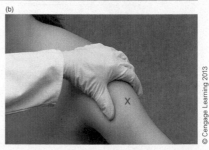

© Cengage Learning 2013

Figure 7-17: The landmark for deltoid injections.

(a)

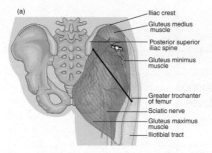

- Iliac crest
- Gluteus medius muscle
- Posterior superior iliac spine
- Gluteus minimus muscle
- Greater trochanter of femur
- Sciatic nerve
- Gluteus maximus muscle
- Iliotibial tract

(b)

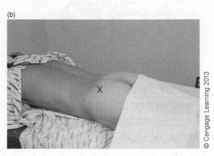

© Cengage Learning 2013

Figure 7-18: The landmark for dorsogluteal injections.

(a)

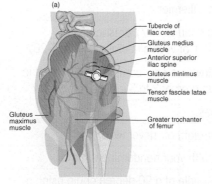

- Tubercle of iliac crest
- Gluteus medius muscle
- Anterior superior iliac spine
- Gluteus minimus muscle
- Tensor fasciae latae muscle
- Greater trochanter of femur

Gluteus maximus muscle

(b)

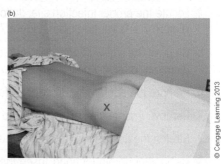

© Cengage Learning 2013

Figure 7-19: The landmark for the ventrogluteal site.

(continues)

(continued)

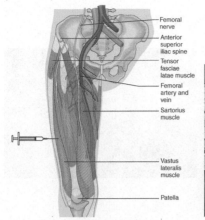

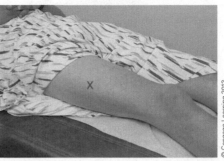

Figure 7-20: The landmark for the vastus lateralis site.

Equipment and Supplies

Appropriate size needle and syringe unit with correct medication Antiseptic wipe	Gauze 2×2 sponge Disposable gloves	Sharps container Medication tray

1. Complete steps 1 to 8 from Procedure 7-1.

2. Identify the patient using two identifiers, identify yourself, and explain the procedure to the patient.

3. Ask patient about drug allergies or latex allergies.

4. Locate the proper injection site; deltoid (Figure 7-17), dorsogluteal (Figure 7-18), ventrogluteal (Figure 7-19), or vastus lateralis (Figure 7-20).

5. Cleanse the site with antiseptic and allow to air dry completely. (Cleanse in a circular motion working outward to an area of 2 to 3 inches.)

6. Prepare the equipment and apply gloves.

7. Remove the needle cap. Pull the cap straight off, never twist.

8. Stretch the tissue to hold the skin taut with your nondominant hand.

9. Using your dominant hand, insert the needle at a 90-degree angle using a quick and smooth motion.

10. Stabilize the needle within the tissue.

11. Aspirate to ensure the needle is not in a blood vessel. If blood enters the syringe, do not inject, but remove the needle immediately. If there is no bloody return into the needle, proceed with the injection process.

12. Inject the medication slowly and steadily.

13. Remove the needle quickly at the same angle of insertion.

14. Place a cotton ball or gauze sponge over the injection site and gently massage the area, if applicable.

15. Engage the safety device on the needle, and dispose of the needle-syringe unit in the sharps container.

16. Place an adhesive bandage over the site and remove gloves and wash your hands.

17. Give related patient educational materials and proper waiting instructions.

18. Perform post-check of the patient and site 20 to 30 minutes after the procedure.

19. Chart the procedure correctly on the progress note and appropriate logs.

05-22-XXXX 3:15 p.m.	*Hepivax 0.5 mL, IM, R. Deltoid per Dr. Jones. MFG: Kline Beecham, Lot#: K449, exp. date: 12/XX. Pt. tolerated well, instructions given to pt. for site care and VIS (04-XXXX) provided and consent form signed and filed. No problems during post check. Sherri Jones, CMA (AAMA)*

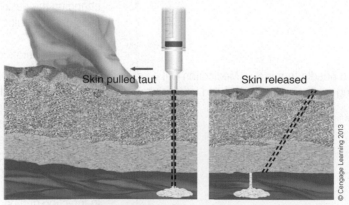

Skin pulled taut   Skin released

© Cengage Learning 2013

Figure 7-21: Use your non-dominant hand to pull the tissue laterally 1–2 inches from the injection site.

Field Tips

When administering a Z-track injection, use your nondominant hand to pull the tissue to be injected laterally 1 to 2 inches away from the injection site (Figure 7-21). Using your dominant hand, insert the needle at a 90-degree angle with a quick and smooth motion. Stabilize the needle within the tissue. Aspirate using the one-hand technique to ensure the needle is not in a blood vessel. If medication is in a blood vessel, remove the needle and prepare a new setup. Wait 10 seconds before removing the needle. Release the tissue *after* removing the needle from the site. Place a cotton ball or gauze sponge over the injection site. *Do not massage the site for a Z-track injection.*

Table 7-12

POSSIBLE PARENTERAL COMPLICATIONS

Incorrect Technique	Consequences	Effects
Failure to change the needle between the vial and patient	Tissue irritation or discoloration Excess pain to the patient	Local reaction to the skin or muscle Discoloration of the skin Increased amount of pain because of needle dullness
Using a needle that is too short	Medication will be deposited into incorrect tissue	Medication will not be absorbed the way the manufacturer intended it to be absorbed, thus changing the desired effects of the medication Abscess Tissue degeneration
Using a needle that is too long	Medication will be deposited into incorrect tissue	Medication will not be absorbed the way the manufacturer intended it to be absorbed, thus changing the desired effects of the medication Could cause damage to the periosteum resulting in infection and bone retardation Needle could break off into the bone

Failing to aspirate on medications that should be aspirated	Deposition of medication directly into a vein or artery	Shock: Medication was not intended to go directly into the bloodstream. May cause patient's heart to beat faster, respiration rate to increase, blood pressure to drop. Patient may become unconscious.
Break in sterile technique	The introduction of micro-organisms into the muscle, subcutaneous tissue, or bloodstream	Blood infection An abscess in the subcutaneous tissue, muscle tissue, or surrounding tissue Tissue degeneration
Choosing a muscle that is underdeveloped	May cause injury to the nearby nerves	Tingling Excruciating pain Paralysis
Injecting a patient with a small-gauge needle when administering a viscid solution	May cause injury to the surrounding tissue	Burning Tissue degeneration Increased pain to the patient

SECTION 7-8

PRESCRIPTION WRITING

Figure 7-22 presents the parts of a prescription.

Parts of a Prescription
1. The physician's name, address, telephone number, and registration number.
2. The patient's name, address, and the date on which the prescription is written.
3. The *superscription* that includes the symbol Rx ("take thou").
4. The *inscription* that states the names and quantities of ingredients to be included in the medication.
5. The *subscription* that gives directions to the pharmacist for filling the prescription.
6. The *signature* (Sig) that gives the directions for the patient.
7. The physician's signature blanks. Where signed, indicates if a generic substitute is allowed or if the medication is to be dispensed as written.
8. Repeat 0 1 2 3 PRN. This is where the physician indicates whether or not the prescription can be refilled.
9. LABEL. Direction to the pharmacist to label the medication appropriately.

LEWIS & KING
L&K 2501 CENTER STREET
NORTHBOROUGH, OH 12345

Name _____ *Juanita Hansen* _____
Address _ *143 Gregory Lane, Apt. 43* _____ Date _ *4/7/XX*
Rx
  Furadantin 50 mg Tabs
  #56
  Sig 1 tab p.o. 4 times/day X 14 days

Generic Substitution Allowed _ *Susan Rice* _____
                                                        M.D.
Dispense As Written _____
                                                        M.D.
Repeat ⓪ 1 2 3 PRN
☑ LABEL

© Cengage Learning 2013

Figure 7-22: The nine parts of a prescription

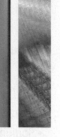

Section Eight
LABORATORY NORMAL VALUES AND PROCEDURES

INTRODUCTION

This section is designed to give quick access to laboratory values and common steps for laboratory procedures.

Section 8-1

COMMON LABORATORY VALUES

Tables 8-1 and 8-2 list normal values for both common chemistry tests and hematology testing.

Table 8-1

COMMON CHEMISTRY TESTS

Test	Abbreviation	Reference Range*	Clinical Significance
Albumin	**ALB**	3.0–5.0 g/dL	Liver, kidney, and nutritional status
Alanine amniotransferase	**ALT**	40 U/L or less	Liver disease
Alkaline phosphatase	**ALP**	30–130 U/L	Hepatobiliary and bone disease
Aspartate amniotransferase	**AST**	40 U or less	Myocardial infarction, liver disease, pancreatitis
Bilirubin • Total	**T Bil, TBili,**	0.2–1.3 mg/dL	Infant jaundice, liver disease and hemolytic anemia
Blood urea nitrogen	**BUN**	8–18 mg/dL	Kidney function

(continues)

(continued)

Test	Abbreviation	Reference Range*	Clinical Significance
Calcium	**Ca**	8.5–10.5 mg/dL	Parathyroid disorders
Creatinine	**creat**	0.4–1.5 mg/dL	Renal function
Electrolytes	**Elect, Lytes**		
• Sodium	**Na⁺**	136–145 mEq/L	Diabetes insipidus, diarrhea, and dehydration
• Potassium	**K⁺**	3.5–5.0 mEq/L	Diuretic therapy, starvation, liver disease
• Chloride	**Cl⁻**	96–110 mEq/L	Renal disease, CHF, anemia, dehydration
Globulin	**glob**	1.5–2.5 g/dL	Rheumatoid arthritis, Hodgkin's disease, and chronic infections
Glucose			
• Fasting blood sugar	**FBS**	70–100 mg/dL	All these tests help to diagnose and follow the treatment of diabetes
• 2 hr post-prandial blood glucose	**2-hr PPBS**	<140 mg/dL	
• Oral Glucose tolerance test	**OGTT**	Fasting: 70–110 mg/dL 1/2 hr: 110–170 mg/dL 1 hr: 120–170 mg/dL 2 hr: 70–120 mg/dL 3 hr: 60–120	
Lactate dehydrogenase	**LDH, LD**	100–225 U/L	Myocardia infarction (MI), pulmonary infarction, liver disease, muscular dystrophy, and pernicious anemia

Lipids
• Total cholesterol
• High-density
  lipoprotein
• Low-density
  lipoprotein
• Triglycerides
	Chol
	
	HDL
	LDL
	
	Trig
		<200 mg/dL
		
		>40 mg/dL
		<130 mg/dL
		
		<150 mg/dL
			Cardiovascular
			and thyroid
			disease

Magnesium	**Mag, Mg**	1.2–2.4 mEq/L	Malnutrition, diar- rhea, pancreatitis
Phosphorous	**P**	2.5–4.5 mg/dL	Parathyroid, renal, and diabetes disorders
Protein (total)	**TP, TPRO**	6.0–8.0 g/dL	Dehydration, mul- tiple myeloma, ne- phrotic syndrome, severe burns
Thyroid tests • Thyroid stimulat- ing hormone • Triiodothyronine • Thyroxin • Uric acid	**TSH** T_3 T_4 **UA**	0.3–4.5 mIU/L 4.5–13.0 µg/dL 4.5–13.0 µg/dL Male 3.5–7.2 mg/dL Female 2.6–6.0 mg/dL	Thyroid disorders Renal failure, gout, leukemia, and lymphomas

*Unless otherwise noted, all reference ranges are for adults.
Please note: The reference ranges are compiled from several sources. Laboratory reference values differ from laboratory to laboratory, according to what test method is used and based on the laboratory's own "normal" patient population.

Table 8-2
COMMON HEMATOLOGY TESTS

Test	Abbreviation	Test Description	Reference Ranges*
Hematocrit	**Hct**	Measures the vol- ume of packed red cells	Males: 42%–52% Females: 36%–45% Neonates: 44%–64%
Hemoglobin	**Hgb**		Males: 13–18 gm/dl Females: 12–16 gm/dl Neonates: 15–20 gm/dl

(continues)

(continued)

Test	Abbreviation	Test Description	Reference Ranges*
Red blood cell count	**RBC Ct.**	Measures the number of RBCs/mm^3	Males: 4.5–6.0 million/mm^3 Females: 4.0–5.5 million/mm^3 Neonates: 4.0–6.6 million/cu mm
White blood cell count	**WBC Ct.**	Measures the number of WBCs/cu mm	Adults: 4500–11,000/ mm^3 Neonates: 9000–25,000/ mm^3
Mean corpuscular volume	**MCV**	Measures the average volume of RBCs	Adults: 82–98 fL
Mean corpuscular hemoglobin	**MCH**	Measures the average hemoglobin content on the RBC	Adults: 26–34
Mean corpuscular hemoglobin concentration	**MCHC**	Measures the average hemoglobin content per unit volume of RBCs	32–36 g/dl
• Neutrophils	**Segs**	Increased in bacterial infections, parasitic infections, and liver disease Decreased in viral infections, humoral diseases, and patients taking chemotherapy	40%–65%
• Eosinophils	**Juvs Eos**	Increased in allergic reactions, parasitic infections, and lung and bone cancer Decreased in infectious mononucleosis, congestive heart failure (CHF), and aplastic anemia	0–2% 1–3%

• Basophils	**Basos**	Increased in allergic reactions, leukemia, hemolytic anemia, and chronic inflammations	0–1%
• Lymphocytes	**Lymphs**	Increased in viral infections, carcinoma, and hematopoietic disorders Decreased in HIV infection, leukemia, and Hodgkin's disease	25%–40%
• Monocytes	**Monos**	Increased in certain bacterial infections	3%–9%
		Decreased when patient is receiving chemotherapuetic agents	
Erythrocyte sedimentation rate	**ESR, sed rate**	Measures how far the RBCs fall in an hour in a fixed volume of blood. Helps to monitor inflammation in the body	Males: 0–20 mm/hr Females: 0–30 mm/hr
Partial thromboplastin time	**PTT**	Monitors patients on anticoagulant therapy and aids in the diagnosis of coagulation disorders	30–45 seconds
Prothrombin time	**PT**	Monitors patients on anticoagulant therapy and aids in the diagnosis of coagulation disorders	10–13 seconds

(continues)

(continued)

Test	Abbreviation	Test Description	Reference Ranges*
International normalized ratio	**INR**	A formula used to help determine clotting function	1–2
Platelet or thrombocyte count	**PLT**	Aids in the diagnosis and evaluation of various bleeding disorders	150,000–400,000/mm³

*Unless otherwise noted, all reference ranges are for adults.
Please note: The reference ranges are compiled from several different sources. Laboratory reference values differ from laboratory to laboratory, according to what test method is used and based on the laboratory's own "normal" patient population.

Section 8-2

CRITICAL LABORATORY VALUES

Following up on patient laboratory results is one of the most important functions of medical assistants and other auxiliary medical staff members. The paper trail, and now computerized drop box, can be overwhelming, especially when there are so many other tasks to complete. It is important to follow-up on all laboratory results, particularly abnormal results. But keep in mind that patients don't know whether their results are normal or abnormal, and until they receive they receive confirmation, they are going to worry. Always do what you can do to alleviate patient fears.

EMR Application

Distribution of laboratory results is much easier with electronic medical records. Centers that share an electronic connection with their reference laboratory can enjoy the convenience of having laboratory results deposited directly into the provider's electronic "Task" or "To Do" box. Results that are critical are flagged so the provider knows to review those results before any others. Once the provider reviews the results, an electronic message or task is sent to the provider's medical assistant or nurse with directions on how to handle the results. It is important not to let these tasks just sit in your electronic "To Do" or "Task" box for a prolonged period of time—especially results that are critical.

Possible Ramifications of Not Handling Critical Laboratory Results in an Efficient Manner

Table 8-3 lists some of the more common critical laboratory results that could put the patient at risk if not handled in an efficient manner. Due to space limitations, only a select few tests are listed.

Table 8-3

RAMIFICATIONS OF NOT HANDLING CRITICAL OR ABNORMAL LABORATORY RESULTS IN AN EFFICIENT MANNER

Test or Classification of Test and Usage	Possible Ramifications of Not Reporting
Clotting factors: One of the most common clotting factor profiles is the **prothrombin time** and **INR.** These tests are frequently performed on patients taking anticoagulants such as warfarin (Coumadin) and heparin. Patients on anticoagulation therapy include patients with a diagnosis of: • Deep vein thrombosis • TIA/stroke • MI	**Low result:** Patients with lower than normal levels may be at a higher risk for developing blood clots. **High result:** Patients with higher results may be more subject to internal and external bleeding.
Electrolyte Panels: Electrolyte panels include sodium, potassium, chloride, and CO_2. Electrolytes are responsible for maintaining homeostasis in the body. **Potassium** and **sodium** are both responsible for maintaining proper water and pH balance. They are also involved in nerve and muscular conduction and excitability.	Possible muscle twitching, heart irregularities or even death.
Calcium levels: Many people think of calcium strictly as a mineral that helps with strong teeth and bones. Calcium is much more. It aids in blood clotting, muscle contraction, and nerve conduction. It is particularly important in cardiac function.	Possible heart irregularities, formation of kidney stones, coma or even death.

(continues)

(continued)

Test or Classification of Test and Usage	Possible Ramifications of Not Reporting
Medication levels: It is imperative to monitor certain medication levels in the patient's bloodstream. Many medications can become toxic to particular organs when levels are too high. Examples of medication classifications that are routinely monitored include: • Anticonvulsants • Tricyclic antidepressants • Drugs used in the treatment of asthma, such as theophylline	**High levels:** Drug levels that are elevated may cause **organ toxicity.** **Low levels:** Drug levels that are too low can put the patient at serious risk of worsening conditions or symptoms that the patient is trying to control. Example: Patients taking Topomax, an anticonvulsant, have a greater risk of developing a seizure if their level is too low.
Complete blood count (CBC): The CBC includes the following: 1. Total white cell count 2. Total red cell count 3. Hemoglobin 4. Hematocrit 5. RBC indicies Monitoring the CBC is particularly important in patients who are taking chemotherapy. Unfortunately, as well as destroying cancer cells, this therapy also destroys the patient's blood cells. Careful monitoring of these patients is essential.	An increase in WBCs indicates infection. Especially important in acute infection. A decrease in WBCs is particularly alarming in patients taking chemotherapy or patients with compromised immune systems. A decrease in the red cell count, hemoglobin, hematocrit, and RBC indices could indicate anemia or blood loss due to hemorrhage.
HIV testing, sexually transmitted infection (STI) testing, etc: Results of these tests should be attended to immediately	Sexually transmitted diseases, particularly in females, that are left untreated may result in a migration of microorganisms to other related structures, causing serious infections in those structures. This can eventually lead to a buildup of scar tissue, which can be a cause of infertility.
Urinary tract infections (UTIs): UTIs are quite common. Females are more at risk to form urinary infections, but males are also likely candidates.	Urinary tract infections left untreated can migrate up into the kidneys, causing infection of the kidneys and attached structures. This can eventually cause serious kidney damage.

Pap smear, prostate specific levels, and cancer screenings:
Any test that screens for cancer is serious. Cancer risks increase with each passing year. As we age, our immune system breaks down and makes us more vulnerable to cancer. However, cancer does not discriminate. It can attack any person at any age.

Abnormal values from any test used to screen for cancer could indicate that the patient has cancer. It is imperative that the patient start treatment as quickly as possible to avoid devastating ramifications.

Section 8-3

MEDICAL LABORATORY PROCEDURES

Blood Cholesterol Testing

Procedure 8-1
BLOOD CHOLESTEROL TESTING

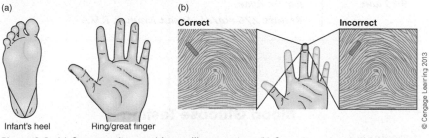

(a)   (b)

Correct   Incorrect

Infant's heel   King/great finger

© Cengage Learning 2013

Figure 8-1: (a) Common sites used for capillary puncture, (b) Correct puncture pattern— across the grain of the fingertip not along the grain.

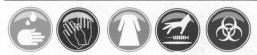

Equipment and Supplies

Hand sanitizer Cholesterol meter and supplies or test kit Control solution	Sterile puncture device	Antiseptic wipe/gauze squares Bandaid Disinfecting solution

1. Review the doctor's order and read instrument manual for your cholesterol meter or kit.

2. Wash hands, apply gloves and run a control if applicable. (If control was out of range, take corrective action.) Record result in control log and remove gloves and wash hands.

(continues)

(continued)

3. Identify the patient using two different identifiers, identify yourself, and explain the procedure.

4. Verify that the patient followed all fasting instructions prior to testing.

5. Wash hands, apply PPE and perform a capillary puncture procedure (Procedure 8-3). Dispose of puncture device and wipe away 1st drop of blood with a gauze pad.

6. Perform capillary puncture and follow manufacturer's instructions for applying the sample to the testing device. Review results once test is completed and record results.

7. Clean and disinfect the work area and properly dispose of used equipment in biohazard waste container.

8. Remove gloves and wash your hands.

9. Document the test results in the patient's chart and the laboratory log.

05/25/XXXX 9:30 a.m.	Capillary puncture, L 4th digit, and cholesterol test per Dr. Ryan. Results: 276 mg/dL. Susan Kramer, RMA ——————

Blood Glucose Testing

Procedure 8-2
BLOOD GLUCOSE

Equipment and Supplies

Hand sanitizer Glucose monitor Glucose test strips	Sterile puncture device Control solution Antiseptic wipe/gauze pads	Adhesive bandage Disinfecting solution

1. Check the provider's order, and assemble the equipment and supplies. Check the expiration date on the reagent strip and control containers.

2. Wash your hands and apply personal protective equipment (PPE).

3. Calibrate the instrument and run a control sample according to the manufacturer's instructions. Remove gloves and wash hands.

4. Identify the patient using two identifiers, identify yourself, and explain the procedure. Verify if the patient is fasting or not.

5. Ask the patient to wash and dry hands and wash your hands and apply new gloves.

6. Cleanse the puncture site with an antiseptic wipe, allowing the site to dry before puncturing.

7. Turn the unit on and check to make certain that the code number on the monitor matches the code number on the reagent strip container.

8. Wait until the blood drop icon appears on the monitor screen before puncturing site. (this may vary in some units)

9. Puncture the site with the sterile puncture device and dispose of it in a sharps container. Wipe away the first drop of blood. (Refer to Figure 8-1 for sites where capillary punctures may be performed and the angle that should be used.)

10. Touch one edge of the test strip to the drop of blood and allow the strip to absorb the blood.

11. Instruct the patient to apply pressure to the puncture site with a clean gauze square.

12. Wait for the reading to appear on the screen.

13. Remove the reagent strip from the monitor and dispose of properly.

14. Remove gloves and wash your hands.

15. Document the test results in the patient's chart and the laboratory log.

| 06-10-XXXX 9:00 a.m. | FBS per Dr. Jones, Result: 78 mg/dL, verified pt. fasted for the appropriate amount of time. Manufacturer: Smith Diagnostics, Lot # 65487, Exp 01/01/XXXX. Melanie Maren, CMA (AAMA) |

Procedure 8-3
CAPILLARY PUNCTURE PROCEDURES

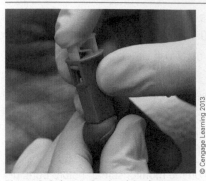

Figure 8-2: Lance the tip of the finger at a right angle to the whorls of the finger print.

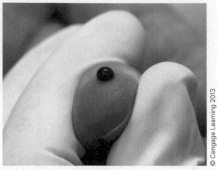

Figure 8-3: Apply gentle pressure to collect a drop of blood.

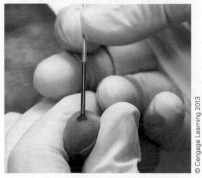

Figure 8-4: Collect the blood specimen into a capillary tube.

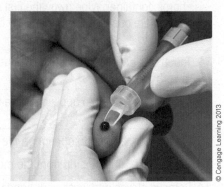

Figure 8-5: Collect the blood specimen into a microtainer tube.

Equipment and Supplies

Hand sanitizer Alcohol wipes	Gauze pads Adhesive bandage Sterile puncture device	Microhematocrit tubes or containers Disinfecting Solution

1. Check the provider's order.

2. Wash your hands and apply PPE. The types of PPE worn during a capillary stick may vary from one facility to another.

3. Assemble all the necessary equipment and label all tubes.

4. Identify the patient using two identifiers and identify yourself.

5. Explain the procedure.

6. Select the fleshy portion of the patient's distal middle or ring finger on the hand. (Refer to Figure 8-1 for specific locations and angles that can be used when performing a capillary puncture.)

7. Apply a warm compress to the area or have the patient run the hands under warm water.

8. Clean the site with alcohol and allow it to air dry.

9. Grasp the finger securely and puncture the fingertip at a right angle to the whorls of fingerprint or foot print. (Figures 8-1 and 8-2.)

10. Dispose of the lancet in the sharps container.

11. Gently squeeze the finger and wipe away the first drop of blood before beginning the sample collection.

12. Secure the finger, and apply pressure by gently squeezing and releasing the fingertip (Figure 8-3).

13. Collect needed samples either in a capillary tube or microcollection tube (Figures 8-4 and 8-5). Mix samples if necessary.

14. Once finished with collection, ask the patient to apply gentle pressure with a clean gauze square, to the puncture site.

15. Check the puncture site and apply a bandage, if necessary.

16. Dismiss the patient.

17. Properly dispose of all used equipment according to OSHA standards and prepare samples for testing.

18. Clean the work area.

19. Remove gloves and any other PPE and wash your hands, and document the procedure in the patient's chart.

11-08-XXXX 12:30 p.m.	*Capillary puncture, R middle finger. 2 heparinized capillary tubes collected for microhematocrit per Dr. Christoper. Hct. 28%. Jessica Hunnicutt, CMA (AAMA)*

Procedure 8-4
ERYTHROCYTE SEDIMENTATION RATE (SEDIPLAST)

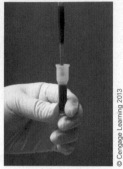

Figure 8-6: Fill the sedivial to the proper level, seal with the lid, and mix well.

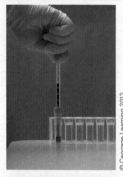

Figure 8-7: Push the Sediplast tube into the sedivial with a firm, twisting motion until the tube fills to the zero line.

Equipment and Supplies

Hand sanitizer
Blood sample from an
  EDTA test tube (lavender
  top tube)
Sediplast kit and rack
	Timer	Disinfecting solution

1. Wash your hands and apply PPE.

2. Assemble the equipment.

3. Mix the tube of blood well for 2 minutes.

4. Remove the stopper from the sedivial and fill with 0.8 mL of blood to the indicated mark. Replace the stopper and mix blood well again inside the sedivial (Figure 8-6).

5. Place the sedivial in the Sediplast rack and place the rack on a level surface.

6. Insert the Sediplast tube through the stopper using a twisting motion while pushing down until tube rests on the bottom of the vial and the blood reaches the zero line (Figure 8-7).

7. Set the timer for 1 hour.

8. Read the results of the ESR at exactly 1 hour.

9. Clean the work area and properly dispose of used equipment in biohazard trash and the tube of blood according to institutional policy.

10. Remove gloves and wash your hands.

11. Record the results in the patient's chart and the laboratory log.

| 02-24-XXXX | *Performed ESR per Dr. Karne. Results: 35 mm/hr.* |
| 2:00 p.m. | *Anne Zeller, CMA (AAMA)* |

Procedure 8-5
ORAL GLUCOSE TOLERANCE TEST

Equipment and Supplies

Hand sanitizer	Glucose meter or chem-	Red-/gray-topped tubes
Phlebotomy equipment	istry analyzer	(number will vary)
Commercial glucose	Alcohol pads/gauze	Timer/stopwatch
tolerance test beverage	squares	Adhesive bandages
		Disinfecting solution

1. Wash hands.

2. Review order and assemble equipment.

3. Identify the patient using two identifiers, identify yourself, and explain the procedure and the length of test to the patient.

4. Wash hands again and apply gloves and any other relevant PPE.

5. Obtain fasting blood and urine specimen.

6. Perform glucose testing on fasting sample either by using a glucose meter or chemistry analyzer. *(If glucose is above 200 mg/dL, the test is usually not performed—it could cause the patient to go into a diabetic coma. Always check with provider).*

7. Remove gloves, wash hands and give patient prescribed amount of commercially prepared glucose test beverage (comes in 50–75, and 100-g dosages).

8. Start timing test when patient finishes beverage.

(continues)

(continued)

---

9. Draw blood and collect urine at the
½ hr interval
1 hr interval
2 hr interval
3 hr interval and so on according to provider's instructions.
(Write patient's name, time of collection, and the time interval of the test
(i.e., ½ hr, 1 hr, etc.)

---

10. Do not dismiss patient until provider releases the patient.

---

11. Clean area with disinfecting solution and put away supplies.

---

12. Document procedure in the patient's chart.

---

13. Document results in appropriate log.

09-09-XXXX	OGTT per Dr. Wise. 7:45 a.m. Blood sample and urine sample collected. FBS 96 mg/dL. 7:55 a.m. 100 g of glucose beverage given. Finished @ 8:00 a.m. 8:30 a.m. Blood sample and urine sample collected. 9:00 a.m. Blood sample and urine sample collected. 10:00 a.m. Blood sample and urine sample collected. 11:00 a.m. Blood sample and urine sample collected. All tubes and urine samples sent to ABC Labs. Pt. tolerated procedure well. Dr. Wise examined pt. following procedure. Gave pt. educational material to take home and read. Pt to call with any questions. C. Krebs, CMA (AAMA)

Field Tip

Chilling the glucose test beverage will help the beverage to taste better. Prior to testing, instruct patient to bring a large bottle of water with them to drink during the testing. Keeping hydrated will help the veins to be more prominent and will assist the patient in providing urine samples throughout the testing.

Procedure 8-6
HEMATOCRIT

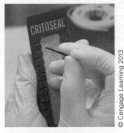

Figure 8-8: Gently press the end of the capillary tube into the sealing clay.

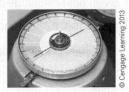

Figure 8-9: Place the tubes across from one another to balance the centrifuge.

Equipment and Supplies

Hand antiseptic	Microhematocrit reader	
Capillary tubes (plain)	Tissue wipes	
Sealing clay or sealing caps	Sterile puncture device	
Microhematocrit centrifuge	Antiseptic wipe/gauze squares	
	Adhesive bandages	
	Disinfecting solution	

1. Wash your hands and apply PPE.

2. Assemble the equipment and supplies.

3. Identify the patient using two identifiers, identify yourself, and explain the procedure.

4. Perform a capillary puncture and wipe away the first drop of blood.

5. a. Hold a heparinized capillary tube to the second drop of blood without touching the skin.
   b. Allow the capillary tube to fill three-fourths full.
   c. After filling the tube to the appropriate level, wipe the outside of the tube with a tissue to remove excess blood.
   d. Seal the end of the tube with clay or a sealing cap (Figure 8-8).
   e. Repeat the procedure with a second tube.
   f. Apply a bandage to the patient's finger.

(continues)

(continued)

6. Place tubes in the centrifuge directly opposite each other with the sealed ends pointed outward and pushed toward the gasket (Figure 8-9).

7. Securely fasten both centrifuge lids.

8. Set the timer for five minutes and adjust the speed if needed.

9. Allow the centrifuge to stop completely before opening both lids.

10. Remove both tubes, place them on the reader, and follow directions to determine the value.

11. Average the results of both tubes.

12. Record the results as a percentage.

13. Properly dispose of the equipment and supplies and cleanse work area with a disinfectant.

14. Remove PPE, wash your hands, and document the procedure.

11-08-XXXX 11:00 a.m.	Microhematocrit per Dr. Leonard. Result: 48% Ken Hardings, CMA (AAMA)

Procedure 8-7
HEMOGLOBIN USING A HEMOGLOBINOMETER

Equipment and Supplies

Hand sanitizer EDTA blood sample or capillary puncture supplies	Hemoglobinometer	Hemolysis sticks Disinfecting solution

1. Wash hands and apply PPE.

2. Assemble equipment.

3. Finger puncture method. Perform finger puncture and place one drop of blood from skin puncture on the glass chamber of hemoglobinometer.

4. Venipuncture: Perform venipuncture and place one drop of well-mixed blood from lavender-topped tube on the glass chamber of hemoglobinometer.

5. Stir blood sample on chamber with a hemolysis stick until blood becomes cherry red and clear.

6. Place coverslip over raised area of chamber.

7. Insert chamber into metal clip.

8. Insert clip into hemoglobinometer.

9. Press button on bottom to activate light source.

10. Look into ocular.

11. Slide handle on side of instrument until the right and left sides match each other.

12. Read results.

13. Report as g/dL.

14. Wash and dry glass chamber.

15. Properly dispose of equipment and disinfect area.

16. Remove PPE and wash hands.

17. Document procedure in chart and in appropriate log.

09-11-XXXX	Finger puncture, L 4th digit for a Hgb per Dr. Sumner.
10:30 a.m.	Result: 7.5 gm/dL. Pt. sent to Memorial Hospital for
	further testing per Dr. Sumner. Kelley Thomas, CMA
	(AAMA)

Rapid Test Kits (CLIA Waived)

Procedure 8-8
MONO TESTING

(a)

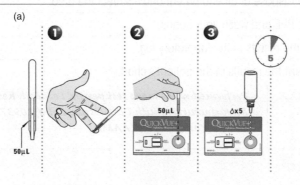

(continues)

(continued)

(b)

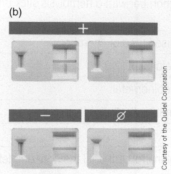

Figure 8-10: Example of the Quickvue+ Infectious Mononucleosis test (b). The top reaction windows show two positive reactions, the bottom left shows a negative reaction; the bottom right shows an invalid test result.

Equipment and Supplies

Hand sanitizer		Mono test kit
Patient specimen		Disinfecting solution
Control (if necessary)		

1. Check the order and assemble the test kit, the patient sample, and all necessary supplies. Read the test kit directions.

2. Wash hands and apply gloves, and any other required PPE.

3. Perform the test (Figure 8-10 illustrates an example for running the QuickVue Mono test from the Quidel Corporation.) You should follow the manufacturer's directions on the kit you are using. Be sure to run a control along with the test.

4. Properly dispose of all equipment and disinfect the area.

5. Remove PPE and wash your hands.

6. Record the results in the laboratory log.

7. Document the results in the patient's chart.

10-10-XXXX 10:00 a.m.	*Performed rapid mono test per Dr. Leonard, Result ⊕, Manufacturer: Smith Diagnostics, Lot # 20937548900. Lillian Karnes, CMA (AAMA)*

Procedure 8-9
PREGNANCY TEST

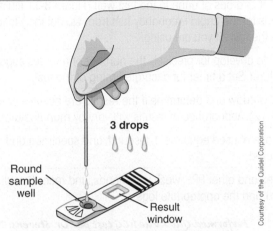

3 drops

Round
sample
well

Result
window

Courtesy of the Quidel Corporation

Figure 8-11: Example of the QuickVue Urine pregnancy test: Add 3 drops of urine to the well.

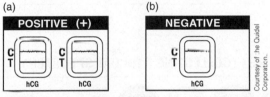

(a)   (b)

POSITIVE (+)		NEGATIVE
C T hCG	C T hCG	C T hCG

Courtesy of the Quidel Corporation.

Figure 8-12: (a) A positive result. (b) A negative result (note the control line).

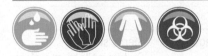

Equipment and Supplies

Hand sanitizer Urine specimen	Human chorionic gonadotropin (hCG) pregnancy test kit and control if applicable	Timer Disinfecting solution

1. Check the order and assemble the test kit, the patient sample, and all necessary supplies. Read the test kit directions.

2. Wash hands and apply gloves, and other required PPE.

3. Perform a control. (Make certain controls are at room temperature.)

(continues)

(continued)

---

4. Open the test unit, and using the dropper provided in the test kit, add the correct number of drops of urine to the test well (Figure 8-11 illustrates the instructions for the Rapid Pregnancy Test from Quidel Inc.) follow the directions on the test kit you are using.

---

5. Allow the test to develop for precisely the number of minutes suggested by the manufacturer. Set a timer for accurate timing of the test.

---

6. Read the test window and determine if the results are positive or negative (Figure 8-12). Appearance of results will vary by manufacturer.

---

7. Properly dispose of used equipment, test unit, and specimen and clean and disinfect the area.

---

8. Remove gloves and other PPE, wash your hands, and record results in the patient's chart and the appropriate logs.

06-01-XXXX 11:30 a.m.	*Performed QuickVue hCG test per Dr. Stevens. Results ⊕, Lot # 123456. Exp 01/01/XXXX. Melanie Maren, CMA (AAMA)*

Procedure 8-10
RAPID STREP TEST (COLLECTING A THROAT SPECIMEN)

Equipment and Supplies

Hand sanitizer Timer	Positive and negative controls Rapid strep kit Patient labeled throat specimen Tongue depressor	Sterile swabs Culture collection system (Culturette) if sending out for a C&S Light source Disinfecting solution

1. Check the order and assemble the test kit, and all necessary supplies. Read the test kit directions.

---

2. Wash hands and apply gloves, and other required PPE.

---

3. Identify the patient using at least two identifiers, identify yourself, and explain the procedure.

---

4. Adjust the light source so the throat is clearly visible.

5. Instruct the patient to stick out the tongue and say "Ahhhh" while you depress the tongue with the tongue depressor.

6. Roll one or two swabs held directly together against the mucous membranes of back of the throat, the crypts of the throat and the tonsillar area, being sure to swab any reddened areas or pustules on both sides of throat.

7. While still holding the tongue down, carefully withdraw the swab from the mouth being sure not to touch the sides of the mouth or the tongue.

8. If sending the specimen to the laboratory for a culture, one of the swabs must be placed in appropriate transport media and accompanied by a laboratory requisition form. If performing a rapid strep test, follow the manufacturer's directions on the rapid strep kit.

9. Properly dispose of used supplies and swabs and clean and disinfect the area.

10. Remove PPE, wash your hands, and document the procedure in the patient's chart and lab log if applicable.

04-22-XXXX 12:30 p.m.	Collected throat swab for C&S per Dr. Samuel. Sent specimen to Qwest Laboratory for testing. Chris Leonard, RMA

Specimen Collection

I, _____ give my permission for ABC Health Center to collect a urine specimen for a

drug screening test, required by _____ as part of my preemployment physical.

List all medications you are presently taking: _____

_____

_____

_____

_____

My signature indicates that I understand that my employment is contingent on a negative drug screening.

Date: _____   Signature: _____

Witness: _____

Figure 8-13: An example of a consent form for drug screening.

CLINICAL LABORATORY	**CHAIN OF CUSTODY FORM**
	SPECIMEN I.D. NO: _____

STEP—1 TO BE COLLECTED BY COLLECTOR OR EMPLOYER REPRESENTATIVE

Employer Name: _____

Address: _____ **OR**

I.D. No: _____

Medical Review Officer Name and Address:
_____
_____
_____
_____

Donor Social Security No. or Employee I.D. No.: _____

Donor I.D. Verified: ☐ Photo I.D. ☐ Employer Representative _____
_{Signature}

Reason for test: (check one)
☐ Preemployment   ☐ Random   ☐ Postaccident
☐ Periodic   ☐ Reasonable suspicion/cause
☐ Return to duty   ☐ Other(specify)

Test(s) to be performed: _____ Total tests ordered ☐

Type of specimen obtained: ☐ Urine ☐ Blood ☐ Semen ☐ Other (specify)

Submit only one specimen with each requisition.

STEP 2—TO BE COMPLETED BY COLLECTOR

For urine specimens, read temperature within 4 minutes of collection.
Check here if specimen temperature is within range: ☐ Yes, 90°–100°F/32°– 38°C

Or record actual temperature here: _____

STEP 3—TO BE COMPLETED BY COLLECTOR

Collection site: _____   Address: _____

City: _____   State: _____   Zip: _____   Phone: _____

Collection date: _____ Time: _____ ☐ a.m. ☐ p.m.

I certify that the specimen identified on this form is the specimen presented to me by the donor identified in step 1 above, and that it was collected, labeled, and sealed in the donor's presence.

Collector's name: _____   Signature of collector: _____

STEP 4—TO BE INITIATED BY DONOR AND COMPLETED AS NECESSARY THEREAFTER

Purpose of change	Released by Signature	Received by Signature	Date
A. Provide specimen for testing			
B. Shipment to laboratory			
C.			

Comments:

STEP 5—TO BE COMPLETED BY THE LABORATORY

Specimen package seal(s) intact when received in lab? ☐ Yes ☐ No. If no, explain.
Laboratory receiver's initials: _____

© Cengage Learning 2013

Figure 8-14: A chain of custody form must be completed and must accompany the specimen to the laboratory. The patient must receive a copy of the form.

Procedure 8-11
COLLECTING A SPECIMEN FOR DRUG TESTING

Equipment and Supplies

Hand sanitizer Urine specimen cup with tight-fitting lid	Cleansing towelettes Consent form	Chain of custody form Thermometer Disinfecting solution

1. Check the order and assemble equipment.

2. Wash hands and apply gloves, and other required PPE.

3. Identify the patient and check a photo ID.

4. Thoroughly explain the collection process to the patient and have the patient sign a consent form (Figure 8-13). This consent is sometimes part of the chain of custody form. The consent form explains the purpose of the test and gives the health care professional permission to collect and handle the specimen. Consent also gives permission to send the specimen for testing and to give the results to the requesting agency.

5. Explain to the patient that prescription and OTC drugs will be detected in the sample and instruct the patient to list all medications or substances taken within the last 30 days.

6. Instruct the patient to remove all outer clothing and empty pockets. Females must leave purses outside the collection area.

7. Ask the patient to wash and dry the hands before collecting the specimen. No water may be running during specimen collection.

8. Explain the collection process to the patient and supply the patient with a specimen container. Sometimes, the health care professional may need to witness the collection procedure (occurs most often in cases in which a crime has been committed).

9. After collection, check the specimen for any signs of alteration such as unusual color or odor.

10. Measure the temperature of the urine within 4 minutes of collection. Variations in temperature could indicate tampering with the specimen.

11. If applicable, transfer the specimen to a transport container while the patient witnesses the transfer. Place an identification label on the container and instruct the patient to initial the label.

12. Check the chain of custody form to ensure all information is complete.

(continues)

(continued)

13. Note the date and time of collection and sign and print your full name.

14. Give the patient a copy of the chain of custody form (Figure 8-14).

15. Seal the specimen in a leak-proof bag.

16. Throw away any trash and disinfect the area. Give the specimen to the laboratory courier.

10-10-XXXX 10:15 a.m.	*Urine specimen collected for drug testing per Dr. Smith's orders. Patient signed consent form. Urine checked for any signs of alteration and temperature. Pt witnessed urine transfer to transport container, pt initialed labeled container, and copy of the chain of custody form provided to patient. Sent specimen to Qwest Laboratory for testing. Pauline Mingus, CMA (AAMA)*

Procedure 8-12
COLLECTING A GENITAL SPECIMEN

Equipment and Supplies

Hand sanitizer	Specimen container, cultures, etc.	Disinfecting solution

1. Gather supplies and check expiration dates on transfer containers or culture tubes.

2. Correctly identify patient.

3. Wash hands and apply PPE. Accept specimens from the provider and place in proper media.

4. Label and date the specimen and identify the origin of the specimen

5. Properly store specimens until they are picked up by courier.

6. Properly dispose of contaminated supplies or equipment in biohazard waste container.

7. Remove PPE and wash your hands.

8. Document the procedure.

9. Sanitize and disinfect the work area.

10-13-XXXX 10:00 a.m.	Vaginal specimens sent to Quest Lab for Chlamydia and herpes testing per Dr. Manton. J. Miller, CMA (AAMA)

Procedure 8-13
COLLECTING A NASOPHARYNGEAL SPECIMEN

Equipment and Supplies

Hand sanitizer Penlight	Tongue blade or nasal speculum Sterile flexible aluminum swab Transport media	Biohazard transport bag (if applicable) Disinfecting solution

1. Check the order and assemble equipment.

2. Identify the patient using two identifiers, identify yourself, and explain procedure.

3. Wash hands and apply gloves and other required PPE.

4. Ask patient tilt the head back.

5. Inspect the nasopharyngeal area

6. Gently open nostril with nasal speculum or by holding back with tongue blade. Insert swab through the nostril straight back into the nasopharynx along the base of the nose (about the distance to the ears). Leave swab in place for a few seconds and slowly rotate swab while you withdraw it from the nostril.

7. Place swab in transport media and label the specimen with the patient's name, collection date and time, and the specimen's origin.

8. Properly dispose of equipment in the biohazard waste container.

9. Clean and disinfect the work area.

10. Remove PPE and wash your hands.

11. Properly store specimen until transport.

12. Document the procedure.

12-08-XXXX 11:20 a.m.	Nasopharyngeal specimen collected and sent to ABC lab for a C&S per Dr. Motika. Rhonda Moore, CMA (AAMA)

Procedure 8-14

COLLECT AND PREPARE A SPUTUM SPECIMEN

Equipment and Supplies

Hand sanitizer Sterile sputum cup with lid/biohazard transfer bag	Cup of water	Microscopic slide Potassium hydroxide (KOH) Disinfecting solution

1. Assemble the equipment and properly label the specimen container.

2. Identify the patient using two identifiers, introduce yourself, and explain the procedure.

3. Wash your hands and put on all of your PPE.

4. Have the patient rinse out the mouth.

5. Carefully remove the lid from the specimen cup and place on the counter without contaminating it.

6. Instruct the patient to take in three deep breaths and to start forcefully coughing.

7. Ask patient to expectorate into the center of the specimen container.

8. Place the lid on the container without contaminating it and tighten it securely. Place it in a plastic bag.

9. Insert the completed laboratory requisition and send to the laboratory for analysis.

Preparing the Smear (if the provider orders a smear to be made with the specimen)

10. Wash hands, apply PPE, and label the slide. Using a sterile swab, smear sputum on a microscopic slide.

11. Squeeze 1 drop of potassium hydroxide over the smear and place a cover slip over it.

12. Place the slide under the microscope on low power for the provider.

13. Clean the area and remove PPE. Throw PPE into biohazard container.

01-03-XXXX 10:00 a.m.	*Sputum specimen obtained for C&S per Dr. Stevens. Substantial amt. blood mixed with sample. Delivered to lab with request. Jessica Hunnicutt, CMA (AAMA)*

Procedure 8-15

INSTRUCT PATIENT HOW TO COLLECT A STOOL SPECIMEN FOR OVA AND PARASITE TESTING

Equipment and Supplies

Hand sanitizer Printed instructions	Appropriate collection containers	Package of O & P Vials Biohazard transfer bag

1. Wash your hands and assemble the equipment.

2. Identify the patient using at least two identifiers, and identify yourself.

3. Give the patient the appropriate collection containers and gloves, and explain that the specimens will be collected at home. Patients are given small O & P vials containing a preservative to hold an aliquot of the original specimen.

4. Instruct the patient to:
   a. Collect the specimen in the wide-mouthed collection container without contaminating the fecal specimen with urine.
   b. Follow the instructions on the vials for preparing each specimen.
   c. Transfer vials into a biohazard transfer bag following collection. Store specimens at room temperature and return specimens to office within two days of collection.

5. Encourage the patient to ask questions and give ample time for answers.

6. Supply the patient with written instructions.

7. Make sure the patient understands the collection process before leaving the office and when and where to return the specimen.

08-12-XXXX 2:30 p.m.	*Provided instructions and appropriate containers for O&P fecal specimen collection. Pt. instructed to return to office with specimen in 2 days, per Dr. Gent's orders.* *Millie Leonard, CMA (AAMA)*

Procedure 8-16

COLLECTING A CLEAN-CATCH URINE SPECIMEN

Equipment and Supplies

Hand sanitizer Gloves for patient and for you	Sterile urine specimen cup with tight fitting lid/transfer bag	Cleansing towelettes (2 for males and 3 for females) Disinfecting solution

1. Wash your hands, apply gloves, and assemble equipment.

2. Identify the patient using at least two identifiers, and identify yourself.

3. Take the patient to a private area near the restroom to explain the collection procedure.

4. Give the patient gloves (optional), towelettes, and a urine specimen cup with the patient's name on it. Make sure the specimen cup has a lid.

5. Explain the collection process.
   Females:
   a. Instruct the patient to spread the labia apart with one hand to expose the urinary meatus, then take one towelette and wipe down either side of the meatus from front to back, and then discard the towelette.
   b. Instruct the patient to take a second towelette and wipe down the opposite side of the meatus from front to back and discard the towelette.
   c. Instruct the patient to take the third towelette and wipe down the middle of the meatus from front to back and discard the towelette.
   Males:
   Instruct the patient to retract the foreskin (if applicable) and cleanse the tip and the urethral opening, from the tip of the penis toward the ring of the glans, with two separate towelettes before beginning to collect the specimen.

6. Females and males:
   Instruct the patient to keep the labia spread apart or the foreskin retracted, and begin to urinate into the toilet. Catch the middle portion of the urine in the specimen cup and finish urinating in the toilet.

7. Have patient place the lid tightly on the specimen container and wipe the outside of the container with a disinfecting wipe paper towel.

8. Instruct patient to leave the sample in the designated area, remove gloves and wash hands.

9. Obtain the specimen, finish labeling the container with the date and time of collection, type of specimen and place in transfer bag with lab requisition form. Store in refrigerator.

10. Clean and disinfect the work area, remove gloves, wash hands and document the specimen collection.

10-10-XXXX 10:30 a.m.	*Instructed patient how to collect a clean-catch midstream urine sample per Dr. Samuals. Specimen sent to Qwest Laboratory for a complete urinalysis and C&S. Lilly Karnes, CMA (AAMA)* ――――

Procedure 8-17
COLLECTING A WOUND SPECIMEN

Equipment and Supplies

Hand sanitizer Disposable gloves/sterile gloves	Skin antiseptic Sterile drapes/ bandaging supplies	Sterile swabs Appropriate transport media Disinfecting solution

1. Complete laboratory requisition form with provider's order.

2. Identify the patient using at least two identifiers, identify yourself, and explain the procedure.

3. Wash your hands, apply PPE and set up a sterile tray. Drape the patient. Wash your hands again and apply sterile gloves.

4. Apply an antiseptic to the affected area. Place the swab in the wound, and saturate with any exudate. Avoid touching the outer edges of the wound when withdrawing the swab.

5. Immediately place the swab in the appropriate transport media and crush the ampule. Clean and dress the area according to the provider's instructions.

6. Properly dispose of contaminated equipment and supplies. Clean and disinfect the area.

7. Remove PPE, wash your hands, and document the collection procedure in the patient's chart.

02-24-XXXX 10:10 a.m.	*Collected wound culture swab from lesion on right forearm, per Dr. Leonard's orders. Specimen sent to Qwest Laboratory for C&S. Lillian Karnes, CMA (AAMA)* ――――

Fecal Occult Blood Test

Procedure 8-18

PATIENT INSTRUCTION, COLLECTING AND TESTING STOOL SPECIMEN FOR OCCULT BLOOD

Equipment and Supplies

Hand sanitizer Test cards and developer	Return envelope	Home care instruction form Disinfecting solution

1. Check order, wash hands and assemble the supplies.

2. Identify the patient using two identifiers, identify yourself, and explain the purpose of the procedure.

3. Explain special dietary instructions that the patient is to follow before collecting the specimen. (This is usually found within the testing supplies!)

4. Explain how to properly label the cards before testing.

5. Explain instructions for collecting the samples, including how many samples the patient is to collect—usually three different samples on three different days.

6. Explain the instructions for sending the samples back to the office.

7. Once the test cards are received in the office, wash your hands and apply gloves before testing begins.

8. Correctly follow the developing instructions, including performing a control on each test. A blue color indicates a positive result.

9. Properly dispose of the test cards and clean the work area with disinfecting solution.

10. Remove gloves, wash your hands, and document the procedure and results in the patient record.

12-13-XXXX 9:45 a.m.	*Hemawipe testing instructions per Dr. Jones. Pt. supplied with testing cards and spatulas to obtain three test samples at home. Verbal and written preparation and collection instructions given. Pt. expressed understanding of procedure and will mail test cards to office in enclosed mailer. Judith Jones, CMA (AAMA)*

12-20-XXXX 10:30 a.m.	Hemawipe test cards received in office today. Test completed. Results: negative for all three specimens. Judith Jones, CMA (AAMA)

Urinalysis Testing

Urinalysis testing is one of the most common tests performed in the medical office. Patients presenting with urinary symptoms should have their urine dipped following an order from the provider. Table 8-4 lists the normal values associated with each test on the dipstick and provides the clinical significance of each positive or elevated result.

Table 8-4

MULTISTIX 10 SG RESULTS

Component	Normal Value	Clinical Significance of Positive or Elevated Results
pH	4.5–8.0	Old specimen; UTI
Protein	Negative/trace	Renal disease, extreme exercise, high fever, dehydration
Glucose	Negative	Diabetes, pancreatic disease, advanced kidney disease
Ketones	Negative	Starvation, low-carbohydrate/high-fat diet, vomiting, uncontrolled diabetes
Blood	Negative	Hemolytic anemias, kidney or urinary tract damage, menstrual contaminant
Bilirubin	Negative	Hepatitis, possible bile duct obstruction
Urobilinogen	0.1–1.0	Liver dysfunction, hemolytic diseases
Nitrite	Negative	UTI, cystitis; used to monitor antibiotic therapy
Leukocytes	Negative	UTI
Specific gravity	1.005–1.030	Kidney function, diabetes insipidus

Procedure 8-19

PHYSICAL AND CHEMICAL URINALYSIS AND PREPARING A MICROSCOPIC SLIDE

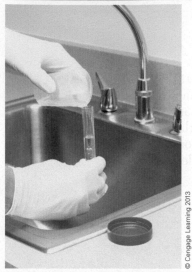

Figure 8-15: Pour the urine specimen into a clear tube.

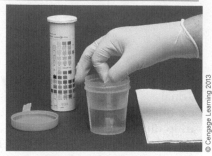

Figure 8-17: Carefully dip the reagent strip into the well-mixed specimen. Note: Make sure all the reagent pads are covered completely by the urine. Do not dip reagent strip into original specimen if there is a chance the specimen will be sent out for a C&S.

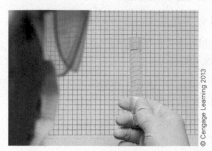

Figure 8-16: Assess the clarity of the urine.

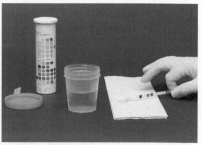

Figure 8-18: Tilt the strip sideways and allow excess urine to drain onto a paper towel.

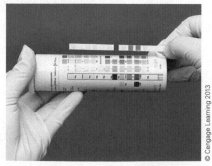

Figure 8-19: Compare the strip to the color chart on the container at the right time intervals.

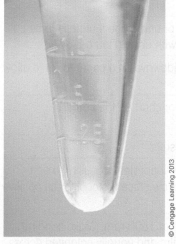

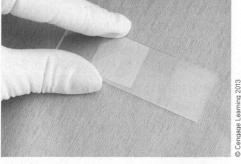

Figure 8-21: Gently place the cover slip over the drop of urine, making sure the drop spreads evenly.

© Cengage Learning 2013

Figure 8-20: A button of sediment forms after centrifugation.

Equipment and Supplies

Hand sanitizer	Centrifuge	Digital refractometer
Urine specimen	Disposable pipettes	Laboratory report form
Urine control sample	Microscopic slides	Laboratory log sheet
Centrifuge tubes/caps	Cover slips	Disinfecting solution
	Reagent strips	

1. Wash hands and apply appropriate PPE.

2. Assemble the necessary equipment.

3. Gently mix the specimen.

4. Pour the specimen into a clear centrifuge tube (Figure 8-15). While holding the specimen in front of a light source, assess and record the color of the urine.

5. Observe the transparency of the urine by holding a printed sheet of paper behind the specimen (Figure 8-16).

6. Note any unusual odor, if present.

7. Measure the specific gravity with either a digital refractometer (following the manufacturer's instructions) or by the reagent strip method.

(continues)

(continued)

8. Dip the reagent strip in the urine specimen, or urine tube if urine is to be cultured, being certain to cover the entire strip with urine (Figure 8-17).

9. After removing the strip from the cup, tilt it sideways on a paper towel to allow excess urine to be removed (Figure 8-18).

10. Hold the strip next to but not against the color chart on the bottle (Figure 8-19).

11. Accurately time all readings and read the results.

12. Record all results on a report form and in the laboratory log, using a pen covered with a disposable plastic sheath. Follow office protocol for all positive results.

13. Centrifuge the urine specimen for 5 minutes at 1500 rpm. (Make certain tubes are covered with plastic caps or parafilm and equally balanced across from each other before centrifuging.)

14. Carefully pour the supernatant off and mix the sediment well (Figure 8-20).

15. Place 1 drop of well-mixed sediment on a glass slide and place a cover slip over the drop of urine (Figure 8-21).

16. Place the slide under the microscope and inform the physician that the specimen is ready to examine.

17. Properly dispose of all equipment and specimens.

18. Remove gloves, wash your hands, and document the procedure.

11-08-XXXX	*Physical and Chemical UA per Dr. Leonard. Amount: 200 mL*
10:00 a.m.	*Color: straw Clarity: hazy. pH: 6G: 1.002 Nitrites: 1+!*
	WBC: Mod. All other results negative. Lyn Collier, RMA

Field Tip

When there is a chance that a urine specimen will be sent out for a culture and sensitivity, never dip the dipstick into the original container as this will contaminate the specimen and possibly alter the results.

Procedure 8-20
PREPARING URINE SEDIMENT

Equipment and Supplies

Hand sanitizer Urine specimen	Urine centrifuge tubes/caps Disposable pipette	Centrifuge Disinfecting solution

1. Wash hands and apply appropriate PPE.

2. Assemble the necessary equipment and supplies.

3. Verify the name on the specimen container with the order or reporting form.

4. Mix specimen well, pour 10 to 20 mL of well-mixed urine into a labeled centrifuge tube and cap with a plastic cap or Parafilm.

5. Centrifuge the sample at 1,500 rpm for 5 minutes.

6. Carefully remove the tubes once the centrifuge has come to a halt.

7. Remove the caps and pour off the supernatant, leaving the sediment. Aspirate the sediment into a transfer pipette and place one drop of urine on a clean slide. Place cover slip over the drop and place on the microscope.

8. Care for equipment and dispose of supplies. Clean and disinfect the work area.

9. Remove PPE and wash your hands.

Procedure 8-21
24-HOUR URINE SPECIMEN TESTING

Equipment and Supplies

Hand Sanitizer
Properly labeled 24-hour
    urine collection
    container (with preservative if required)
	Wide-mouth urine
	    collection container
		Patient education
		    materials
		Disinfecting solution

(continues)

(continued)

1. Wash hands.

2. Assemble the necessary supplies and equipment.

3. Check the order and identify the type of 24-hour urine collection requested.

4. Check to determine if any preservative needs to be added to the container.

5. Properly label the container.

6. Apply appropriate PPE and add preservative to the 24 hour collection container, if necessary.

7. Patient Instructions
   a. At the beginning of the 24-hour collection period, void your first urine into the toilet. (Record the date and time of first collection on the label provided on the bottle.)
   b. Collect all urine specimens over the next 24 hours in the wide-mouth collecting container and pour into 24- hour collection container.
   c. Void last urine exactly 24 hours after first urine void and pour into collection container.
   d. Record the date and time of last collection on the label.

8. Explain how to properly preserve the urine over the 24-hour period (usually by refrigeration or preservative tablet).

9. Instruct patient to return the specimen when collection process is finalized.

10. Document the 24- hour urine collection education and any supplies given to patient.

11. Upon return of specimen:
   a. Double check beginning and ending times of collection with the patient.
   b. Record on lab requistion form.

12. Wash hands and apply PPE and follow the lab's instructions for properly preparing and preserving the urine for lab pickup.

13. Dispose of any waste and clean and disinfect the work area.

14. Remove PPE and wash your hands and document the procedure.

| 11-08-XXXX 9:30 a.m. | 24-hour urine collection instructions given to patient per Dr. Smith. Pt supplied with properly labeled urine containers and written instructions. Pt. expressed understanding of procedure and will return urine specimen to office upon completion. Lucy Frank, CMA (AAMA) |

Venipuncture

Before performing venipuncture, you should be familiar with the different color-topped tubes and the additives in those tubes. You should also be familiar with the different tests that correspond with the tubes. Figure 8-22 lists the more common tests, tubes, and their additives. Always double-check the laboratory manual for specifics.

Order of Draw

Health care workers should also be familiar with the order of draw when performing phlebotomy. The current recommendations from the CLSI are listed in Table 8-5. These change from time to time, so check the CLSI website to ascertain that no changes have taken place. The recommended order of draw is the same for both evacuated tube and syringe methods.

Vein Selection

Figure 8-23 illustrates the major veins used for blood draws in the antecubital area as well as arteries that should be avoided.

Hemogard Closure	Rubber Stopper	Additive	Additive Function	Laboratory Use
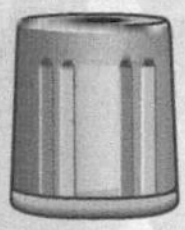	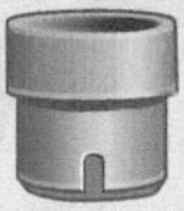	EDTA (ethylenedi-aminetetra-acetic acid)	Binds calcium to prevent clotting	Hematology testing: CBC, differential, and ESR
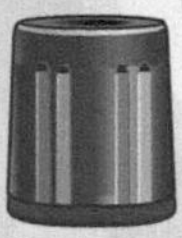	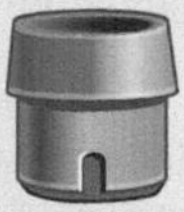	No additive	Promotes blood clot formation	Serum testing: hormone studies, organ panels, medication levels, and HIV testing
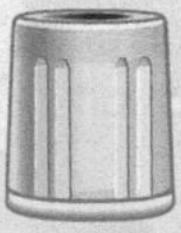	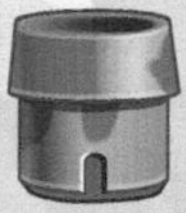	Clot activator and gel for serum separation	Serum separation; allows technician to pour off serum	Serum testing, same as for the red top

Figure 8-22: Common vacuum tube color guide.
*Please note: Each tube containing an additive of any kind must be inverted a specified number of times immediately following blood collection. Refer to the manufacturer's directions for the correct number of inversions.

Hemogard Closure	Rubber Stopper	Additive	Additive Function	Laboratory Use
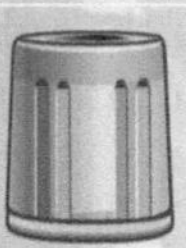	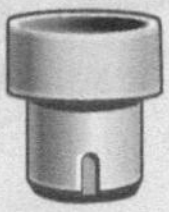	Potassium oxalate and sodium fluoride	Binds calcium and stabilizes glucose	Glucose testing and alcohol levels
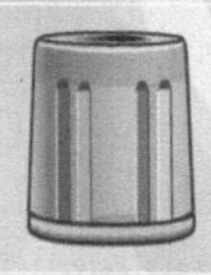	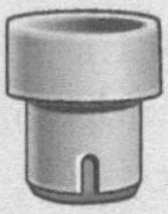	Sodium citrate	Binds calcium to prevent clotting	Coagulation studies: PT, PTT, and INR
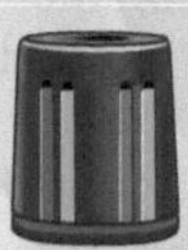		Sodium heparin	Inhibits formation of thrombin and prevents clotting	Plasma studies for trace elements
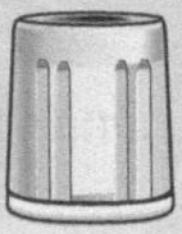	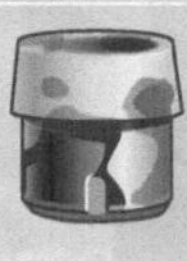	Lithium heparin and gel for plasma separation	Heparin prevents the release of potassium by platelets during clotting, and the gel separates the plasma from the red cells	STAT chemistry plasma studies: electrolytes, arterial blood gases, etc.
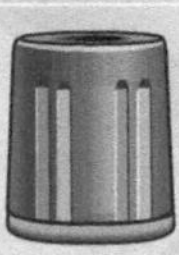	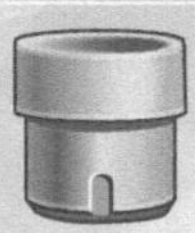	Lithium or sodium heparin	Inhibits formation of thrombin and prevents clotting	Chemistry plasma studies: electrolytes, arterial blood gases, etc.
	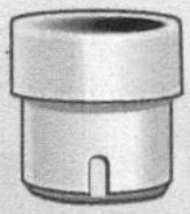	Sodium polyanetholesulfonate (SPS)	Binds calcium to prevent clotting and inhibits bacterial growth	Blood or body fluid cultures
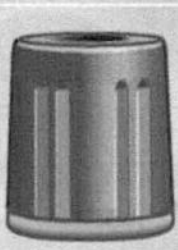	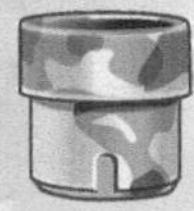	Thrombin activator	Results in faster clot formation	STAT serum chemistry testing

Figure 8-22: (continued)

TABLE 8-5

CLSI RECOMMENDED ORDER OF DRAW

Order Of Draw	Tube Color
Sterile culture bottles or tubes	Yellow
Coagulation tubes	Light blue
Serum tubes with or without a clot activator and with or without separator gel	Plain red Red and Gray speckled
Heparin tubes with or without gel	Light green Green speckled Green
EDTA tubes	Lavender
Glycolytic inhibitor	Gray

Source: NCCLS (Now CLSI): "Order of Draw," H3-A5, Vol. 23, No. 32, 8.10.2.

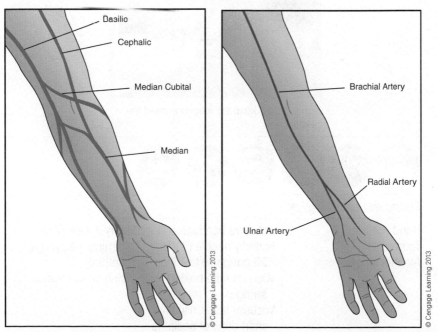

Figure 8-23: (a) Surface veins used for venipuncture. (b) Major arteries of the arm that should be avoided during a venipuncture.

Field Tip

In order to reduce complications during and following a blood draw, health care workers should select the median cubital vein in the antecubital fossa as their first choice, cephalic vein as their second choice, and the basilic vein as their last choice. The basilic vein should only be used when there are no other options. This is because the basilic vein has more nerves in the surrounding area, which may result in complications in the event a nerve is nicked.

Field Tip

To reduce the risks for reflux or backflow during a phlebotomy procedure, make certain that the patient's arm remains in a downward position throughout the blood draw.

Procedure 8-22
VENIPUNCTURE (BUTTERFLY METHOD)

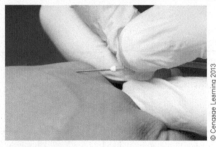

Figure 8-24: Grasp the wings and insert the needle.

Equipment and Supplies

Hand sanitizer Tourniquet Alcohol wipes	Adhesive bandage Butterfly needle (21 to 23 gauge, ½ to 1 inch) Vacuum tube holder/syringe Vacuum tubes, usually short draw or pediatric size	Safety device (if performing the syringe method) Disinfecting solution

1. Check the provider's order and complete the laboratory requisition form.

2. Wash your hands and apply PPE. Remember that the types of PPE worn during a blood draw may vary from one facility to another.

3. Assemble all the necessary equipment and label all tubes.

4. Identify the patient using two identifiers, identify yourself, and explain the procedure.

5. Verify compliance of fasting instructions and other restrictions (e.g., the need to draw blood from one side or another because of a mastectomy or the presence of a shunt).

6. Visually inspect the patient's skin and veins in both arms or hands. Always ask if the patient has a preference. Patients usually know which veins produce the best results.

7. Select the appropriate arm or hand and apply a tourniquet 3 to 4 inches above the elbow or wrist when drawing from the hand. The tourniquet should not remain in place longer than 1 minute.

8. Ask the patient to make a fist.

9. Place the fist of the patient's other hand under the elbow when drawing from the arm, or under the wrist when drawing from the hand.

10. Palpate the vein and selected final site.

11. Cleanse the site with alcohol using a circular motion.

12. Allow the area to air dry, or dry wipe the area with a clean/sterile cotton ball.

13. Pull the skin taut.

14. Grasp the wings of the butterfly and insert the needle bevel up, at a 5- to 10-degree angle (Figure 8-24).

Evacuated Tube Method

Once blood enters the tubing, push the tube onto the needle inside the tube adapter and allow it to fill completely. Remove the tube and invert additive tubes to mix before pushing in additional tubes. When the last tube is filling, release the tourniquet. When the tube is completely full, withdraw the tube and then withdraw the needle. Engage the safety device.

Syringe Method

Once blood enters the hub of the needle, start pulling back on the plunger. Fill the syringe completely and ask the patient to relax the hand. Release the tourniquet, withdraw the needle, engage the safety device. Place needle in a sharps container. Fill the tubes using a safety transfer device and immediately invert them to mix.

(continues)

(continued)

15. Place a dry cotton ball over the site and instruct the patient to apply firm pressure to the site for 2 to 5 minutes.

16. Discard used equipment according to OSHA standards.

17. Check the puncture site and apply a pressure bandage.

18. Dismiss the patient.

19. Clean the work area with a disinfectant.

20. Remove gloves and wash your hands.

21. Document the procedure in the patient's chart.

02-12-XXXX 11:25 a.m.	*Phlebotomy (butterfly method) R. antecubital for PT, PTT, and INR per Dr. Price. 1 blue top sent to ABC Laboratory. Patient c/o slight pain during procedure but feels fine now. Advised to apply ice upon returning home per Dr. Price. Addision Miller, CMA (AAMA)—*

Procedure 8-23
VENIPUNCTURE (EVACUATED TUBE METHOD)

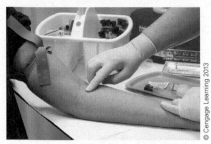

© Cengage Learning 2013

Figure 8-25: Palpate for the vein in an up-and-down direction.

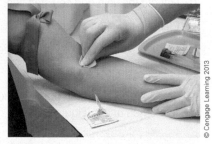

© Cengage Learning 2013

Figure 8-26: Cleanse the site with alcohol, moving in a circular motion.

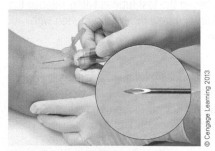

© Cengage Learning 2013

Figure 8-27: Insert the needle using a 15- to 30-degree angle with the bevel up.

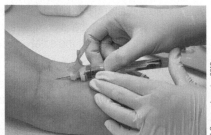

© Cengage Learning 2013

Figure 8-28: With your nondominant hand, push the vacuum tube onto the needle, allowing it to completely fill.

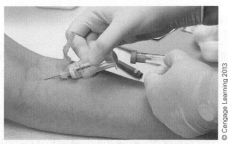
Figure 8-29: Change tubes as needed until all tubes have been collected.

Equipment and Supplies

Hand sanitizer	Gauze squares	Vacuum tube holder
Tourniquet	Adhesive bandage	Disinfecting solution
Alcohol wipes	Multisample safety needle (20 to 22 gauge, 1-½")	
	Vacuum tubes	

1. Check the provider's order and complete the laboratory requisition form.

2. Wash your hands and apply PPE. Remember that the types of PPE worn during a blood draw may vary from one facility to another.

3. Assemble all the necessary equipment and label all tubes.

4. Identify the patient using two identifiers, identify yourself, and explain the procedure.

5. Verify compliance of fasting instructions and other restrictions (e.g., the need to draw blood from one side or another because of a mastectomy or the presence of a shunt).

6. Visually inspect the patient's skin and veins in both arms or hands. Always ask if the patient has a preference. Patients usually know which veins produce the best results.

7. Select the appropriate arm or hand and apply a tourniquet 3 to 4 inches above the elbow. The tourniquet should not remain in place longer than 1 minute.

(continues)

(continued)

8. Ask the patient to make a fist.

9. Place the fist of the patient's other hand under the elbow to assist with the flow of blood in a downward direction. (This helps to prevent reflux)

10. Palpate the vein and selected final site (Figure 8-25).

11. Cleanse the site with alcohol using a circular motion (Figure 8-26).

12. Allow the area to air dry, or dry wipe the area with a clean/sterile cotton ball.

13. Pull the skin taut to anchor the vein.

14. Using a 15- to 30-degree angle, insert the needle with the bevel up (Figure 8-27) and tube label down.

15. Using the hand that anchored the vein, grasp the flanges of the holder and push the tube until the needle punctures the stopper and blood flows into the tube (Figure 8-28).

16. Allow the tube to fill to the desired level before changing the tube. Withdraw the tube and mix the additive tubes immediately.

17. Change tubes until all tubes have been collected (Figure 8-29). Instruct the patient to open the hand.

18. Release the tourniquet and remove the tube before removing the needle.

19. Place a dry cotton ball above the site, withdraw the needle, and ask the patient to apply firm pressure to the site for 2 to 5 minutes.

20. Engage the safety device and dispose of needle into sharp's container. Discard the used supplies and equipment according to OSHA standards.

21. Check the puncture site and apply a pressure bandage.

22. Dismiss the patient.

23. Clean and disinfect the work area.

24. Remove gloves and wash your hands.

25. Document the procedure in the patient's chart.

02-12-XXXX 10:30 a.m.	*Phlebotomy (evacuated tube method) R. antecubital for CBC and CMP per Dr. Smith. 2 red tops and 1 lavender top sent to ABC Laboratory. No Complications. Carson O'Brien, CMA (AAMA)*

Procedure 8-24

VENIPUNCTURE (SYRINGE METHOD)

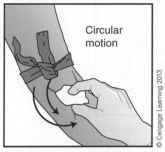

Figure 8-30: Cleanse the area with the alcohol and either wipe dry or allow to air dry.

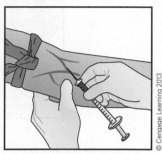

Figure 8-31: Pull the skin taut and insert the needle.

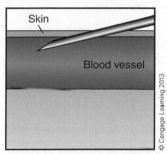

Figure 8-32: The correct route of entry.

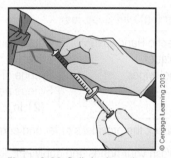

Figure 8-33: Pull slowly on the plunger and withdraw blood.

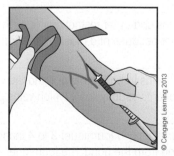

Figure 8-34: Release the tourniquet.

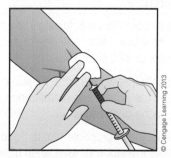

Figure 8-35: Apply a cotton ball slightly above the puncture site but not directly over needle.

(continues)

(continued)

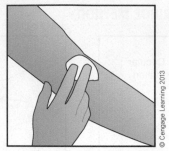

Figure 8-36: Instruct the patient to apply firm pressure to the site until bleeding has stopped.

Equipment and Supplies

Antiseptic Handwash Tourniquet Alcohol wipes	Gauze squares Adhesive bandage Syringe (10 to 20 cc) Syringe needle (21 to 22 g, 1-½")	Transfer device Vacuum tubes Disinfecting solution

1. Check the provider's order and complete the laboratory requisition form.

2. Wash your hands and apply PPE. Remember that the types of PPE worn during a blood draw may vary from one facility to another.

3. Assemble all the necessary equipment and label all tubes.

4. Identify the patient using two identifiers, identify yourself, and explain the procedure.

5. Verify compliance of fasting instructions and other restrictions (e.g., the need to draw blood from one side or another because of a mastectomy or the presence of a shunt).

6. Visually inspect the patient's skin and veins in both arms or hands. Always ask if the patient has a preference. Patients usually know which veins produce the best results.

7. Select the appropriate arm or hand and apply a tourniquet 3 to 4 inches above the elbow or wrist when drawing from the hand. The tourniquet should not remain in place longer than 1 minute.

8. Ask the patient to make a fist.

9. Place the fist of the patient's other hand under the elbow when drawing from the arm, or under the wrist when drawing from the hand. This keeps blood flowing in a downward direction—avoiding reflux.

10. Cleanse the site with alcohol using a circular motion (Figure 8-30).

11. Allow the area to air dry, or dry wipe the area with a clean/sterile cotton ball or gauze.

12. Pull the skin taut to anchor the vein (Figure 8-31).

13. Insert the needle using a 15- to 30-degree angle and make certain that the bevel is upward. (Figure 8-32).

14. When blood appears in the hub of needle, slowly pull back on the plunger at a steady rate using the opposite hand (Figure 8-33).

15. Allow the syringe to fill completely.

16. Instruct the patient to open the hand.

17. Release the tourniquet (Figure 8-34).

18. Place a dry cotton ball above the site, withdraw the needle, and ask the patient to apply firm pressure to the site for 2 to 5 minutes (Figures 8-35 and 8-36).

19. Push the sheath over the needle and carefully remove it from the syringe. Discard the needle into the sharps container.

20. Carefully transfer the blood from the syringe to vacuum tubes using a safety transfer device.

21. Immediately mix each filled tube according to the manufacturer's instructions.

22. Discard used equipment according to OSHA standards.

23. Check the puncture site and apply a pressure bandage.

24. Dismiss the patient.

25. Clean the work area.

26. Remove gloves and wash your hands.

27. Document the procedure in the patient's chart and in the laboratory log.

02-24-XXXX 10:30 a.m.	Phlebotomy (syringe method), L. antecubital for CBC and ESR per Dr. Leonard. 2 lavender tops sent to ABC Laboratory. ⊖ Complications. Abisha Hood, CMA (AAMA)

Section Nine

X-RAY AND DIAGNOSTIC EXAMINATIONS (PREPARATION)

INTRODUCTION

This section will benefit those who are not familiar with x-ray, ultrasound, computed tomography (CT), and magnetic resonance imaging (MRI) examinations, as well as other common diagnostic procedures. A list of terms and definitions, common patient preparations, and descriptions of these examinations will aid the medical assistant and other ancillary health team members in providing valuable advice to patients.

This section also includes standard information that will need to be obtained before scheduling the examinations. Because of differences in health insurance, precertification of procedures may be necessary. If the procedure is not fully covered by the patient's health insurance, a waiver must be obtained from the patient, with his or her signature, stating that any fee not covered by the insurance company will be paid by the patient.

The examination preparation instructions are general because medical facilities often change these instructions. Therefore, it is wise to check with the facility for specific instructions.

Section 9-1

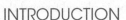

X-RAY EXAMINATIONS

Information Needed When Ordering X-Ray Procedures

1. Name and age of patient or date of birth
2. Patient's telephone number and address
3. Patient's Social Security number and insurance information
4. Name of x-ray/procedure to be ordered and who ordered it
5. Diagnosis code(s)
6. Symptoms or signs of the medical condition

Most insurance companies require precertification before certain procedures such as CT and MRI scans. It is generally the responsibility of the ordering provider's office to precertify radiological procedures. It is important to check with the insurance company before sending a patient for x-ray procedures.

Positioning Terms and Abbreviations

1. *Supine position:* Patient is placed on his or her back with the face pointing upward.

2. *Prone position:* Patient is placed with the face pointed downward and to the side.

3. *Oblique:* Patient is positioned in a semilateral position or at a 45-degree angle.

4. *Lateral:* The beam goes from one side of the body to the other.

5. *Right lateral (RL):* The right side of the body is positioned next to the film, and the x-ray tube is placed toward the left side of the body so the radiation will travel from the left side of the body to the right side.

6. *Left lateral (LL):* The left side of the body is positioned next to the film, and the x-ray tube is placed toward the right side of the body so the radiation will travel from the right side of the body.

7. *Posteroanterior view (PA):* The x-ray tube is placed toward the posterior portion of the body, with the film toward the anterior aspect of the body.

8. *Anteroposterior view (AP):* The x-ray tube is placed toward the anterior portion of the body with the film toward the posterior aspect of the body.

Disclaimer: All patients having x-ray examinations should be provided with lead shielding, when permitted, particularly in the gonadal region. All patients should have consent forms explained and signed, when indicated. Pregnant women must sign a release form stating that she is aware of the risks associated with the x-ray procedure.

X-ray Preparations

IMPORTANT NOTE: The preparation procedures in Tables 9-1 and 9-2 list only general information; always double-check with the x-ray facility before providing specific instructions to the patient. (Procedures vary from one facility to another.)

Table 9-1

X-RAY EXAMINATION PREPARATION INSTRUCTIONS

Prep A	Ten-day rule for females ages 12 years and older: Day 1 of menses to day 10 of menses is considered a safe time to take x-rays. Inquire about birth control. If the patient is past day 10 of cycle, a urine pregnancy test should be performed before taking the x-ray. (If the test is positive, x-rays should not be taken.)
Prep B	Remove false teeth, necklaces, earrings, and other body piercings before taking the x-ray.

Prep C	Remove necklaces, earrings, and other body piercings before taking the x-ray.
Prep D	Do not apply any deodorants, lotions, perfumes, or powders to breasts or underarms before x-ray.
Prep E	Nothing by mouth after midnight.
Prep F	Fluids only the day before the x-ray; take laxatives as directed.
Prep G	Laxative or cathartic given the night before or the morning of the examination.
Prep H	Do not take vitamins that contain iodine 4 weeks before testing, per provider's orders. Patient will be given one to two capsules containing radioactive iodine before testing.
Prep I	Ask if the patient is allergic to iodine, if so, consult provider.

Table 9-2
X-RAY VIEWS

Type	Description	Prep
Cervical spine	Various views are taken on C1–T1.	A
Thoracic spine	Various views are taken on T1–T12.	A
Lumbar spine	AP and lateral views are taken on T12–L1 and a lateral spot of L5 and S1 is also taken.	A
Extremities	Anterior, posterior, and oblique views are taken on the extremities involved.	A
KUB (flat abdomen)	Views allow visualization of the kidneys, ureters, and bladder.	A
Sinus films	Visualization of the sinuses	A, B
Chest x-ray	Posterior and left lateral views are taken of the chest.	A, C
Mammogram	X-ray views are taken of the breast from multiple angles.	A, D
Barium swallow (upper GI)	X-ray views of the esophagus only; may be ordered with upper GI series, although both tests cannot be obtained on the same day	A, E
Upper GI series	X-ray views of the stomach and small intestine; may be ordered with barium swallow and/or small bowel follow-through	A, E

(continues)

(continued)

Type	Description	Prep
Barium enema (lower GI)	X-ray views of the large colon only; may be ordered with air contrast, which means gas is inserted into the colon to distend the bowel	A, E, F
IVP (intravenous pyelogram)	X-ray views of the kidneys, ureters, and bladder; intravenous contrast is used	A, E, G, I
Thyroid uptake or thyroid scan	Evaluates overall function of the thyroid and detects any abnormalities	A, H, I

Viewing sections vary from one facility to another.

Ultrasound

Ultrasound uses high-frequency sound waves to produce an image of an organ or tissue for diagnostic examination. Tables 9-3 and 9-4 describe ultrasound preparations and examinations.

Table 9-3
ULTRASOUND PREPARATIONS

Prep A	Nothing by mouth after midnight
Prep B	No carbonated beverages the day before the procedure
Prep C	Low-fat meal the night before the test
Prep D	One to two quarts of water 2 hours before the examination. Do not urinate before the ultrasound is performed.

Table 9-4
ULTRASOUND EXAMINATIONS

Type	Description	Prep
Abdominal	Can view liver, gallbladder, spleen, or pancreas	A, B, C
Renal ultrasound	Able to view kidneys and bladder	A, B
Pelvic ultrasound	Able to view bladder, ureters, ovaries, fallopian tubes, and uterus	B, D
Echocardiogram	Used to evaluate the electrical and structural activity of the heart	None
Thyroid ultrasound	Distinguishes cystic from solid thyroid nodules	None

Computerized Tomography (CT Scan)

CT scanning combines special x-ray equipment with sophisticated computers to produce multiple images or pictures of the inside of the body. These cross-sectional images of the area being studied can then be examined on a computer monitor, printed, or transferred to a CD. Tables 9-5 and 9-6 list CT preparations and procedure types.

Table 9-5

CT PREPARATIONS

Prep A	Nothing by mouth 4 hours before test
Prep B	Ten-day rule for female patients ages 12 years and older: Days 1–10 of menstrual cycle is considered a safe time to take x-rays. If the patient's last menstrual period is past the 10-day mark, a urine pregnancy test should be performed before taking the x-ray. If test is positive, *do not perform the test.*
Prep C	Patient is given an oral contrast agent, either the night before or several hours before the x-ray is obtained, or intravenous contrast may be administered.
Prep D	Ask if patient is allergic to seafood (iodine).

Table 9-6

TYPES OF CT PROCEDURES

Type	Prep
Brain CT	A, B, C, D
Body CT	A, B
Chest CT	A, B, C, D
Abdomen/pelvic CT	A, B, C, D

Magnetic Resonance Imaging (MRI)

MRI uses a powerful magnetic field, radiofrequency pulses, and a computer to produce detailed pictures of organs, soft tissues, bones, and many other internal body structures. The images can then be examined on a computer monitor, transmitted electronically, printed, or copied to a CD. MRI does not use ionizing radiation (x-rays).

Preparations

The patient needs to remove all items that may be affected by a magnet, such as watches, jewelry, credit cards, keys, bobby pins, and coins. It is important to inform the facility about implanted devices such as:

- Cardiac pacemaker or implantable defibrillator
- Catheter that has metal components that may pose a risk for burn injury
- Ferromagnetic metal clip placed to prevent bleeding from an intra-cranial aneurysm
- Implanted or external medication pump (such as that used to deliver insulin or a pain-relieving drug)
- Cochlear (inner ear) implant
- Neurostimulation system

The facility will determine if the patient can safely undergo an MRI with implanted devices.

Positron Emission Tomography (PET Scan)

A PET scan is a type of nuclear medicine imaging that uses small amounts of radioactive material to diagnose or treat a variety of diseases, includ-ing many types of cancers, heart disease, and certain other abnormalities within the body. It is often used in combination with CT imaging.

Preparations

Patients should be instructed to remove all metal objects including jewelry, eyeglasses, dentures, and hairpins. Generally, for a whole-body PET/CT scan, the patient will be NPO because eating may alter the dis-tribution of the PET tracer.

Barium Series (Barium Swallow or Barium Enema)

Barium series may be limited to a barium swallow, also referred to as an upper gastrointestinal exam (UGI)or barium enema or lower gastroin-testinal exam (LGI). Generally the tests will need to be separated by a few days. A barium enema should be done before the barium swallow.

A UGI examines the pharynx, esophagus, stomach, and first part of the small intestine (also known as the duodenum). Images are produced using fluoroscopy and an orally ingested barium.

An LGI evaluates the right (ascending) colon, the transverse colon, the left (descending) colon, the sigmoid colon, and the rectum. The ap-pendix and a portion of the distal small intestine may also be included.

Preparations

UGI: Patients should be instructed to remove all metal objects, including jewelry, eyeglasses, dentures, and hairpins. The patient should be NPO after midnight on the day of the procedure.

LGI: Patients should be instructed to drink clear liquids only the day before the procedure. No solid foods are allowed. The patient should be NPO after midnight on the day of the procedure.

Section 9-2

OTHER DIAGNOSTIC PROCEDURES

This section will address other radiological procedures that are sometimes performed in the radiology suite.

Cardiac Catheterization

Cardiac catheterization is a procedure performed under fluoroscopy called angiography. It is used to evaluate the coronary arteries, cardiac chambers, and cardiac valves. A radionuclide substance is injected into a major artery (usually the femoral artery) to determine whether there is an obstruction caused by plaque formation (atherosclerosis). The pressures of the chambers of the heart are recorded.

Preparations

Elective cardiac catheterizations are done as an outpatient procedure. A complete history will be obtained, a physical examination will be performed, and an electrocardiogram (ECG) and laboratory studies will be done before the scheduled testing. The patient is NPO after midnight on the day of the procedure. Light sedation is administered for this procedure.

Cardiac Stress Testing

Stress testing of the heart is used to provide information about how the heart is responding on exertion. There are different types of stress testing, and the type used is determined by a provider.

Treadmill Stress Test: This is the most common method of cardiac testing. It usually involves walking on a treadmill or pedaling a stationary bike at increasing levels of difficulty while monitoring heart rate, blood pressure, and ECG.

Dobutamine or Adenosine Stress Test: This test is used in people who are unable to exercise. A drug is administered to make the heart respond as if the person were exercising. This allows the provider to determine how the heart responds to stress, even though no exercise is required.

Treadmill Stress Echocardiogram: An echocardiogram (often called an "echo") is a graphic outline of the heart's motion. A stress echo can accurately visualize the motion of the heart walls and pumping action when the heart is stressed; it may reveal a lack of blood flow.

Nuclear Treadmill Stress Test: In this test a small amount of radioactive substance (thallium) is injected to determine the uptake of thallium in the heart. If there is a decreased uptake of thallium, it may determine structural problems of the heart.

Preparations

Facilities that perform cardiac stress testing will have specific directions for the patient to follow. Generally, the following preparations are recommended:

- Patient should have water only for 4 hours before the test.
- Patient should have no caffeine for 12 hours before the test.
- Patient should wear comfortable clothing.

There is no sedation for cardiac stress testing.

Colonoscopies

A colonoscopy is a procedure used to evaluate the colon and rectum for abnormalities such as inflamed tissue, abnormal growths, and cancer. Current recommendations for persons 50 years of age and older is to have the first colonoscopy at age 50. Follow-up recommendations for repeat procedure interval is determined after the initial results are completed.

Preparations

The large intestine and rectum must be completely empty of stool for an accurate study. A bowel cleanse is performed using oral or rectal laxatives the day before the procedure. Patients will be instructed to follow a clear liquid diet for 1 to 2 days before the procedure. The patient will not be able to ingest any liquids that are purple or red, because the dye from the liquids may interfere with evaluation of the bowel and rectum. The patient should be NPO after 12 midnight the day before the procedure. Sedation is provided for this procedure.

Bone Density Testing

Bone density testing is used to assess the strength of the bone and determine the likelihood of fractures in persons at risk for osteoporosis. The test is also referred to as bone densitometry or bone mineral density (BMD) scan. The test is a noninvasive procedure. BMD analysis is recommended for women between ages 50 and 65 with risk factors for osteoporosis and for all women over the age of 65. In addition, men and women taking certain medications or having certain diseases should discuss testing with their provider.

Preparation for Bone Density Testing

There is no specific preparation for a bone density test. If the patient has had a barium enema or contrast material injected for a CT scan or nuclear medicine test, the contrast materials may interfere with the test.

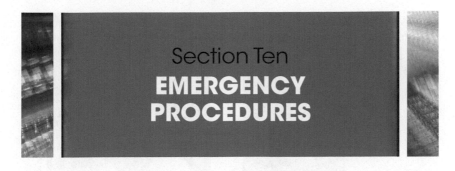

Section Ten
EMERGENCY PROCEDURES

INTRODUCTION

This section provides a review of basic emergency procedures in the event an emergency occurs.

Section 10-1

BLEEDING CONTROL

Bleeding occurs when there has been damage to a blood vessel. In external bleeding, there can be damage to veins or arteries to produce visible blood. Arterial bleeding is more life threatening than venous bleeding.

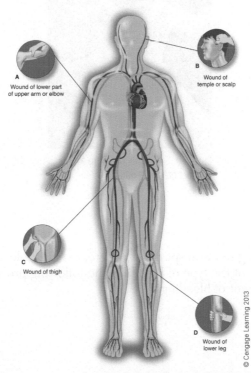

A
Wound of lower part
of upper arm or elbow

B
Wound of
temple or scalp

C
Wound of thigh

D
Wound of
lower leg

© Cengage Learning 2013

Figure 10-1: Common arteries that can be used to control bleeding.

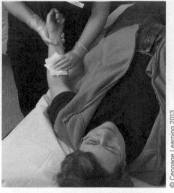

Figure 10-2: Apply direct pressure using a sterile bandage whenever possible.

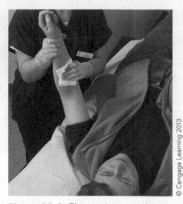

Figure 10-3: Elevate the arm above the level of the heart.

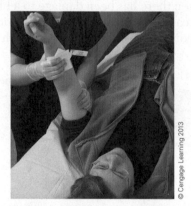

Figure 10-4: Apply pressure to the nearest pressure point.

Arterial bleeding tends to spurt out, whereas venous bleeding is continual. Regardless of the type of bleeding, the following procedure reviews basic management of bleeding.

Procedure 10-1
BLEEDING CONTROL

Equipment and Supplies

Several sterile 4×4s	Roller gauze	Gloves

1. Apply gloves.

2. Apply direct pressure to the bleeding site unless there is a foreign object protruding from injury (Figures 10-1 and 10-2).

3. Continue to apply pressure to the site for a minimum of 2 minutes.

4. If bleeding persists, do not remove initial dressing; apply second dressing and continue to apply pressure.

5. Elevate the affected area above the level of heart to slow bleeding (Figure 10-3) and apply pressure to the closest major artery in the area to further slow down or stop the bleeding (Figure 10-4).

6. Once bleeding is under control, remove gloves, wash hands, and follow provider's order in regards to closing the wound.

12/12/XXXX 9:25 a.m.	Pt. entered urgent care with a towel saturated with blood wrapped around his L. wrist. "Sliced wrist while using a band saw." Escorted pt. immediately to the treatment room. Alerted physician. Towels were removed. Pressure bandage applied by patient was saturated with blood. Applied several 4 × 4s over the existing pressure bandage and elevated the arm above the level of the heart. While continuing to apply pressure to the site, used other hand to gently compress the brachial artery just above the elbow. Approximately 10 minutes later, the physician instructed me to release my fingers that were compressing the artery and to remove the dressing and bandages. The bleeding appeared to be under control. Set the pt. up for a laceration repair per Dr. Ditullo. Physician took over the management of the wound from that point. Samantha Keir, CMA (AAMA)

Section 10-2

SHOCK MANAGEMENT

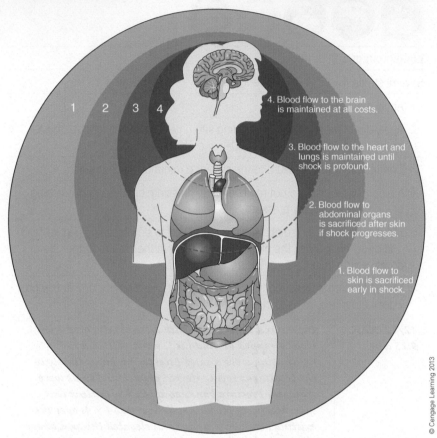

4. Blood flow to the brain is maintained at all costs.

3. Blood flow to the heart and lungs is maintained until shock is profound.

2. Blood flow to abdominal organs is sacrificed after skin if shock progresses.

1. Blood flow to skin is sacrificed early in shock.

© Cengage Learning 2013

Figure 10-5: When blood volume diminishes, as in cases of shock, the body tries to compromise by sacrificing blood supply to the less-significant organs in order to preserve blood for the vital organs such as the heart and brain.

There are many different types of shock. The most common type of shock is caused by a major hemorrhage but shock can also be caused by heart conditions such as heart attack, dehydration, anaphylaxis, and burns. It is important to be familiar with signs of shock, which include low blood pressure, rapid and weak pulse rate, rapid and weak respirations, dizziness, and possible unconsciousness. It is also very important to respond appropriately and quickly when symptoms are present. Procedure 10-2 lists steps that should be taken when a patient goes into shock from severe bleeding.

Figure 10-5 illustrates the events that occur within the body during shock.

Procedure 10-2
SHOCK MANAGEMENT

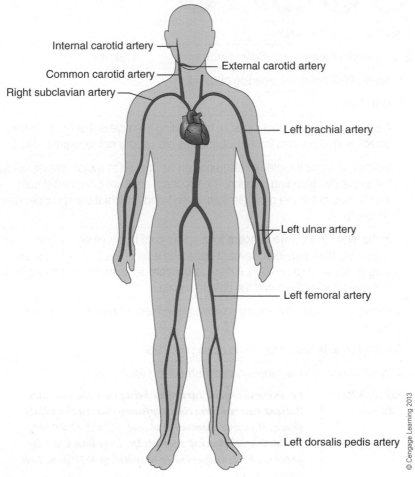

Internal carotid artery

External carotid artery

Common carotid artery

Right subclavian artery

Left brachial artery

Left ulnar artery

Left femoral artery

Left dorsalis pedis artery

© Cengage Learning 2013

Figure 10-6: Pressure points.

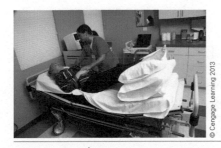

© Cengage Learning 2013

Figure 10-7: Elevating the patient's legs will help the blood to flow back down toward the brain.

(continues)

(continued)

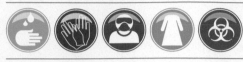

Equipment and Supplies

Several sterile 4×4s	Roller gauze	Gloves

1. Apply PPE if patient is bleeding outwardly.

2. Call 9-1-1.

3. If applicable, apply direct pressure to bleeding site unless there is a foreign object protruding from injury. (Tourniquets are usually not recommended.)

4. Indirect pressure for internal bleeding can be applied to major arteries below the suspected bleeding location. The two main pressure points most commonly used are in the groin (femoral artery) and (brachial artery) upper arm (Figure 10-6).

5. In the event there is **no concern** for a spinal cord injury, place the patient in supine position with legs elevated above the level of the heart (Trendelenburg position) (Figure 10-7). If there **is concern** for a spinal cord injury, keep the spine immobilized and the patient supine.

6. Keep patient warm by placing a blanket over them. Continue to reassure them!

7. Follow provider's lead regarding calling the EMS.

8. Wash hands, remove gloves, and document the encounter.

02/16/XXXX 6:25 p.m.	*Pt. entered urgent care after being in a car collision. Patient started sweating profusely during the vitals check. Skin was clammy and cool. Vitals: BP 88/40, P 106. Placed blanket over pt. Dr. Legg had EMS dispatched. Pt. transported to hospital @ 6:50 p.m. Rosa Garcia, RMA*

Section 10-3

BANDAGING

Bandaging is a skill that is used in most ambulatory care settings. Bandaging can range from very simple to very complex. Table 10-1 describes the different types of dressings that are available and their use. Always check with the provider for specifics.

Table 10-1

TYPES OF DRESSINGS

Types and Examples	Properties	When to Use	Pros	Cons
Gauze	Plain cotton material	Should only be used on minor wounds or as a secondary dressing	Absorbs drainage	Sticks to skin May disrupt the wound bed when removed May inhibit the healing process
Hydrocolloids	Main component is cellulose, which turns into a gel during exudate absorption and helps to keep the wound moist	Used on wounds with light to heavy drainage or on wounds that are granulating	Promotes autolytic debridement Adheres to moist skin	May promote hypergranulation Can cause the edges of the wound to become macerated
Hydrogels	Polymer gel composed of absorbent polymers with a gel structure that has a high water content	Used on wounds that are sloughing off or that have necrotic tissue Should not be used on wounds with moderate to heavy exudates Very useful on burns	Rehydrates tissue Minimally absorbent Cool and soothing to tissue	May be slippery and difficult to keep in place May cause maceration of skin around wound edges

(continues)

(continued)

Types and Examples	Properties	When to Use	Pros	Cons
Alginates	Composed of calcium alginate Works by exchanging calcium on the dressing with sodium from fluid coming from the wound Turns the dressing into a gel, promoting a moist environment	Good for clean exudating wounds Aids in debridement	Highly absorbent May be slightly hemostatic	Can dry a wound with limited drainage Can dry out the dressing May leave fibers from the dressing in the wound
Collagens	Contains a collagen, which helps to stimulate the formation of collagen in the wound bed	Absorbs exudates Provides a moist environment	Attracts macrophages and fibroblasts Encourages autolytic debridement	Collagen gels are heat sensitive and may become altered with excessive heat Some people may be allergic to products in the gel
Foams	Made of a polyurethane foam pad	Good for wounds with large amounts of drainage	Very absorbent Breathable, Less frequent bandage changes Reduces skin maceration	Could promote wound drying May not adhere well to deeper wounds
Transparent films	Clear film dressing	Used as a secondary dressing Great to secure intravenous lines	Permits visibility of the wound Promotes autolytic debridement Contours to body parts Waterproof so patients can shower	May experience difficulty in applying and removing Zero absorbency May be irritating to tissue

Terms That Are Used in Wound Care

Terms used for exudates include the following:

Serous: Fluids that contain serum; may appear as a clear fluid or may also be yellow

Sanguineous: A discharge that contains blood

Serosanguineous: A discharge that contains both serum and blood

Purulent: A discharge containing pus

Guidelines for Applying Dressings

Guidelines for applying and caring for dressings include:

1. Wash your hands thoroughly before bandaging.
2. Use sterile technique and sterile products when applying dressings to wounds that are open.
3. Use an ointment only if directed to do so by the provider.
4. Encourage patients to change dressings that appear soiled.
5. Avoid ripping or tearing a bandage away from a wound. This could reinjure the site. Instead, soak the bandage with normal saline for several minutes. Always pull a dressing toward the wound when removing.
6. Document the following after removing a dressing: appearance of the dressing and bandage and wound. Record any unusual drainage and the color of the drainage, and report any unusual odors coming from the area.

Guidelines for Applying Bandages

Bandaging tips include:

1. Always place a sterile dressing over an open wound before applying a bandage.
2. Use sterile technique when applying a dressing and institute medical asepsis when removing a dressing.
3. The area should be clean and dry before bandage application.
4. Always wrap distal to proximal.
5. Bandages should extend 1 to 2 inches beyond the dressing.
6. Pad bony surfaces and joints to prevent friction.
7. Bandage body parts in their normal positions, slightly flexed to avoid muscle strain or damage.
8. Leave fingers and toes open when applying a bandage to the extremities so that circulation may be evaluated.
9. Check for signs of poor circulation, which include blueness around the nail beds, pallor, skin temperature changes, tingling sensation, and numbness.

Different Types of Bandaging Techniques

Figure 10-8 illustrates the different types of bandaging techniques that can be used in an emergency situation. Always check with the provider for any specifics.

(a) A recurrent bandage may be used on the head.

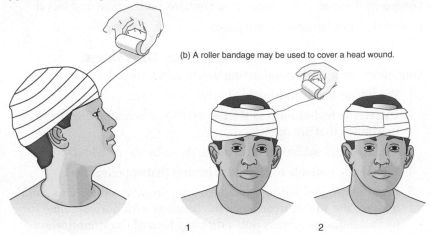

(b) A roller bandage may be used to cover a head wound.

1   2

(c) A triangular bandage may also be used to cover a head wound.

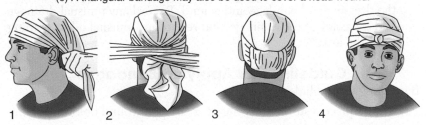

1   2   3   4

(d) A cravat may be used to hold a dressing in place on the head.

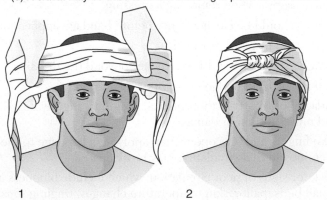

1   2

(e) A double cravat may be used to cover and secure an ear injury.

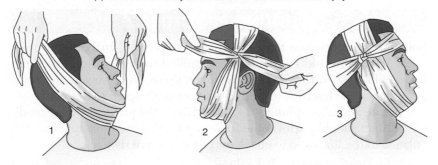

(f) A figure eight bandage is used to immobilize a joint.

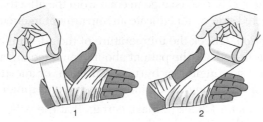

(g) A spiral bandage may be used to cover an extremity.

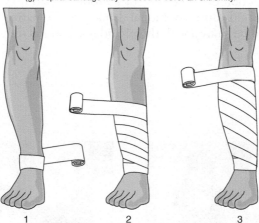

(h) A reverse spiral turn may be used when extra padding is essential.

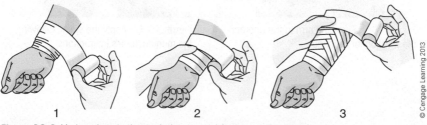

Figure 10-8: Various bandaging techniques used for traumatic wounds.

Section 10-4

SPLINTING PROCEDURES

Splinting is a procedure that is performed to prevent further damage or injury to the affected extremity. Uncontrolled movement to a fractured limb could cause further damage to the soft tissue, blood vessels, or nerves surrounding the fracture, as well as cause extensive pain to the victim.

Before and after splinting an injured limb, the provider or the medical assistant should perform the following CSM mnemonic to check circulation of the limb and to check for possible nerve damage.

- C for *circulation:* Check the distal pulse of the limb to make certain that blood is reaching below the point of injury and check for capillary filling of the nail bed. A change in color from the affected side versus the unaffected side could indicate an impairment in circulation.

- S for *sensation:* Check the temperature of the affected limb with the opposite limb and ask the patient about overall feeling and pain status. Paresthesia (tingling or burning sensation) or anesthesia (a lack of feeling or no feeling) could indicate nerve entrapment or damage.

- M for *movement:* Check to make certain that the patient can move the digits on the affected limb.

An interruption of blood flow or a problem with how the extremity is positioned could cause additional damage to the patient, so the CSM findings should be shared with the provider as soon as they are obtained.

Procedure 10-3
SPLINTING AN ARM

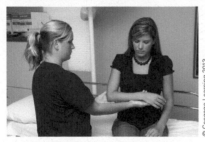

Figure 10-9: Place the arm in the appropriate position for splinting.

© Cengage Learning 2013

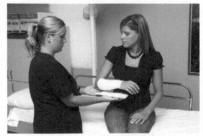

Figure 10-10: Apply the splint, following the manufacturer's instructions.

© Cengage Learning 2013

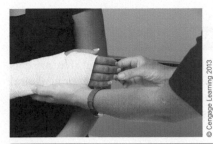

Figure 10-11: Check the distal pulse point, sensation, and movement after applying the splint.

© Cengage Learning 2013

Equipment and Supplies

Splint	Sling

1. Gather supplies and wash your hands.

2. Identify the patient using two identifiers, identify yourself, and explain the procedure.

3. Follow the steps on the commercial splint for preparing the splint.

4. Place the arm in the position that will be used for splinting (Figure 10-9). Be sure to stabilize the injured area by stabilizing the joint above and below the injury.

5. Check the pulse point distal to the injury.

6. Check for sensation and movement while the arm is in the splint position.

7. Apply the splint following the manufacturer's instructions (Figure 10-10). If the arm is to be totally immobilized, place the arm with the splint in a sling as well.

8. Check distal pulse point, sensation, and movement after applying the splint (Figure 10-11).

9. Apply ice to help reduce swelling.

10. Wash your hands and document the procedure.

05/14/XXXX 12:30 p.m.	Pt. fell off of his porch hitting his R forearm on the grill. ⊕ Tenderness, ⊕ swelling, ⊖ discoloration. Pt. had good strong pulse, movement, and sensation before splinting. Splinted R forearm with commercial air splint and placed arm in a sling. Checked circulation, sensation, and movement once again after splinting. Good strong pulse, color was slightly pink, and temperature was warm. Pt. still able to move fingers. Applied ice to forearm per Dr. Woo. Martin Ford, RMA ———

Section 10-5

BURNS

Burns are very concerning because of the complications that may arise as a result of a burn. There are three types of burns: thermal, chemical, and electrical. Before assessing a burn, one must understand how to classify burns. Table 10-2 describes the various types of burns.

Table 10-2
TYPES OF BURNS

Type	Degree/Thickness
Thermal burn: Caused by heat, such as a hot surface or flames	**First-degree burn:** A superficial burn involving the first layer of the skin
Chemical burn: Caused by contact with acids or alkalis	**Second-degree burn:** Extend into the dermis, or second layer of skin. Also referred to as a partial-thickness burn.
Electrical burn: Occurs after contact with electrical wiring. An electrical burn can be caused by a lightning strike. Hard to assess outwardly. Internal injuries not visible to the naked eye could be present.	**Third-degree burn:** Involves all three layers of the skin and is also referred to as a full-thickness burn

Rule of Nines

Another factor that helps to assess the severity of a burn is the percentage of body surface area involved in the burn. The *Rule of Nines* formula is used most often in the field by medics who need to determine very quickly how much of the body is affected. Table 10-3 and Figure 10-12 present the Rule of Nines.

Table 10-3
BURN AREA FORMULA FOR ADULTS

Body Part	Burn Area (%)
Each arm	9
Face	4½
Each leg	18
Back of head	4½
Upper and lower back	18
Genitals	1
Chest and abdomen	18

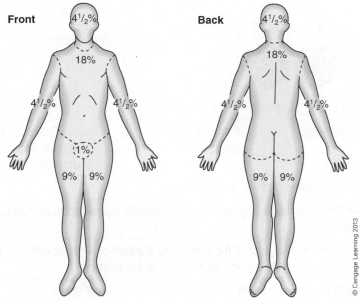

Figure 10-12: The Rule of Nines is used to estimate the percentage of body surface area burned (adult example).

When Patients with Burns Should Be Sent to the Emergency Department

The following criteria may be used to assess the seriousness of a burn. Patients who exhibit any of the signs or symptoms in the following list or match the following criteria are usually sent on to the emergency department.

1. Patients with breathing problems (be prepared to assist with the breathing emergency)
2. Patients with burns in certain locations (burns located on the head, neck, hands, feet, and genitals are considered severe)
3. Patients with multiple burns or burns that cover a large surface area
4. Patients of certain ages (the pediatric patient and older adults are more susceptible to complications from burns)
5. Patients with full-thickness burns (all full-thickness burns are considered critical burns)

Procedure 10-4
TREATMENT OF BURNS

Equipment and Supplies

Sterile dressings	Sterile 4×4s Sterile saline	Silver sulfadiazine or Silvadene ointment (if ordered by provider)

1. Gather supplies and wash your hands.

2. Identify the patient using two identifiers, identify yourself, and explain the procedure.

3. Assess the seriousness of the burn using the Rule of Nines to estimate the percentage of body surface area burned (adult example).

4. Use the following treatments if outside of a health care facility:

Treatment of Superficial Burns
   A1. Apply cool water or sterile saline to the affected area.
   A2. Apply a nonstick sterile dressing to protect the area.
   A3. Provide patient with ample amount of fluids to drink.
   A4. Do NOT apply butter or ointments because this will hold in the burn and cause more pain.

Treatment of Partial Thickness Burns
   B1. Remove any jewelry because edema might be severe.
   B2. Provide patient with ample amount of fluids to drink.
   B3. Remove clothing; flood the area with water for a minimum of 15 minutes or place compresses saturated in cool saline over the burn. (Dry chemicals should be brushed off before flushing the patient's skin. Some dry chemicals are activated by water.)
   B4. Cover the burned area with non-stick sterile dressing and treat the patient for shock.
   B5. Caution patient to refrain from breaking blisters and peeling the skin.

Treatment of Full-Thickness Burns
   C1. Contact emergency medical services (EMS) for immediate transport.
   C2. Cover the burned area with sterile dressings and treat the patient for shock.
   C3. Do NOT try to remove clothing that is adhered to the burn as surgical care will be needed to remove burned fabric.
   C4. If more than 10% of the body surface area (BSA) is involved, the burn is considered a major burn and requires surgical intervention.

5. If inside a health care facility, ensure that the patient is comfortable. Check with provider to determine if sterile 4×4s dipped in sterile saline can be applied to area for temporary relief.

6. Determine the patient's last tetanus shot.

7. If provider orders an ointment such as Silvadene be applied to the skin, use sterile technique to apply the ointment and cover the burn with a sterile dressing.

8. Remove gloves, wash hands, and document the procedure.

Section 10-6

FOREIGN BODY AIRWAY OBSTRUCTION (FBAO)

Choking occurs when a foreign object becomes lodged in the trachea. The universal sign for choking is hands clutched to the throat. If the person does not give this signal, look for these indications: inability to talk; difficulty breathing; skin, lips, and nails cyanotic. Table 10-4 presents the steps for responding to a patient with an FBAO.

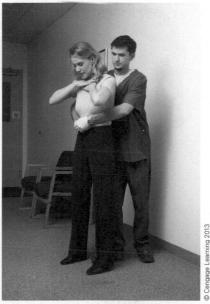

© Cengage Learning 2013

Figure 10-13: The proper placement of the rescuer's hands when giving abdominal thrusts to relieve an obstructed airway.

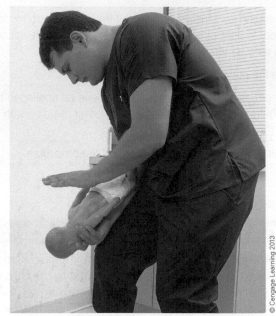

Figure 10-14: When infants have an obstructed airway, the rescuer starts by administering back blows to the infant.

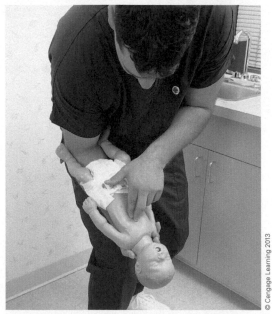

Figure 10-15: The rescuer then gives the infant chest compressions to assist in expelling the object from the infant's airway.

Table 10-4

STEPS FOR RESPONDING TO A PATIENT WITH A FOREIGN BODY AIRWAY OBSTRUCTION

Age group	Adult (puberty through adulthood)	Child (age 1 year to puberty)	Infant (birth to 1 year of age)
Activation of 9-1-1	Immediately	If you are **alone,** perform 2 minutes of cardiopulmonary resuscitation (CPR) before activating 9-1-1	If you are **alone,** perform 2 minutes of CPR before activating 9-1-1
Procedure type	Abdominal thrusts	Abdominal thrusts Use less force than with an adult	Back blows followed by chest thrusts, 5 and 5 (Figures 10-14 and 10-15)
Number of times to perform procedure	No limit; perform abdominal thrusts until the obstruction is relieved or patient loses consciousness (Figure 10-13)	No limit; perform abdominal thrusts until the obstruction is relieved or patient loses consciousness	5 back blows followed by 5 chest thrusts until the obstruction is relieved or patient loses consciousness
If the FBAO is not relieved:	Begin CPR: 30 compressions to 2 breaths	Single rescuer: 30 compressions to 2 breaths If 2 health care providers are present, the ratio is 15 compressions to 2 breaths	Single rescuer: 30 compressions to 2 breaths If 2 health care providers are present, the ratio is 15 compressions to 2 breaths.

Section 10-7

CARDIOPULMONARY RESUSCITATION FOR THE HEALTH CARE PROVIDER

American Heart Association (AHA) Recommendation for Cardiopulmonary Resuscitation (CPR) 2010

In 2010, changes were made by the AHA regarding CPR for all ages. The current emphasis is starting **chest compressions** first, rather than the previous technique of starting with breathing. There should not be delays in starting chest compressions. Table 10-5 lists the steps for administering CPR.

Acronym for CPR sequence: CAB

C = Compressions

A = Airway

B = Breathing

Table 10-5

STEPS FOR PROVIDING CARDIOPULMONARY RESUSCITATION

Age groups	Adult (puberty through adulthood)	Child (age 1 year to puberty)	Infant (birth to 1 year of age)
Activation of 9-1-1	Immediately	If you are **alone,** perform 2 minutes of CPR before activating 9-1-1.	If you are **alone,** perform 2 minutes of CPR before activating 9-1-1.
Chest compressions to breathing ratio	30:2	Single rescuer 30:2 If 2 health care providers are present, the ratio is 15:2.	Single rescuer 30:2 If 2 health care providers are present, the ratio is 15:2.
Depth of chest compression	2 inches (Figure 10-16)	About 2 inches	About 1½ inches
Rate of compressions/ minute	At least 100/ minute	At least 100/ minute	At least 100/ minute

| Defibrillation/ Automated External Defibrillation (AED) | Attach as soon as available | Attach as soon as available | Attach as soon as available; no absolute indication to use in this age group |

Figure 10-16 illustrates the proper way to perform chest compressions in adult CPR, and Figure 10-17 illustrates the proper way to open the airway when providing rescue breaths.

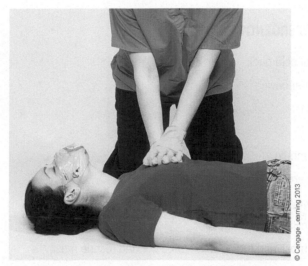

Figure 10-16: The proper hand positioning for CPR on an adult victim.

(a)   (b)

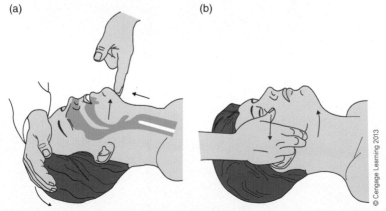

Figure 10-17: (a) When there is no sign of head or neck injuries, the rescuer may use the head tilt/chin lift procedure to open the airway. (b) When head or neck trauma is suspected, the rescuer should use the jaw thrust maneuver to open the airway.

Section 10-8
CRASH CART EQUIPMENT RECOMMENDATIONS

Every office is required to have basic emergency equipment available until Emergency Medical Personnel (EMT-B, EMT-P) help arrives. Individual offices may have more advanced equipment and medication available. Table 10-6 lists the basic emergency equipment that should be available in every office.

Table 10-6
BASIC EMERGENCY EQUIPMENT

Chemical cold pack
CPR barrier device
Eye wash
Gloves
Nasal cannula
Non-rebreather mask
Oral airways
Oxygen cylinder and regulator
Oxygen mask and tubing with connector and rescue mask
Suction machine with suction gauge and suction catheter
Tape

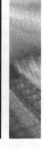

Section Eleven
HUGS IN THE HALLWAY

INTRODUCTION

The pace of today's health care professional is at an all-time high. There are faxes to collect, e-mails to return, and computer programs to master. A patient needs a referral, the insurance company is not going to accept that code, and "Yes, I will schedule that test." And we wonder why we have grown weary with health care. The warm spirit of tenderness that attracted us to the industry is often replaced with a cold triteness.

Many may question how the content in this section relates to the technical information that makes up the majority of this handbook. The authors want readers to understand that there is much more to medicine than performing technical tasks.

This section, Hugs in the Hallway, is devoted to health care professionals all over the country. Its purpose is to remind health care workers of the "awesomeness" of the positions that you hold. You have been empowered with authority that most people do not have. You see and touch parts of patients' bodies that the patients themselves may have never seen or touched. You are entrusted with confidential information that no one else has ever heard. Patients literally put their lives into your hands.

We intend to rejuvenate and warm the spirit of those whose spirit has grown cold. We hope to enlighten those just entering the profession of the unique opportunities that occur daily in this profession. Finally, we remind you that you too someday will be the one who is hurting, that you too will long for empathy from a stranger you just met, that you too one day will exchange your laboratory coat for a patient gown.

SETTING THE SCENE FOR HUGS IN THE HALLWAY

The title "Hugs in the Hallway" came to me years ago when I worked for a family practice in rural Ohio. The clinic stands in a pasture of green fields surrounded by rich farmland on all sides. The sereneness of the beautiful landscape outside the clinic helped to make the frenzied pace on the inside a little more bearable.

My position title was hall assistant. I saw patients who were not going to see the doctor. Patients coming in for laboratory work, injections, and pre-admission testing were just a few of the types of patients I saw in the hallway. Many of the patients who frequented my hallway suffered from chronic illness. Others suffered from terminal illness.

I was not one to give lots of hugs, but I found myself giving many of my patients a hug at the end of their visits. It was a bit awkward at first but seemed to become automatic as the months rolled on. It became my trademark!

Patients started looking forward to their hugs. Some patients' eyes would fill with tears as they acknowledged that they hadn't been hugged in years. Other patients requested a hug at both the beginning and end of each visit. And on those occasions when I forgot to extend a hug, the patients themselves initiated one.

What will be your trademark in health care? Will your patients remember you as a kind, caring, compassionate member of the health care team? Or will they remember you as someone who is cold and insensitive?

—Michelle E. Heller, CMA

STORIES FROM THE CLASSROOM
Bree's Story

I met Bree when I was still in the process of building the medical assisting program at Carrington College. I went out to lunch and Bree was my waitress. Bree picked a hair off of my shoulder and we began talking.

Bree is a very lively, outgoing, and loving person who exudes energy. We discussed that she is a single mom of a 2-year-old little boy and works full time. Bree told me she was kind of lost and didn't really know what direction she wanted to go in her life. She also said that she had been a volunteer firefighter and emergency medical technician (EMT) and was interested in a career in the medical field. I explained the Medical Assisting program to her and gave her my card.

As a result of our conversation, Bree left work and went straight to Carrington and enrolled in the program within the hour. Bree was the very first student at the Reno campus. Bree graduated with the highest grade point average in her class and received an award for perfect attendance.

Bree has been the heart and soul of the first class. Her spirit resonates with all who come in contact with her. She is our greatest cheerleader. After graduation, Bree was hired at a medical center as a laboratory assistant. She works in the emergency department (ED) and the intensive care unit doing stat draws and processing laboratory specimens. Our MA program will always be a part of Bree and has enriched and fulfilled her life, giving her a purpose and direction.

—Kim Hockaday

Blood Drawing Practice

I had one medical assisting student who was "scared to death" of needles and was afraid of hurting other students during blood drawing practice. I explained to her that obtaining blood from the "patients" would really be helping them find out if they were in good health. She was a sweet young lady, and when she would try to draw on one of the other students, her hand would shake so badly that the other "student patient" would look horrified, start backing up, and almost run from her. As she proceeded to come near the "patient," I would have to intervene and hold her hand as she practiced her blood draw. I repeated this several times before she could actually do it by herself. She finally perfected her skill and ended up being my assistant with the other students for blood draws. The funny part about this story is that she ended up working at our local American Red Cross facility—drawing blood. She had mastered her fear and become proficient in this skill as a medical assistant.

—Susanna Hancock

I Love My Job

I've heard it said, "There is only one in three who can say 'I love my job'." I am that one in three who can say, "I love my job." I enjoyed being a Medical Assistant Instructor-Director. I was going to work every day and getting paid for something I loved doing. As I taught my students, I was always watching for the lights to come on in their eyes when they finally "got it." As I expounded on the anatomy and physiology of the human body and monitored them as they practiced the clinical skills needed to pass their classes, I impressed upon them that I wanted them to be good enough to work on my family and theirs someday and continue to be accurate, efficient, and proud of their work. I wanted them to be the BEST MA that any physician could hope to employ.

At graduation, with tears of joy, I watched each of them cross the stage, hug me, and receive their diplomas. I had many mixed emotions. I felt sadness, I felt relief, I felt victorious, and I felt proud. I knew they had all worked hard to please me and accomplish their goal.

I have been retired for 6 years now and miss the day-to-day interaction with my students. However, I see many of them still in the medical field and it warms my heart each time I see them and they say to another staff member, "This is my teacher."

I sent one student as an extern to help two nutrition doctors set up their office. A few years later the doctors decided to move, so the student's husband said, "Why don't you buy the clinic?" Now she and her family run this very successful clinic. What a great accomplishment for a newly graduated MA! My students of yesteryears are now the medical professionals of today. It feels so good to have been just a small part of their new careers and their success.

—Susanna Hancock

We Can All Make a Difference

From an educator's perspective, every class is special and every student is unique, but every once in a while one class or one student creates a lasting impression—validating the reason you are in education.

This particular class started out like any other—a blend of different ages and coming from varying walks of life. Through the months of the program, the entire instructional team and staff were mesmerized by the sensitivity of this special group of students.

Danny was a young man who was married and had a child. Danny and his wife separated early in the training program, leaving him nowhere to live. Often, Danny had to sleep in his car. Sometimes he would come in late, with a wrinkled uniform, looking unkempt. Danny was very likable, but at times other students would complain about his unkemptness and tardiness. Miss Stout, Danny's instructor, would hear none of it. She knew Danny's potential and had inside information that his classmates didn't have. She encouraged students to put themselves in Danny's place and urged them to think of ways to assist him.

The students took Miss Stout's advice and teamed up to help Danny. Some invited him into their homes; others helped him with gas money or provided him with lunch. When Danny faced termination from school because of his attendance, the students bought him an alarm clock and gave him pep talks to help him finish the race with a victory.

Toward the end of the program, Miss Stout set up several interviews for Danny and his classmates. Everyone knew he didn't have the money to purchase interview attire, so all the students and staff members pitched in and bought him a suit and dress shoes for the interviews. On the day of Danny's first interview, one classmate cut his hair and another shaved his face. There were lots of emotions that day when Danny walked out of the bathroom, freshly shaven—looking great in his new suit. There wasn't a dry eye in the entire class.

Eventually, we lost touch with Danny and weren't sure what happened to him. Miss Stout left the institution, and we didn't have Danny's new contact information. A year or so following graduation, he showed up asking for Miss Stout. I told him that Miss Stout was no longer with the institution, but that she and I had continued our friendship. He said, "Will you tell Miss Stout that she made a huge impact in my life, and because of her my life is much better? Will you thank her for not giving up on me?"

I told Danny that I would be happy to relay the information to Miss Stout. He went on to state that he was working for a veterinarian group and was in charge of the computer operations for three different centers. (The veterinarians felt that Danny's medical assisting training was applicable to some of the tasks he would be performing in their office.) He had a new home and was able to care for his daughter because of his new career. I reassured Danny I would share the information with Miss Stout.

The bond that was formed by that special group of students made a lasting impression on all of us. Danny's classmates reached beyond the borders of the classroom; they also commissioned other classes and staff members to get involved. Helping Danny became an institutional effort from which everyone benefited!

—Michelle E. Heller, CMA

STORIES FROM THE FIELD

Hannah's Story

Working in a pediatric office in the first year of being a CMA, I had a new patient: a 5-year-old girl with special needs, who came in for a well-child check. As the little girl clenched her doll tightly, I sensed something more than fear in her. She was brought in by her grandmother, who informed me that they'd been to several doctor's offices and each visit had been unsuccessful because the little girl's special needs caused them to leave before being seen by the physician. A bit perplexed, I squatted down to the little girl, and said, "Hi Hannah, my name is Ann. I like your baby doll, and I think she likes me because she keeps looking at me."

Hannah gave me a glare and said nothing.

I said, "Let's make this a good day today at the doctor's office. I'd like you to help me with some things."

"Help you with what?" Hannah asked, in a very angry tone.

I said, "Let's see . . . I need to hear your heart, but first will you listen to mine?"

I showed her my stethoscope, put it in her ears, and she listened to my heart. She was so excited, she said "I hear it, I hear bum bum bum bum . . ."

"Yes, that's right," I said.

I removed the stethoscope from her ears, listened to her heart, obtaining the apical pulse rate. Next, I said, "Let's use the arm hugger (blood pressure cuff) to give my arm a hug and then I'll let it hug your arm."

Hannah's grandmother stood off in the corner of the room with her hand up to her mouth as if to say, "Oh no, oh no."

I placed the cuff around my arm and handed the bulb to Hannah. I said, "Okay Hannah, squeeze the ball five times and give my arm a hug."

Hannah squeezed with all her might, watching the cuff hug me tighter and tighter. Then I said, "Okay, now let's let the air out."

I unscrewed the valve.

"Hannah, you did it, you used the arm hugger!" I said.

Her grandmother cheered and said, "Hannah, you've never done that before, that was really good!"

"Now it's my turn. Can I put the hugger on your arm?" I asked.

I obtained Hannah's blood pressure for the first time in her medical history. Her grandmother stood there with tears, saying, "You have no idea the miracle you just had. Normally Hannah gets violent toward medical staff (as part of her illness), and the only way to calm her down is to leave the office." Her grandmother must have thanked me a dozen times in a row.

I said, "Hannah, thank you for helping me today. Now will you help the nice doctor too?"

She said, "Okay, I will."

And that she did.

—Ann Zeller, CMA (AAMA), AAS, GxMO

You Saved My Life!

My patient, Nancy, had high blood pressure and was told by her physician, Dr. Frazier, to come in weekly for blood pressure checks. One week, Nancy and her husband, John, came in together for her weekly check. I was on duty that day. As I brought Nancy and John back to the examination room, Nancy commented, "My husband, John, has been having headaches, chest pain, and pain radiating down his left arm! Will you check his blood pressure?"

I said, "No problem! After I finish with you, I'll check John's."

Nancy's blood pressure results were normal, and she was very happy.

"Now check John's," said Nancy.

John refused, telling Nancy not to be so pushy, and that I had more important things to do than check his blood pressure. "I am not a patient here, Nancy! Quit pushing Deborah to do this."

I told John that I was never too busy to check anyone's blood pressure, especially his. I realized I had to butter John up to gain his approval to check his blood pressure. John finally agreed. Before checking his blood pressure, I asked him several cardiac screening questions. I specifically asked John if he had a history of heart problems. He answered "No."

"What day did your chest pains start?"

He said, "Three days ago, when I was mowing my grass."

"Can you show me where your pain is located?"

He pointed to the left side of his chest, near his heart. I checked his blood pressure and noted the reading, which was 210/100. I told John and Nancy that I would be right back as I needed to speak with the doctor.

I quickly notified Dr. Frazier of John's blood pressure results. She ordered me to get set up for an ECG! We both entered the examination room where John and Nancy waited for his results. Dr. Frazier talked with John while taking his blood pressure to confirm the results.

Suddenly, Dr. Frazier said, "Deb, get the ECG, stat!"

I asked John to undress from the waist up and lie down on the examination table. I placed the electrodes on his chest area and ran the recording. John was experiencing a heart attack. Dr. Frazier called 911 and stabilized John until the paramedics arrived. In less than 5 minutes the ambulance crew rushed in, took John's vital signs, placed him on the gurney, and rolled him out to the ambulance. John was taken to the (Emergency Department) for evaluation.

The next day, Dr. Frazier told me she had received a phone call from the hospital stating that John had to have emergency five-way heart bypass surgery. They commented, "Had he waited any longer, he would not be here today." Dr. Frazier commended me on my professionalism, empathy, and quick thinking. I thanked the doctor for her kind words. I voice a silent prayer thanking God for helping me to do what needed to be done to help John.

Four weeks passed following John's visit and I wondered how he was doing. During the fifth week, Nancy came in for her weekly blood pressure check. While checking her pressure I asked her, "How is John getting along now following his heart surgery?"

She said, "I will let John tell you himself, he'll be right in after parking the car."

As I finished Nancy's blood pressure check, John entered the examination room. He grabbed me and hugged me tightly saying, "If it wasn't for your persistence that day, I wouldn't be here today. Deborah, YOU SAVED MY LIFE!"

This story is one of many reasons I love being a medical assistant— the opportunity to serve others!

—Deborah A. Hood, A.T.S, CMA (AAMA), GxMO

Patient Management

One day, when I was employed as the receptionist in my first family practice office, I was standing at the reception window when a man came in and threw a $20 bill across the counter at me. He stood with a scowl on his face and said, "Here's your money that you dunned me for."

I called him by name and said, "Please wait; let's talk about this for a minute."

I got a pad and pencil. This showed him I really cared enough to write down what he told me. He said, "That woman in there (pointing to the insurance office) sent me a letter saying that I owed this money and I had to pay it right now."

I asked him if I could look at the letter he received, and he threw it across the desk. Now it was evident that he was very frustrated. I reviewed the letter, which included a Medicare EOB showing what Medicare would pay and the portion the patient needed to pay. I asked him if he had an insurance supplement. He said he did. I smiled and told him all he had to do was give us his insurance information and we would be glad to bill it for him. His face softened as he pulled out his wallet to give us his insurance information.

Following the incident, the patient was always kind and courteous to the entire staff. We made a friend out of him. If we had become angry or defensive because he yelled at us, the end result may have been different. Think before you act or speak. Why is the patient upset? Find out first. Be genuinely interested in the patient's concern. Write it down. Offer solutions to the patient. Be kind and caring.

I've heard that one patient will tell 10 others about the service they encounter, good or bad. It is the receptionist's responsibility to keep the environment light and positive. After all, the receptionist is the window to the practice.

—Susanna Hancock

The Power of Laughter

While working in a cardiovascular surgeon's office, I took care of an older gentleman who had just undergone quadruple bypass surgery. Unfortunately, because of improper wound care, all of his incision lines became infected. He was coming in weekly for wound checks and dressing changes. The wounds were healing nicely!

The healing process was slow, however, and as the weeks went by I noticed he was becoming depressed. His daughter was concerned about the depression as well. He had been put on antidepressants, but his daughter said there was no change in his mood. His wounds were preventing him from being outdoors doing the things he loved to do.

This particular visit, as I was performing his dressing changes, he asked me for a tissue. I handed the tissue box over to him to allow him to pull one out, and just as he was about to grab one, I pulled the box away and said, "How do you make a tissue dance?"

He gave me a nasty look and said very sharply, "I don't know."

I stated retorted, "You put a little boogie in it."

I was waiting for another sharp reply, but instead he began to laugh.

A few days later I received a phone call from his daughter. She shared with me that the laughter at his last visit had turned him around, and that that was the first time he had laughed in months. She thanked me over and over again. I was shocked that such a silly little joke could help so much.

—Judy Mackey

Estrogen Therapy

In our family practice office, a female patient was trying estrogen transdermal patches as her therapy for menopause. She came in one day to have her patch checked and stated that she didn't think it was working correctly. I asked her to explain how she was applying the patch. She stated that she taped the patch to her skin and that each time she took a shower it would fall off. I told her she shouldn't have to tape the patch on, that it had an adhesive backing and all she had to do was remove the backing.

She laughed and said, "Oh, that's the reason they aren't staying on."

I explained that in order for the medication to be absorbed properly the tabs needed to be removed from the adhesive backing, which explains why she didn't notice any effect. The next time she came in, she told me a funny story. She stated that she had removed the adhesive back and applied the patch as I had instructed. One night she woke up and couldn't find her patch anywhere. Then, laughing she stated, "When my husband rolled over—there was my patch on his back!"

I jokingly asked if his voice was any higher. She said "No," and we both had a good laugh.

Educating patients regarding how to take their medication is a critical task. When educating patients on patch administration, it is vitally important to explain where the medication is located within the patch, and how and where it is to be applied to the body. Remember that the patient doesn't have the medical knowledge that you have. Be cognizant of the patient's knowledge. Observe the patient's body language, noting facial expressions, nods, or gestures for confirmation whenever you introduce a new procedure or medication.

—Susanna Hancock

"You Want My Picture?"

It was only my second day at work when I met John. There he was in his muddy bib overalls looking impatiently at his watch. Upon entering the room I saw the look of disappointment in his eyes.

"Where is Martha?" he asked.

"Martha no longer works here Mr. Johnson. I will be drawing your blood today."

"Where's Vicki?" he insisted. "She can usually get my blood."

"Vicki is with other patients right now, Mr. Johnson. You have nothing to fear. I have drawn lots of blood over the past few years."

"Well you might have drawn lots of blood, but you haven't drawn blood from many people with veins like mine," he replied.

The gruffness of his voice and the stern look on his face said it all. It was obvious he'd had many bad experiences, and he was quite certain that I would only add to the list.

"What kind of problems have you experienced in the past?" I inquired.

"My veins roll! There are only a couple of people who can ever get my blood and that's Martha and Vicki. The hospital can't even get my blood! They stick and they poke. Why the last time I was hospitalized, one of the lab girls stuck me six times before she was able to get my blood."

"I am sorry to hear that, Mr. Johnson. We have a two-stick rule in this office. If I can't get your blood after two attempts, I will ask someone else to draw your blood. I certainly understand your concern with your past history. Do you have a preference as to which arm I should try?" I asked.

"They usually have the best luck with my right arm," he replied.

"All right, Mr. Johnson. The right arm it is."

I prepared Mr. Johnson's arm for the blood draw. I felt each vein in the antecubital area. They were large but rolled easily upon palpation. I anchored the vein and inserted the needle. The vein immediately rolled. I tried to reposition the needle several times but to no avail.

With great disappointment, Mr. Johnson said, "You didn't get it, did you?"

"No, I am afraid that I didn't, Mr. Johnson. I am really sorry! I do see what you mean about your veins rolling. I have an idea though that I think will work. If you will permit me to try one more time, I will get another assistant in here to help me steady your vein while I draw your blood."

Reluctantly, Mr. Johnson agreed to one last attempt.

"If you don't get it this time, you can just forget it. I am not a pincushion!"

I asked Helen if she was available to help me. She said that she drew Mr. Johnson's blood on a previous occasion and missed, but that she would be happy to assist me in any way that she could.

Mr. Johnson suffered from coronary artery disease and had a history of deep vein thrombosis. His veins had little lumen left and felt hard upon insertion. I felt that if Helen could just hold the vein steady, it would give me a better opportunity to get the needle into the right spot to retrieve the specimen.

Helen carefully anchored the vein well above and below the area that I wanted to stick, while I inserted the needle at a 45-degree angle. The needle went directly into the center of the vein and the vein did not roll. I pushed the tube in and blood immediately started flowing into the tube. What a relief! I released the tourniquet and withdrew the needle. Mr. Johnson actually grinned when the procedure was over.

"That technique seemed to work very well, Mr. Johnson," I explained. "Lots of people's veins roll. Usually, just by anchoring the vein really well with the non-drawing hand, it steadies the vein enough. But your vein is really tough! Even with a tight anchor from the non-drawing hand, it was able to roll. Helen anchored the vein with both hands to steady it while I inserted the needle. The next time you come in, we will try that technique again."

"Well, all right," he said with hesitation in his voice. It was apparent he still didn't fully trust me.

The next week, Mr. Johnson came in again for his blood draw. I asked Helen if she could again assist me with the draw. Mr. Johnson was still not convinced we would be able to get his blood on the first try, but we did.

For the next several weeks, Mr. Johnson came in once or twice a week. We used the same technique for each draw and got blood on the first try. He grew more trusting each week.

One afternoon I told Mr. Johnson I would be taking pictures for our Tri-County Hall of Fame Board the following week. I asked him if he would allow me to take his picture for the board.

"You want my picture to hang on your board?" he asked with surprise.

"Why yes, Mr. Johnson. I would be honored to have your picture on our board!"

"What is the purpose of the board?" he asked.

"This hallway is a bit depressing. There are no windows and the atmosphere is bleak. Every time patients come back here, it is usually to get a needle stuck in their arm. I thought it would be nice to take pictures of our special patients who frequent the hallway and hang them on a board in the hallway. You are one of those special people, Mr. Johnson."

"Do I have to wear a suit?"

"No, just a smile!" I said jokingly.

The next week, I received a phone call from Mr. Johnson.

"Do you have your camera with you today?" he asked.

"Yes, I do," I said.

"I will be there around 3 o'clock, okay?" he asked with anticipation in his voice.

"That will be fine, Mr. Johnson. I will see you then."

At 3 o'clock, the front office buzzed me to tell me that Mr. Johnson was here but didn't have an appointment. I said that was okay and asked them to send him back.

When I looked up, I couldn't believe it. There was Mr. Johnson in a beautiful blue warm-up suit, freshly shaven, with his hair cut and groomed.

"You look very handsome, Mr. Johnson!" I exclaimed.

"Why, thank you," he proudly stated.

"Your blue suit matches your blue eyes," I said.

I asked him to sit down and give me a big smile. As I looked through the camera and saw Mr. Johnson's smile, it dawned on me that something very special had taken place. We finally connected. The bond that you can only know when your heart touches the heart of another person blossomed that day.

It is the little things that can make a big difference with your patients. No, it wasn't the picture itself that made the difference with Mr. Johnson. The true connection began on the first visit. The picture was merely the icing on the cake.

—Michelle E. Heller, CMA (AAMA)

INDEX